IAP-NNF
Textbook of
Neonatal Resuscitation

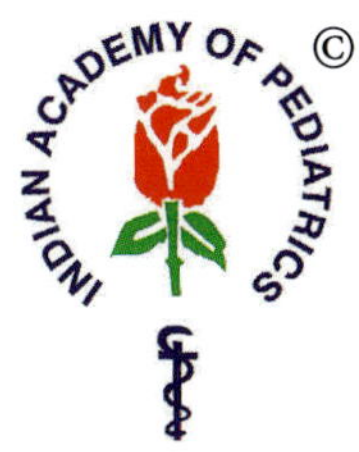

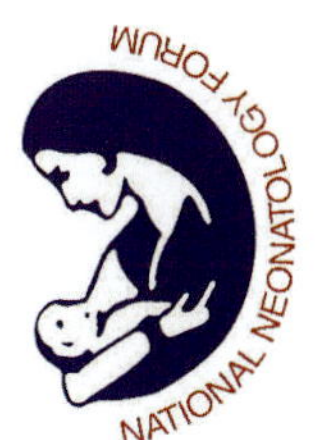

IAP-NNF
Textbook of
Neonatal Resuscitation

Editors

Piyush Gupta
MD FIAP FNNF FAMS FRCPCH
Principal and Professor
Department of Pediatrics
University College of Medical Sciences
New Delhi, India
President, Indian Academy of Pediatrics (2021)

Siddarth Ramji
MD FNNF
Former Director–Professor
Department of Neonatology
Dean
Maulana Azad Medical College and
Associated Lok Nayak Hospital
New Delhi, India
President, National Neonatology Forum (2022)

An Official Publication of
Indian Academy of Pediatrics (IAP) and
National Neonatology Forum (NNF)

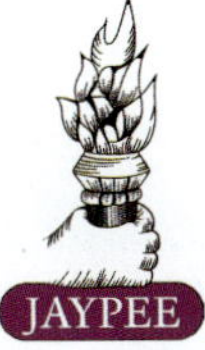

JAYPEE BROTHERS MEDICAL PUBLISHERS
The Health Sciences Publisher
New Delhi | London

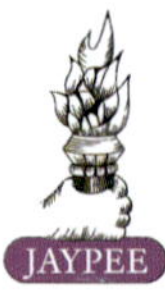 **Jaypee Brothers Medical Publishers (P) Ltd.**

Headquarters
EMCA House
23/23-B, Ansari Road, Daryaganj
New Delhi 110 002, India
Landline: +91-11-23272143, +91-11-23272703
+91-11-23282021, +91-11-23245672
Email: jaypee@jaypeebrothers.com

Overseas Office
J.P. Medical Ltd
83 Victoria Street, London
SW1H 0HW (UK)
Phone: +44 20 3170 8910
Email: info@jpmedpub.com

Corporate Office
4838/24, Ansari Road, Daryaganj
New Delhi 110 002, India
Phone: +91-11-43574357
Fax: +91-11-43574314
Email: jaypee@jaypeebrothers.com

EU GPSR Authorised Representative
Logos Europe, 9 rue Nicolas Poussin
17000, La Rochelle, France
Phone: +33 (0) 6 67 93 73 78
E-mail: Contact@logoseurope.eu

Website: www.jaypeebrothers.com
Website: www.jaypeedigital.com

IAP-NNF Textbook of Neonatal Resuscitation

First Edition: 2023, **Reprint:** *2024, 2025,* **2026**

ISBN: 978-93-5696-096-1

Printed at: Samrat Offset Pvt. Ltd,

Contributing Authors

Abhishek S Aradhya MD DM
Neonatal Director
Ovum Hospitals
Ovum Woman and Child Specialty Hospital
Bengaluru, Karnataka, India
abhishekaradhyas@gmail.com

Abiramalatha T MD DM
Associate Professor
Department of Neonatology
KMCH Institute of Health Sciences and Research
Coimbatore, Tamil Nadu, India
abiramalatha@gmail.com

Akash Bang MD DNB-MNAMS PGDMLS IDPCCM
Additional Professor
Department of Pediatrics
All India Institute of Medical Sciences
Nagpur, Maharashtra, India
drakashbang@gmail.com

Aparna C MD DM
Clinical Director, Neonatology
Senior Consultant, Neonatology and Pediatrics
KIMS Cuddles
Hyderabad, Telangana, India
appubanu@gmail.com

Ashish Mehta MD DCh FNNF
Director and Consultant Neonatologist
Arpan Newborn Care Centre Pvt Ltd
Ahmedabad, Gujarat, India
ashish.arpan11@gmail.com

Chandrakala BS
Professor and Head
Department of Neonatology
St John's Medical College Hospital
Bengaluru, Karnataka, India
bms_chandra@yahoo.co.in

Deepak Chawla MD DM
Professor
Department of Neonatology
Government Medical College
Chandigarh, India
drdeepakchawla@hotmail.com

Dheeraj Shah MD FIAP FAMS
Director-Professor
Department of Pediatrics
University College of Medical Sciences
and Guru Teg Bahadur Hospital
New Delhi, India
dshah@ucms.ac.in

Harish Chellani MD DCH FNNF
Professor and Former Head
Department of Pediatrics
Vardhman Mahavir Medical College
and Safdarjung Hospital
New Delhi, India
chellaniharish@gmail.com

Piyush Gupta MD FIAP FNNF FAMS FRCPCH
Principal and Professor of Pediatrics
University College of Medical Sciences
and Guru Teg Bahadur Hospital
New Delhi, India
prof.piyush.gupta@gmail.com

Prakash Amboiram MD
Professor and Head
Department of Neonatology
Sri Ramachandra Medical College and Research Institute
Sri Ramachandra Institute of Higher Education
and Research (SRIHER)
Chennai, Tamil Nadu, India
draprakash1@gmail.com

Praveen Kumar MD DM
Professor
Neonatal Unit
Department of Pediatrics
Postgraduate Institute of Medical Education and Research
Chandigarh, India
drpkumarpgi@gmail.com

Rashna Dass Hazarika MD Fellow PID MECS
Senior Consultant
Pediatrics and Neonatology
Nemcare Superspeciality Hospital
Guwahati, Assam, India
rashnadass@gmail.com

Rhishikesh Thakre
DM MD DNB DCH FCPS FIAP FNNF
Director
Neo Clinic and Hospital
Aurangabad, Maharashtra, India
rptdoc@gmail.com

Reeta Bora MD DM
Professor and Head
Department of Pediatrics and Neonatology
Assam Medical College
Dibrugarh, Assam, India
bora64reeta@gmail.com

Satvik C Bansal MD
Assistant Professor
Department of Pediatrics
GR Medical College
Gwalior, Madhya Pradesh, India
drsatvikbansal@gmail.com

Shashi Kant Dhir MD DM
Professor and Head
Department of Pediatrics
Guru Gobind Singh Medical College
Faridkot, Punjab, India
drshashikantdhir@gmail.com

Siddarth Ramji MD FNNF
Former Director–Professor
Department of Neonatology
Maulana Azad Medical College and
Associated Lok Nayak Hospital
New Delhi, India
siddarthramji@gmail.com

Somashekhar Nimbalkar
MD FNNF CPH PGDPH
Professor and Head
Department of Neonatology
Pramukhswami Medical College
Bhaikaka University
Anand, Gujarat, India
somu_somu@yahoo.com

Sugandha Arya MD
Professor
Department of Pediatrics
Vardhman Mahavir Medical College
and Safdarjung Hospital
New Delhi, India
sugandha_arya@hotmail.com

Suksham Jain MD DM
Professor and Head
Department of Neonatology
Government Medical College and Hospital
Chandigarh, India
dr.sukshamj@gmail.com

Suman Rao PN MD DM
Professor and Head
Department of Neonatology
St John's Medical College Hospital
Bengaluru, Karnataka, India
raosumanv@gmail.com

Sushma Nangia MD DM
Director–Professor and Head
Department of Neonatology
Lady Hardinge Medical College and
Kalawati Saran Children's Hospital
New Delhi, India
drsnangia@gmail.com

Tejo Pratap Oleti MD DM
Consultant and Head
Department of Neonatology and Pediatrics
Fernandez Hospital, Hyderabad, Telangana, India
tejopratap@gmail.com

Umamaheswari Balakrishnan MD MRCPCH
Professor and Senior Consultant
Department of Neonatology
Sri Ramachandra Medical College
Sri Ramachandra Institute of Higher Education
and Research, Chennai, Tamil Nadu, India
drumarajakumar@gmail.com

US Jagdish Chandra DCH FIAP FNNF
Senior Consultant
Department of Pediatrics
Sai Suprashant Clinic
Hyderabad, Telangana, India
drusjagdishchandra@yahoo.com

VC Manoj MD MSc FRCPCH FNNF
Professor and Head
Department of Neonatology
Jubilee Mission Medical College and Research Institute
Thrissur, Kerala, India
manojvaranattu@gmail.com

Vikas Goyal MD
Consultant Pediatrician
Vinayak Hospital, Kutch, Gujarat, India
drgoyalvikas@yahoo.co.in

Foreword

It is with immense pride and a sense of deep gratification that I write the foreword for the *IAP-NNF Textbook of Neonatal Resuscitation*. As the former President of the Indian Academy of Pediatrics (IAP) and one of the pioneers of the Neonatal Resuscitation Program in India, I am honored to witness the remarkable progress we have made in this vital field.

IAP-NNF Textbook of Neonatal Resuscitation represents a significant milestone in the pursuit of excellence in neonatal care worldwide. I commend the IAP and the NNF for their visionary approach in recognizing the need for a textbook specifically tailored for the Indian context, acknowledging the unique challenges and resources available within our healthcare system. This initiative will undoubtedly have a profound impact on the quality of neonatal resuscitation practices throughout the country, saving countless lives and improving outcomes for our precious newborns.

I extend my sincere gratitude and appreciation to the Editors-in-Chief, Dr Piyush Gupta and Dr Siddharth Ramji, authors and contributors for their exemplary dedication and tireless efforts in bringing this textbook to fruition.

As the President of the International Pediatric Association, I am honored to endorse the *IAP-NNF Textbook of Neonatal Resuscitation* whole-heartedly. Together, let us strive towards a world where every newborn has the opportunity to thrive and fulfil their limitless potential.

Naveen Thacker
President, 2023–2025
International Pediatric Association (IPA)

Foreword

I am extremely happy to write a foreword to this first ever *Textbook of Neonatal Resuscitation* produced in a collaborative effort by IAP and NNF. When a little 'bundle of joy' is born after an uneventful 40 weeks of intrauterine life, with a birth weight of around 3.5 kg, and cries immediately after birth; it is the greatest joy for the doctor and parents alike. Though most babies make this transition from intrauterine to extrauterine life without difficulty, some 10% of newborns have a challenging birth and require assistance, and a smaller proportion of those may even require intense resuscitative measures at birth. Although more advanced resuscitative interventions such as chest compression or medications are necessitated less than 1% of the time; these are life-saving skills that every birth attendant should be trained in, along with having access to clean and functional equipment and supplies.

A baby that receives timely medical care from trained professionals in the shortest time has the best chance of survival. To make rapid strides towards our goal of reducing India's neonatal mortality rate to a single digit by 2030, Both IAP and NNF have been working tirelessly over the last three decades to train all birth attendants across the country in the art of neonatal resuscitation. The next step in this regard was to have our own textbook of neonatal resuscitation which will give uniform, appropriate, scientifically backed and evidence-based guidelines on the subject. Thanks to the herculean efforts put in by the Editors-in-chief, Dr Piyush Gupta and Dr Siddarth Ramji along with a large team of subject experts across the country, we have our own textbook ready to be used as single reference book on neonatal resuscitation. Starting from pre-resuscitation team briefings and checklists to the physiologic changes that occur during and after birth, communication and teamwork skills used by effective resuscitation teams, the steps in resuscitation and the grounding ethical principles; every possible issue in neonatal resuscitation has been dealt with in a format that is easy to read, understand, and implement.

Key points at the end of every chapter along with self-assessment questions are a major highlight of the book. The illustrative cases used throughout will help readers visualize the clinical scenario as though they are present in the delivery room and make them a part of the medical decision-making process. I am sure that this textbook will help doctors, nurses, and every birth attendant in acquiring the knowledge and skills essential for neonatal resuscitation and enable them to provide optimal care and assistance to neonates in the smooth transition from intrauterine to extrauterine life.

Upendra Kinjawadekar
National President 2023
Indian Academy of Pediatrics (IAP)

Foreword

It is a moment of pleasure and pride to be associated with this Make in India, *Textbook of Neonatal Resuscitation*. This is indeed a high-quality evidence-based comprehensive, yet simple and practical book. The uniform structured organization of each chapter with liberal use of diagrams, flowcharts, and tables make it a pleasure to read. The book is suitable for basic and advanced practitioners, as well as researchers, trainers, and planners. The organization of the book into logical sections makes it easy for the readers to quickly find what you need.

The successful completion of such a mammoth task in a time-bound manner was possible only because of the leadership and coordination of the two well-known masters—Professor Piyush Gupta and Professor Siddarth Ramji. Using their complementary expertise, they have been able to bring out a state-of-the-art book which is possibly the best one in the current times. I am sure this will become the standard textbook of neonatal resuscitation not only in India, but the entire Southeast Asian region and the developing world.

Apart from its academic brilliance, this textbook brings the collaboration of Indian Academy of Pediatrics and National Neonatology Forum to the fore. It is one important step to harmonize and standardize the NRP training across the country and across the cadres. The next step for both the organizations is to take this collaboration further to streamline and ensure uniformity in quality of trainings and certification methods. We also need to ensure regular timely updates to the book with the emergence of new evidence. Another task for the collaboration would be to ensure harmonization of resuscitation trainings and manuals under various national and state programs for different cadres of health workers, with this evidence-based text.

Praveen Kumar
Head, Division of Neonatology
Postgraduate Institute of Medical Education and Research
Chandigarh, India; and
National President 2023
National Neonatology Forum (NNF)

Message

It is with a sense of great pride and pleasure that I announce the launch of the *IAP-NNF Textbook of Neonatal Resuscitation*, a comprehensive and updated guide for neonatal resuscitation in India. This IAP-NNF textbook is based on existing latest evidences and recommendations in the field of neonatal resuscitation.

Our country has much different conditions than developed countries. We do not have sophisticated gadgets at the majority of health centers and thus a book with adaptations according to our limited resources was need of the hour. *IAP-NNF Textbook of Neonatal Resuscitation* bridges this gap and is a valuable resource for all healthcare professionals who are involved in the delivery and immediate care of newborns, such as pediatricians, obstetricians, nurses, midwives, and paramedics.

This book encompasses the essential knowledge and practical skills on the subject, antenatal counseling, equipment preparation, initial steps, ventilation, chest compressions, medications, preterm care, post-resuscitation care, ethics, quality improvement, and much more. It also includes special considerations for preterm babies, resuscitation outside the delivery room, and quality improvement.

It is also the official textbook for the IAP-NRP-FGM project, which aims to train about 200,000 birth attendants in neonatal resuscitation in 10 years. NRP is the most prestigious project of IAP through which we have been able to make a positive impact on neonatal survival rates in India. The ultimate objective of this project is to have one person at every delivery who is trained in neonatal resuscitation and thus further reduce the neonatal mortality due to birth asphyxia in our country.

I appreciate the interest and support of IAP-NNF textbook committees in this important initiative. Together, we can make a difference in the lives of newborns and their families.

Vineet K Saxena
Hon Secretary General, 2022–2023
Indian Academy of Pediatrics

Message

Almost one-third of all newborn deaths and stillbirths are preventable. This has been shown in various meta-analyses and systematic reviews that improving skills of healthcare providers (HCP) around childbirth can reduce stillbirths and neonatal deaths by almost 30%.

National Neonatology Forum (NNF) India has always emphasized on training neonatal resuscitation to all levels of healthcare providers be it a doctor, nurse, or trained birth attendant. It had over the decades rolled out its own Neonatal Resuscitation Program of India. This NR India program had the latest evidences from ILCOR along with local practical adaptations. NNF India and Indian Academy of Pediatrics (IAP) in association with American Academy of Pediatrics (AAP) had jointly initiated IAP-NNF-AAP NRP FGM; Neonatal Resuscitation Program—First Golden Minute in 2009. Lakhs of healthcare providers (HCP) across all the states have been trained under this initiative.

A need for an updated textbook on neonatal resuscitation from India was mentioned in the joint memorandum of understanding (MoU) between NNF and IAP. National level joint collaborative efforts to involve neonatal resuscitation experts and prolific writers have resulted in bringing out this textbook. It is imperative henceforth for all involved in care of newborns around childbirth in India to update themselves according to this new textbook.

I take pride in congratulating Dr Siddarth Ramji and Dr Piyush Gupta on completion of this onerous groundbreaking task. The authors aptly deserve all the accolades on contributing for such a high level of academic treatise with latest scientific evidences. NNF and IAP will jointly undertake NR India program to train healthcare workforce as per this new textbook.

NNF India and IAP should continue to utilize the services of such an expert dedicated liaison group for collating recent evidences, jointly undertake research in gap areas and bring out updated editions of this textbook at regular interval of 5 years.

May the fruits of this mammoth effort be accessible to all families and benefit all the newborns of India.

Surender Singh Bisht
Secretary General, 2023–2024
National Neonatology Forum

Preface

Neonatal resuscitation is a key intervention for reducing asphyxia-related neonatal mortality. An essential pre-requisite is availability of healthcare providers with the requisite skills for neonatal resuscitation. This in-turn requires a standardized training program for imparting the skills for neonatal resuscitation which should be able to address the needs of healthcare providers working across a range of healthcare settings—primary to tertiary. However, resuscitation of newborn in the delivery room poses two challenges: (i) large variability in the skill sets of healthcare providers, and (ii) the large variation in the resources available in the health settings where births take place. This has led to the emergence of separate neonatal resuscitation programs that addressed the needs of healthcare providers in adequately resourced settings and for those involved in care of the newborn at birth working in resource-constrained settings. As the 'science of neonatal resuscitation' started shifting to evidence-based medicine, it became incumbent for all the neonatal resuscitation programs to harmonize with the emerging global guidelines to provide the best for all newborns while they were adapted to address the regional needs.

A decade ago, the National Neonatology Forum, brought out the first NRP-India book which was adapted for the country. However, over time, the need for a uniform and harmonized *Textbook of Neonatal Resuscitation* for the country was recognized by both the National Neonatology Forum (NNF) and the Indian Academy of Pediatrics (IAP). It was this shared vision that has given shape to this first edition of *IAP-NNF Textbook of Neonatal Resuscitation*. This textbook will serve not only as the standard resource book for the national basic and advanced neonatal resuscitation training programs, but also as a ready reckoner for those interested in the science of neonatal resuscitation. The book is a blend of a workbook for training (each chapter having practical practice guidelines and a self-assessment section) and a standard textbook providing information beyond the objectives of skill transfer of a training course. In addition to the core chapters focused on the neonatal resuscitation process, the book has chapters dealing with ethical issues in neonatal resuscitation (e.g., termination of resuscitation and end-of-life care), neonatal resuscitation in resource-constrained settings, evolution of international guidelines and the current evidence for neonatal resuscitation practices, gaps in knowledge and research priorities, and quality considerations in neonatal resuscitation.

It is our fervent hope that this textbook will meet the needs of all healthcare providers involved in newborn care and would provide the policy makers with a national technical consensus guideline to refer to while planning for resources needed at each delivery point in the country and for the post-resuscitation care of newborns. It is envisaged that the subsequent editions of this book will keep pace with the emerging evidence in neonatal resuscitation to enable all healthcare professionals to remain updated so that all our newborns receive the care that will optimize the best outcomes for them.

Piyush Gupta
Siddarth Ramji

Contents

SECTION 5: Postresuscitation Care

SECTION 6: Evidence-base for Neonatal Resuscitation Practices

SECTION 7: Evolution of Neonatal Resuscitation Practices

SECTION 8: Ethical Issues and Research in Neonatal Resuscitation

SECTION 9: Beyond Resuscitation Issues

Introduction to Neonatal Resuscitation

Anatomy and Physiology Related to Resuscitation

Harish Chellani, Sugandha Arya

Lessons to Learn

- Anatomy and physiology of fetal circulation
- Normal transition of fetal circulation to neonatal circulation
- What happens during abnormal transition
- Fetal/newborn response to abnormal transition
- Differences in newborn and adult resuscitation

Approximately 85% of newborns breathe spontaneously at birth and have normal transition from fetal to neonatal circulation. Amongst those needing resuscitation, almost two-thirds will start to breathe following drying and tactile stimulation and the remaining after positive-pressure ventilation (PPV). Only 0.1–0.3% of newborn would require more advanced resuscitative interventions such as chest compression or medications.[1] This chapter will cover normal transition from fetal to neonatal circulation and fetal/newborn response to abnormal transition. This will help to understand the rationale and sequence of resuscitation described in the subsequent chapters.

FETAL CIRCULATION

Gas exchange in the fetus takes place at the level of the intervillous spaces of the placenta. The oxygenation of fetal blood is facilitated by the higher oxygen affinity of fetal hemoglobin (HbF) compared to adult hemoglobin (HbA). The umbilical artery has a PO_2 of about 15–25 mm Hg, and that in the umbilical vein being 30–35 mm Hg. Even though the umbilical vein has a low partial pressure of oxygen, due to the high affinity of HbF to oxygen, the oxygen saturation achieved is between 65 and 70%.[2]

In the fetus, the circulation is characterized by a circuit that has low-systemic resistance and high-pulmonary resistance, with shunts at the level of ductus venosus, ductus arteriosus (DA), and foramen ovale (FO). Almost two-thirds of the blood from the umbilical vein (receiving blood from the placenta) is shunted via the ductus venosus

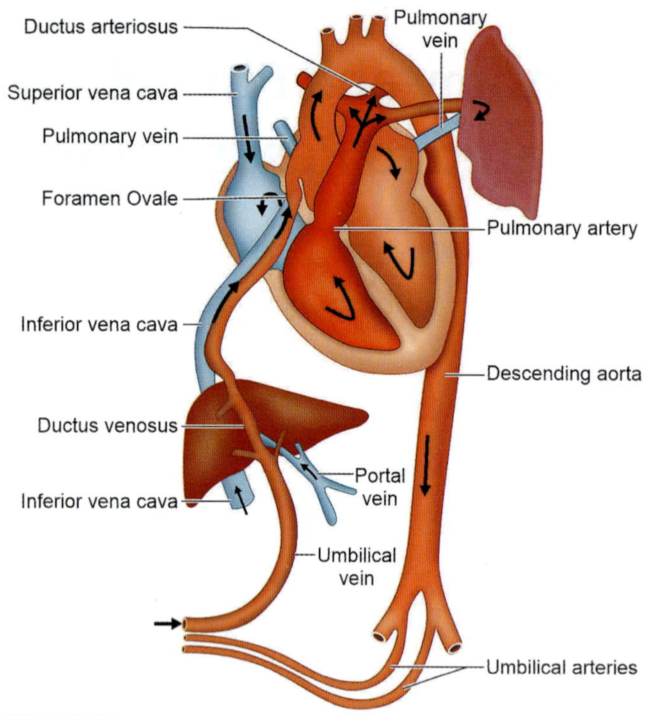

FIG. 1.1 Fetal blood circulation.

and the inferior vena cava (IVC) to the right atrium. Almost half of the oxygenated blood from the umbilical vein is shunted across the foramen ovale (FO) into the left atrium (*Right to Left Shunt*). This highly oxygenated blood passes directly to the fetal brain and heart.[3] The rest of the blood from the IVC mixes with the blood from the super vena cava (which has a PO_2 of 12–14 mm Hg) and enters the right ventricle and the pulmonary artery. Since the pulmonary vascular resistance is high and systemic resistance is low, most of this blood is shunted into the descending aorta via the DA (*Fig.* **1.1**).

NORMAL TRANSITION FROM FETAL TO NEONATAL CIRCULATION

After birth, a series of events culminate in a successful transition from fetal to neonatal circulation **(Table 1.1)**. The placenta is no longer a source of oxygen supply or CO_2 elimination, and the baby must depend on its lungs for oxygen supply and CO_2 removal. This transition usually happens within minutes after birth. The major changes during this transition are:

TABLE 1.1: SUMMARY OF MAJOR PHYSIOLOGIC TRANSITION AT BIRTH		
	Intrauterine	*Extrauterine*
Temperature regulation	Maternal	Self
Gas exchange	Placenta	Lung alveoli
Lungs	Fluid filled	Air filled
Pulmonary vessels	Constricted	Dilated
Pulmonary vascular resistance	High	Low
Pulmonary blood flow	Low	High
Foramen ovale	Is open; right to left shunt of blood from right atrium to left atrium	Closed due to increased left atrial pressure
Ductus arteriosus	Is patent; right to left shunting of blood from pulmonary artery to aorta (bypasses lung) and to the placenta	Closed due to increase in arterial oxygen and decrease in prostaglandins
Ductus venosus	Carries oxygenated blood from the placenta to the right atrium	Constricted due to reduction in umbilical venous flow

- *Absorption of fetal alveolar fluid* into pulmonary lymphatics and its replacement by air following the baby's initial breaths. Since room air contains 21% oxygen, filling the alveoli with air provides oxygen that can diffuse into the blood vessels surrounding the alveoli.

- *Closure of the umbilical vessels* by clamping the cord removes the low resistance placental circuit and increases baby's systemic blood pressure and thus decreases the right to left shunt across the foramen ovale and the ductus arteriosus and facilitates in increased flow to the newborn's lungs.

- *Decrease the pulmonary vascular resistance* resulting from air filling the alveoli after birth and the consequent increase in oxygen levels in alveoli which dilate the pulmonary blood vessels. This increases the blood flow into the lungs. The increase in oxygen levels also results in constriction of the ductus arteriosus (*Fig.* **1.2**).

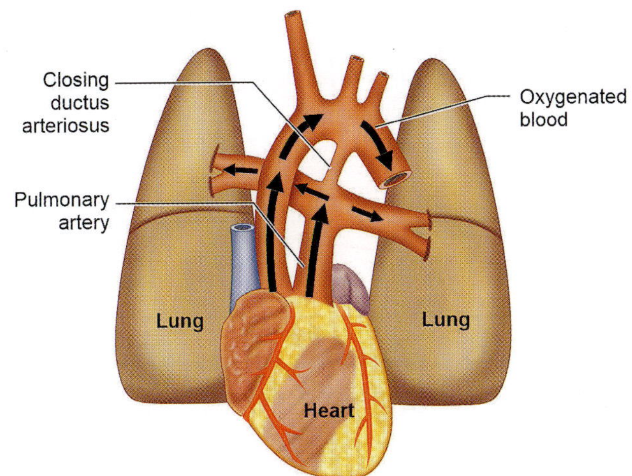

FIG. 1.2 Changes in pulmonary circulation after birth due to ductus closure.

The first few steps of transition from fetal to neonatal circulation occur within a few minutes of birth. However, the complete sequence of events may take hours or days. A healthy term newborn usually achieves oxygen saturation of >90% in about 10 minutes. Complete absorption of fluid in the lungs may take up to few hours and pulmonary pressures may gradually reduce over many months.[1]

WHAT CAN GO WRONG DURING TRANSITION AT BIRTH?

The fetus/newborn may encounter difficulties either before labor, during labor, or after birth. Problems before and during labor reflect a compromise in placental blood flow. Difficulties after birth usually reflect problems with the baby's airway and/or lungs. Normal transition may be disrupted by the following:

- Lungs do not fill with air because the baby does not breathe or has inadequate spontaneous breaths. Also, foreign material may block the airway. Therefore, oxygen may not reach the baby's blood.

- The expected increase in systemic blood pressure may not occur either because of excessive blood loss or neonatal hypoxia. These conditions may cause poor cardiac contractions or bradycardia and result in hypotension.

- Pulmonary arterioles may remain constricted because of inadequate gaseous distension of the lung or lack of oxygen. These result in decreased blood flow into the lungs and thus reduce oxygen supply to the tissues.[4]

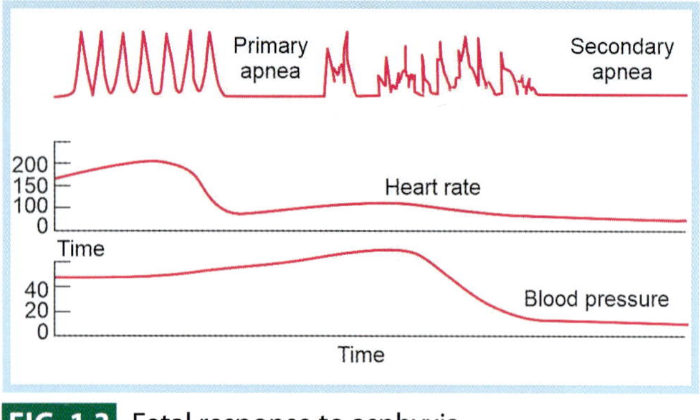

FIG. 1.3   Fetal response to asphyxia.

FETAL/NEWBORN RESPONSE TO ASPHYXIA

The pathophysiology of fetal/newborn response to asphyxia has been described in animal models. Dawes described the breathing response to acidosis in different animal species. It was observed that when there is asphyxia, animals typically have a relatively short period of apnea followed by gasping. The gasping pattern then increases in rate until breathing ceases again for a period of secondary apnea. The physiologic effects that occur with worsening asphyxia are shown in *Figure* **1.3**. Dawes also noted that primary apnea, could be reversed with stimulation, while the latter period, secondary apnea, required assisted ventilation to effectively establish spontaneous breathing. The first sign of improvement was noted to be an increase in heart rate.[5]

The first response to asphyxia is primary apnea, which is associated with bradycardia but normal blood pressure. If asphyxia continues, primary apnea is followed by irregular gasping efforts and then secondary apnea ensues. Secondary apnea is associated with bradycardia and hypotension (*Fig.* **1.3**). A baby who is apneic at birth may be either in primary apnea or secondary apnea. ***However, it must be assumed that all newborns who are apneic at birth are in secondary apnea and interventions must begin immediately and one must be prepared to carry out advanced resuscitation.***

During primary apnea, maintaining airway patency and tactile stimulation is adequate to restore breathing. If resuscitation is ineffective, gasping and secondary apnea occurs. During this period, tactile stimulation may not be sufficient and assisted ventilation (PPV) is required. Prolonged asphyxia leads to acidosis and cardiac arrest requiring chest compression (CC) and/or drugs. When the normal transition is interrupted, the oxygen supply to tissues is decreased, and the baby may exhibit one or more of the clinical signs listed in **Table 1.2**.

HOW IS NEWBORN RESUSCITATION DIFFERENT FROM ADULT RESUSCITATION?

In adults, the most common cause of cardiac arrest is coronary artery disease. Due to sudden arrhythmia or myocardial ischemia, heart is not able to circulate blood effectively. Due to poor circulation to the brain, adult patient becomes unconscious and breathing stops. Initially the oxygen and carbon dioxide levels in blood are usually normal and the lungs remain filled with air. Hence cardiac compression, airway, and breathing approach (C-A-B approach) is used for adult resuscitation.

TABLE 1.2: CLINICAL SIGNS OF ABNORMAL TRANSITION

Clinical sign	Cause
Poor respiratory drive—apnea, gasping	Due to insufficient oxygen delivery to the brain, muscles, and other organs
Respiratory distress—tachypnea, chest-indrawing	Due to delayed resorption of lung fluid
Poor muscle tone	Due to insufficient oxygen supply to the brain
Bradycardia	Due to insufficient oxygen supply to the heart muscle or brainstem
Hypotension	Insufficient oxygen to the heart muscle or blood loss
Persistent cyanosis or low oxygen saturation	Due to insufficient oxygen in blood

The emphasis is on initiating chest compressions at the earliest followed by effective ventilation during resuscitation.

In contrast, in most asphyxiated newborns the heart is normal. The most common cause of cardiopulmonary arrest is respiratory in origin due to ineffective gas exchange which may occur before, during, or after birth. It is characterized by respiratory failure due to inability to establish or sustain breathing at birth. Hence airway, breathing, and circulation approach (A-B-C approach) is used for newborn resuscitation. The primary focus of newborn resuscitation is to establish effective ventilation.[1]

Another major factor affecting newborn, resuscitation is thermal wellbeing. If the newborn is hypothermic, the response to resuscitative efforts is likely to be suboptimal. Hence the sequence of events for newborn resuscitation is T-A-B-C, where T is thermal care and takes a priority over ABC.

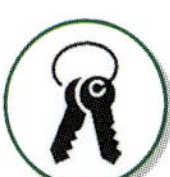 ## KEY POINTS

1. Most newborn infants undergo successful transition at birth from fetal to neonatal ventilation and circulation. However, a few have delayed transition due to asphyxia and need resuscitative assistance at birth to help make this transition.

2. Successful transition at birth is dependent on establishment of the lungs as the organ of gas exchange.

3. The key respiratory transition events include initiation of breathing, clearance of fluid from the lungs and airways, and increase in pulmonary blood flow.

4. The major cardiovascular change at birth is the transition from fetal to neonatal circulation which includes establishment of significant pulmonary blood flow (which is dependent on increasing oxygenation of the neonatal blood), closure of foramen oval and ductus arteriosus.

5. The newborn infant's primary need at birth is establishing effective ventilation.

▉ REFERENCES

1. Weiner GM (Ed). Textbook of Neonatal Resuscitation, 8th edition. Elk Grove Village (IL): American Academy of Pediatrics and American Heart Association; 2021.

2. Berger TM. Neonatal resuscitation: foetal physiology and pathophysiological aspects. Eur J Anaesthesiol. 2012;29(8):362-70.

3. Katheria A, Finer NN. Newborn resuscitation. In: Gleason CA, Juul SE (Eds). Avery's Diseases of the Newborn, 10th edition, vol. 1. Philadelphia (PA): Elsevier; 2018. p. 274.

4. Hooper SB, Kitchen MJ, Polglase GR, Roehr CC, Te Pas AB. The physiology of neonatal resuscitation. Curr Opin Pediatr. 2018;30(2):187-91.

5. Dawes GS. Foetal and Neonatal physiology: a comparative study of changes at birth. Chicago: Yearbook Medical Publishers; 1968.

 # Self Assessment

1. Successful transition from fetal to neonatal circulation requires:
   a. Increased pulmonary blood flow
   b. Clamping of cord
   c. Closure of the foramen ovale and ductus arteriosus
   d. All of the above

2. Which of the following suggests inadequate respiratory transition at birth?
   a. Gasping
   b. Apnea
   c. Tachypnea
   d. All of the above

3. A healthy term newborn achieves oxygen saturation >90%:
   a. At birth
   b. At 5 minutes after birth
   c. At 10 minutes after birth
   d. At 30 minutes after birth

4. State true or false:
   a. Gasping respiration is a physiologic transition. (..........)
   b. Lungs are fluid filled in fetal life. (..........)
   c. Most babies are pink at birth. (..........)
   d. Drugs are rarely required during newborn resuscitation. (.........)
   e. A newborn not responding to tactile stimulation is in secondary apnea. (..........)
   f. The commonest cause of cardiopulmonary arrest in newborns is cardiac in origin. (..........)
   g. To restore effective ventilation is the primary goal in neonatal cardiopulmonary resuscitation. (..........)

Answers

For answers, go to the end of the Book, Page no. 321

Preparing for Resuscitation and Familiarizing with the Equipment

US Jagdish Chandra

Lessons to Learn

- Importance of Preparation
- How to anticipate birth asphyxia and identifying risk factors?
- How to prepare personnel for resuscitation?
- Documenting neonatal resuscitation in delivery room
- Description of a newborn corner
- Description of the equipment needed for neonatal resuscitation
- Conducting a post-resuscitation debriefing session
- Behavioral skills required for neonatal resuscitation

IMPORTANCE OF PREPARATION

Nearly 10% of infants need some assistance to begin breathing at birth, with approximately 0.1% of term babies and 15% of preterm babies needing extensive resuscitation and about 0.2–0.3% developing moderate or severe hypoxic-ischemic encephalopathy.[1-3] Newborn infants with birth asphyxia can suffer from short to long-term neurological complications. Severe asphyxia has been linked to cerebral palsy, mental retardation, epilepsy, and learning disorders.[4,5] Mortality in infants with hypoxic-ischemic encephalopathy ranges from 6–30%, and significant morbidity, such as cerebral palsy and long-term disabilities, occurs in 20–30% of survivors. The probability of sequelae is low if a newborn infant is resuscitated promptly and correctly and starts breathing spontaneously within 20 minutes.[6]

The goal of neonatal resuscitation is to prevent the morbidity and mortality associated with hypoxic-ischemic tissue injury to vital organs namely, the brain, heart, kidney and to reestablish adequate spontaneous respiration, and cardiac output.[7-9] The first "*Golden minute*" is crucial for the intact survival of an asphyxiated baby. Global evidence suggests that the risk of neonatal death increases by 16% for every 30 seconds delay in initiating ventilation in the first 6 minutes after birth, and 6% for every minute of delay thereafter.[10] Therefore, it is clear the first minutes after birth are critical to reducing neonatal mortality.

Anticipation, early recognition of the problem, initiation of appropriate resuscitation measures using the correct technique and assessment of the effectiveness of ventilation are critical for successful neonatal resuscitation. The most common causes of failed resuscitation are failure to recognize the problem promptly, not reacting quickly and ineffective ventilation of the lungs due to incorrect technique or nonfunctioning/malfunctioning equipment. Delayed or ineffective action makes resuscitation more difficult and increases the risk of brain damage.

ANTICIPATING BIRTH ASPHYXIA AND IDENTIFYING RISK FACTORS

Most often the transition from intrauterine life to extrauterine life happens without difficulty. However multiple maternal, placental, mechanical, and fetal conditions exist that can jeopardize a smooth transition signaling the need for intervention.

Anticipating a risk requires timely and accurate communication between the obstetric team and the neonatal resuscitation team so that the latter is apprised about the risk status for each delivery. The need for resuscitation should always be anticipated and every birth should be treated as a potential emergency. *A healthy pregnancy, uneventful antenatal period and a normal delivery do not rule out the chances of the baby developing problems and needing resuscitation.* Factors that affect newborn care can be assessed by reviewing the medical record, interacting with the obstetrician and the mother. There are several risk factors in the mother or fetus, which can predispose to asphyxia at birth or need for special care and management in the baby. The number and severity of risk factors are indicative of the magnitude of risk. Prior information and assessment of the risk factors helps in better preparation in terms of personnel required and additional equipment which may be needed and the smooth flow of resuscitation.

Antenatal Assessment of Risk

To assess risk for neonatal resuscitation, the following information should be sought from the obstetrician prebirth:

- What is the expected gestational age?
- Is there a single or are there multiple fetuses?
- Are there any other risk factors?

Table 2.1 lists some of the important perinatal risk factors that are associated with birth asphyxia and increase the risk for the newborn of needing resuscitation at birth.

PREPARATION OF PERSONNEL FOR RESUSCITATION

It is desirable that for every birth of a term newborn infant without any antenatal risk factors, there should be a healthcare provider

TABLE 2.1: PERINATAL RISK FACTORS ASSOCIATED WITH NEED FOR NEONATAL RESUSCITATION AT BIRTH

Maternal	Fetal	Intrapartum
• Antepartum hemorrhage (placental abruption, placenta previa) • Pregnancy-induced hypertension, chronic hypertension • Maternal intrapartum pyrexia • Prolonged rupture of membranes—i.e., >18 hours/maternal infection • Multiple pregnancy • Diabetes mellitus • Rhesus isoimmunization • Previous fetal/neonatal deaths • Poly/oligohydramnios • Chorioamnionitis • Maternal infection • Chronic illness (e.g., anemia, congenital cyanotic heart disease) • No antenatal care • Maternal age <16 or >35 years	• Preterm/post-term • Intrauterine growth restriction • Antenatally diagnosed congenital abnormalities (e.g., congenital diaphragmatic hernia and congenital heart disease, etc.) • Intrauterine infection • Reduced fetal movement before onset of labor	• Cardiotocographic (CTG) abnormalities • Reduced fetal movements • Abnormal presentation—e.g., breech • Cord prolapse • Meconium-stained liquor • Forceps/vacuum delivery • Emergency cesarean section • Precipitate labor • Prolonged first or second stage of labor • Maternal sedation (within 4 hours) • Maternal general anesthesia

trained to provide positive pressure ventilation (PPV). If a delivery is anticipated where there are risk factors, then the delivery should be attended by a healthcare provider who is trained in advanced neonatal resuscitation (intubation, chest compression, etc.). In cases of an anticipated delivery with risk factors there should be at least two or more personnel trained in advanced neonatal resuscitation available at the time of birth of the baby whose primary responsibility should be management of the newborn.[11]

If the delivery room has only one healthcare provider who is trained and capable of initiating basic resuscitation—assess and support airway, and initiate ventilation and if required be able to assist during chest compressions, they should be able to call for additional help if required. Situations that may demand additional help could include multiple births or a newborn needing resuscitative assistance beyond PPV, e.g., intubation, chest compression, or need for medication. The contact details of personnel for providing additional help when required, should be displayed prominently in the delivery room of such health facilities. Ambulance to transport such babies should be available to shift the baby if the need arises for urgent referral of complicated birth asphyxia cases to higher level healthcare facilities.

Identifying the Team and Team Leader

Neonatal resuscitation requires multiple tasks to be performed as part of the resuscitation process. While individual care providers

TABLE 2.2: Requirements for Effective Team Work	
Leader	• Must assess patient status • Assign work to team members • Direct team members for action • Supervise, analyze, and coordinate • Provide feedback to team members • Periodically summarize key information and progress • Invite inputs from the team
Task allotment	• Should be aware of one's role and responsibility • Perform and confirm the task • Coordinate within the team
Communication	• Should be clear, concise, and precise • Address team members directly by name • Recipient should confirm the instruction by feedback
Mutual respect	• Calm, cordial environment • Nonthreatening and nonhurried • Must be supportive and respectful to one another • Knowledge sharing must be encouraged • During communication use words such as "please", "thank you", "sorry", etc.

may have the required skills, no single individual can perform all the tasks required. Hence, it is very crucial to have a team involved in the resuscitation process. However, to have favorable outcomes, the team must work in a coordinated and efficient manner. There is sufficient evidence to suggest that inefficient teams result in unfavorable outcomes. The selected team members must have the skills to provide effective resuscitation and to work as a coordinated team. The team leader selected must have a thorough knowledge of the neonatal resuscitation protocol, be an effective communicator, be able to delegate responsibilities to various team members considering the skill sets, they possess and be able to effectively utilize the resources available to them. He/she should also be able to hand over leadership to another team member if he/she gets involved in a procedure. **Table 2.2** outlines the requirements for effective teamwork.

Predelivery Team Briefing

If risk factors are present, the team should be assembled and tasks assigned by the team leader to the team members as per their expertise and capabilities. The clinical situation should be reviewed and possible outcomes and emergency plan of action discussed. Tasks such as receiving the baby and doing initial assessment, performing PPV, intubation, chest compression, administering medication, and documentation should be assigned to different persons who are briefed and ready. In addition to individual skills each team member must effectively follow the instructions and participate as a team.

This helps in smooth execution of resuscitation and avoids confusion. Team members should arrange and check all the equipment and supplies required and discuss the emergency measures to be taken like additional expert help or shift to higher facility. The 2020 International Consensus on cardiopulmonary resuscitation concluded that "briefing or debriefing may improve short-term clinical and performance outcomes for infants and staff. The effects of briefing or debriefing on long-term clinical and performance outcomes are uncertain".[11]

Communication

Good communication is key to effective teamwork. Sharing information between team members requires that instructions are heard and understood. Instructions must be directed to the concerned team member by name making direct eye contact and must be spoken clearly. If the recipient of the instruction repeats the instruction given, the sender is assured that the instruction given has been effectively conveyed.

DOCUMENTATION

Documentation of the events is an important and integral part of neonatal resuscitation. Documentation keeps a track of the events, action taken, and time taken by the baby to respond to each of the resuscitation measures thereby making planning easy and executing the resuscitation without confusion. Documentation is also important from the medicolegal aspect. The emergency circumstances of carrying out a resuscitation procedure can make it challenging for accurate recording of events and procedures. A well-designed recording chart which follows the neonatal resuscitation algorithm can make the task of recording events as they occur easier. Retrospective recording of events should be kept to as minimal as possible. Hence it would be desirable that the team member documenting the events should be an experienced healthcare provider and not be entrusted with multitasking.

NEWBORN CARE CORNER

Every delivery room/area must have a designated area for resuscitating a newborn baby which must be at least 3 m^2 with clear floor area. All healthcare providers must be familiar with this area and its upkeep. **Table 2.3** outlines the requirement of a newborn care corner.

EQUIPMENT FOR RESUSCITATION

Table 2.4 provides the list of equipment/supplies/medication that must be available for neonatal resuscitation (*Fig.* **2.1**).

Supplies and equipment required for resuscitation must be readily available and accessible for every birth in an organized area

TABLE 2.3: Newborn Care Corner Requirements	
Environment	• Radiant warmer • Well-lit • Draught free area
Equipment	• All equipment/supplies/medication listed in **Table 2.4** • Infant weighing machine • Clearly visible clock (with seconds hand)/timer • All equipment/supplies/medication to be available and functional 24×7 • All supplies/medications checked regularly for their availability by a designated individual using an equipment checklist must
Asepsis	• Hand washing facility (24 hours water supply, elbow/foot operated taps, hand wash detergent, etc.) • Availability of gowns, gloves, and mask • Disposable supplies
Documentation	Standard forms for documenting newborn resuscitation

earmarked for neonatal resuscitation such as the "Newborn Care Corner". This improves the performance of the resuscitation team and would help to minimize delays in the resuscitation process. It is of utmost importance that all equipment be cleaned/disinfected/sterilized before each use, and their function checked periodically and before and after each delivery to ensure that they are ready for use. A brief description regarding some of the important equipment for resuscitation is provided here.

Self-inflating Bag (*Fig.* **2.2**)

A neonatal self-inflating resuscitation bag with mask is the most commonly used device for ventilating an asphyxiated newborn who are <5 kg in weight. It is generally made of silicone or similar approved material. It generally has three main components—the bag, pressure release valve, and a face mask. The tidal volume immediately after birth in the newborn infant ranges from 6–7 mL/kg. During resuscitation, it is generally recommended to maintain a tidal volume between 4 and 8 mL/kg and ventilate at a rate of 40–60 breaths/minute. Ventilation with low tidal volume can result in hypercarbia and atelectotrauma. On the other hand, ventilation

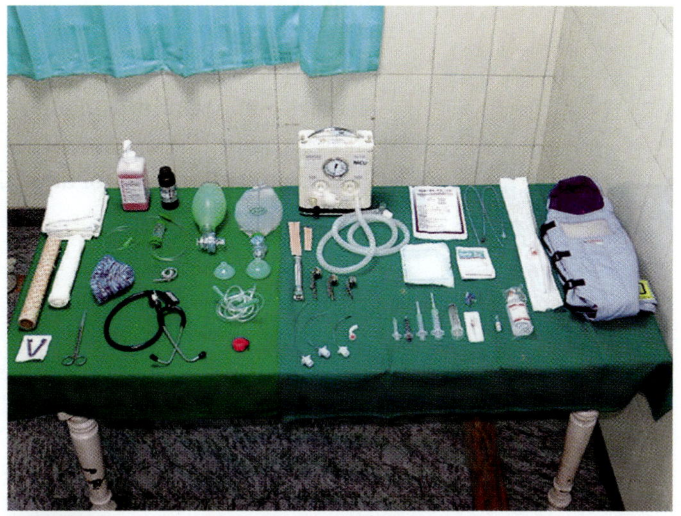

FIG. 2.1 Equipment required for newborn resuscitation.

TABLE 2.4: EQUIPMENT REQUIRED FOR NEONATAL RESUSCITATION

	Term neonates	Additional requirements for preterm neonates
For temperature maintenance	• Radiant warmer (preheated) • Pair of clean prewarmed sheet • Room thermometer • Clinical (digital) thermometer	• Plastic wrap (<32 weeks) • Cap • Thermal mattress (<32 weeks)
For airway clearance	• Suction device set at 80–100 mm Hg (central, electric) • Suction catheters (size,10F,12F) • Mucous extractor • Oropharyngeal airway (size 0, 1) • Shoulder roll	• Oropharyngeal airway (size 00)
For ventilation and oxygenation	• T-piece resuscitator or self-inflating bag (250 mL; 200–320 mL) or flow inflating bag • Face mask (size 0, 1/50–60 mm outer diameter) • Flow meter (up to at least 10 L/min) • Oxygen source • Oxygen blender/oxygen-air mix (set to 21%) • Pulse oximeter with neonatal probe • Feeding tube (size 8F) • Laryngoscope with batteries and straight blade (size 0,1) • ET tubes (size 2.5, 3, 3.5, 4 mm) • Stylet (optional) • Scissors • Laryngeal mask (size 1) (optional) • End-tidal CO_2 detector (optional)	• Face mask (Size 00, 0/35–50 mm outer diameter) • Oxygen blender/oxygen-air mix (set to 21–30%) • Feeding tube (size 5F, 6F) • Laryngoscope straight blade (size 0, 00)
Circulation	• Syringes (1 mL, 2 mL, 5 mL, 10 mL, 20 mL, and 50 mL) • Umbilical catheterization set (umbilical catheters 3.5, 4.0, and 5.0, sterile blade, gloves, cord ties, mosquito forceps, alcohol sponges, povidone iodine, 3-way stopcock) • Adhesive tape • Sterile gauze • Needles—25, 21, and 18-gauge • Stethoscope • Electronic cardiac monitor and ECG leads	
Drugs	• Epinephrine (1:10,000) • Normal saline (0.9%)	
Miscellaneous	• Gloves • Timer • Extra laryngoscope bulb • Extra laryngoscope batteries • Cord scissors • Cord clamp, tie • Measuring tape	Transport incubator

with high tidal volume can result in volutrauma. Therefore, it is recommended that the volume of neonatal resuscitation bags should be around 250 mL (200–320 mL).[12] The bag also has a patient nonbreathing valve with a pressure limiting valve so that it does not exceed an airway pressure of 45 cmH$_2$O and can generate an airway pressure of at least 30 cmH$_2$O. The face mask is generally translucent and made of silicone or similar approved material. It is generally round and available in 2 sizes—size 1 (for term babies) with an outer diameter of 50–60 mm, and size 0 (for preterm and low birth weight babies) with an outer diameter of 35–50 mm (*Fig.* **2.3**). The inlet valve of the compressible bag may have a nipple for connecting an oxygen tube.

In contrast to a self-inflating bag, the ***flow-inflating bag*** (anesthesia bag) only inflates when compressed gas flows into the bag (*Fig.* **2.4**).

T-piece Resuscitator (*Fig.* **2.5**)

It is a flow-controlled pressure limited ventilator device. Compressed gas is delivered at one port of T-piece. A preset peak inspiratory pressure (PIP) and positive end-expiratory pressure (PEEP) is set. It has a maximum pressure relief control, which is a safety feature like the pressure relief valve in a self-inflating resuscitation bag. With a T-piece device, gas flows into a face mask or endotracheal tube through a "patient supply line". Inflation is achieved by interrupting the escape of gas through an outlet hole on the T-piece using a thumb so that the pressure rises and is displayed by a manometer.

Suction Devices

DeeLee mucus extractor is usually made of plastic with two tubes—one goes into mouth of healthcare provider and other (usually 8F/10F size) into the baby's mouth (*Fig.* **2.6**). Suction can also be provided by an *electric suction machine or a central vacuum system or a foot operated suction device.* The maximum vacuum should not be >100 mm Hg. They usually have one or two suction jars of 1 L capacity and a

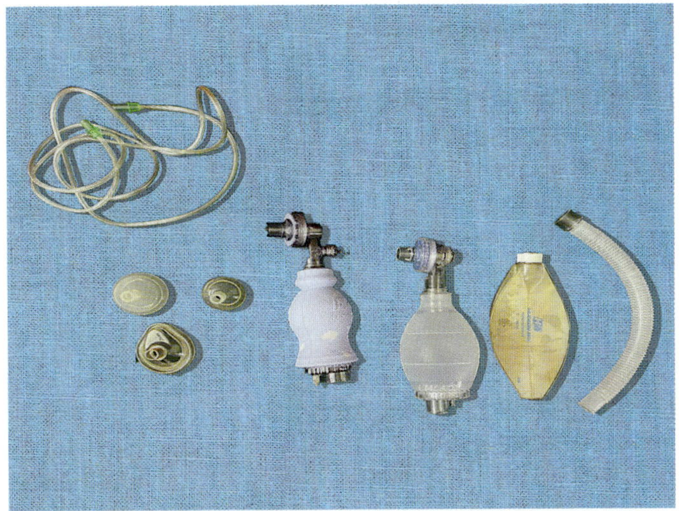
FIG. 2.2 Self-inflating bag, reservoirs, and masks.

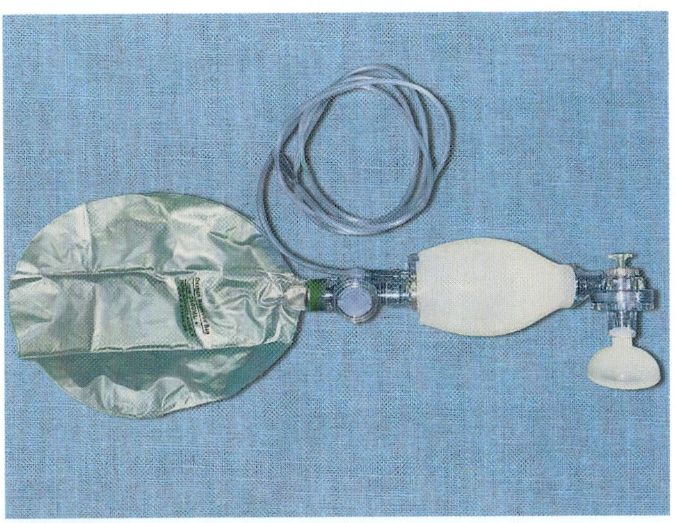
FIG. 2.3 Self-inflating bag with reservoir.
Source: Sweta Kumari, Piyush Gupta.

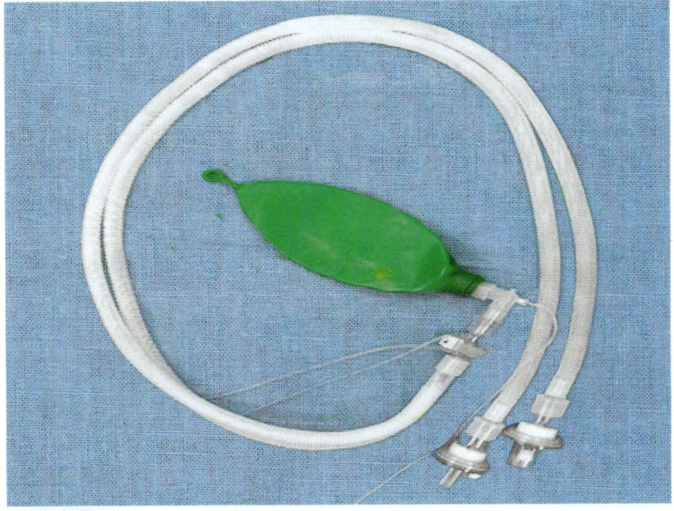
FIG. 2.4 Flow-inflating bag.

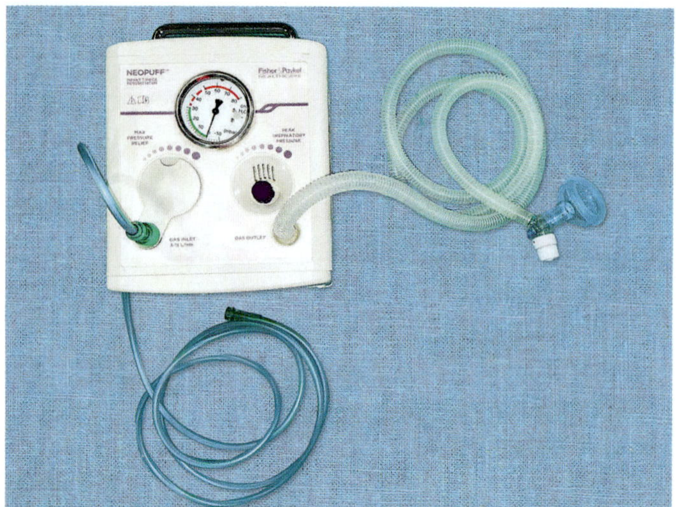

FIG. 2.5 T-piece resuscitator.
Source: Sweta Kumari, Piyush Gupta.

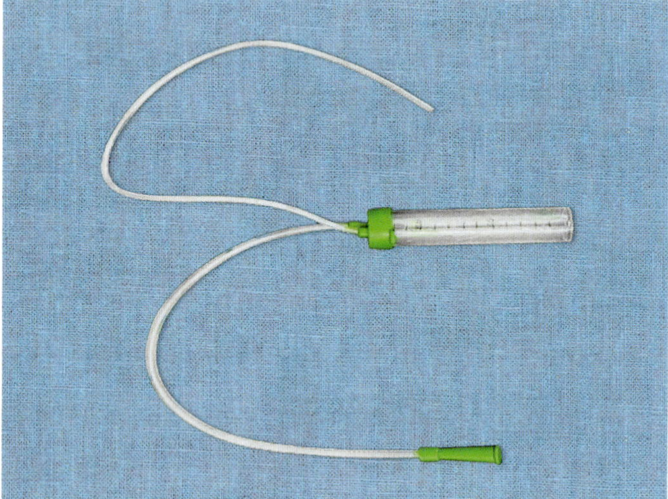

FIG. 2.6 DeeLee's mucous extractor.

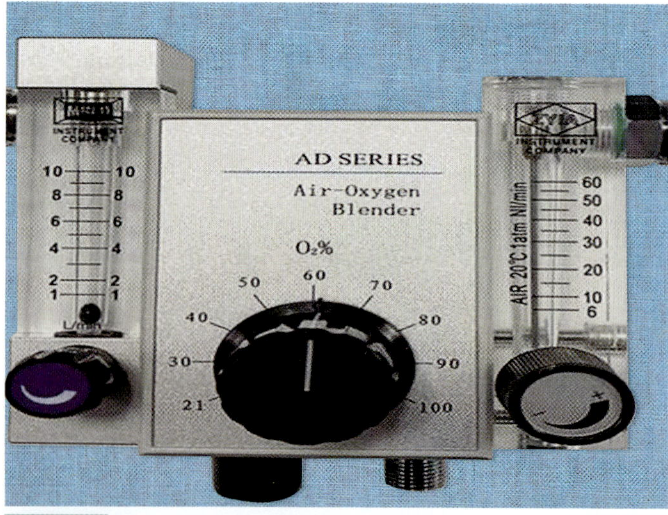

FIG. 2.7 Air-oxygen blender.

connecting tube of noncollapsible material to which an 8F or 10F size suction catheter can be connected.

Oxygen Blender (*Fig.* **2.7**)

An oxygen blender can regulate the delivered inspired oxygen concentrations ranging from 21–100% oxygen. In the absence of a blender, an air-oxygen mix can be used to deliver oxygen concentration to neonates needing resuscitation. **Tables 2.5 and 2.6** provide the oxygen and air flows at a total flow of 8 L/min and 10 L/min respectively, to provide different inspired oxygen concentrations (FiO_2).

Pulse Oximeter

Pulse oximeter is a device to noninvasively measure the oxygen saturation of hemoglobin. The visible red part and the invisible infrared part of the spectrum are specifically absorbed by the oxygenated hemoglobin and reduced hemoglobin fraction respectively. The relative proportional presence of these two fractions is calculated as the percentage of the oxyhemoglobin fraction to the total hemoglobin and is displayed as oxygen saturation percentage on the monitor (*Fig.* **2.8**).

Medication and Supplies

All supplies and medications should be checked for their date of expiry and those which have crossed their expiry date should be discarded.

▪ POSTRESUSCITATION DEBRIEFING

A quick debriefing should be conducted immediately after resuscitation with the team members to review and introspect the actions taken. It provides an opportunity to give inputs and identify areas which could be improved. This helps in better coordination among the team members. The process involves discussion on the following points—need for preparing for resuscitation, asking for the risk factors, and analyzing the information available, how was the preparation and was it done well, whether

TABLE 2.5: Oxygen Air Flows at 8 l/min to Provide Inspired Oxygen Concentrations between 21 and 100%		
Approximate oxygen (%)	**Oxygen flowmeter (L/min)**	**Air flowmeter (L/min)**
21	0	8
30	1	7
40	2	6
50	3	5
60	4	4
70	5	3
80	6	2
90	7	1
100	8	0

TABLE 2.6: Oxygen Air Flows at 10 l/min to Provide Inspired Oxygen Concentrations between 21 and 100%		
Approximate oxygen (%)	**Oxygen flowmeter (L/min)**	**Air flowmeter (L/min)**
21	0	10
30	1	9
40	2	8
50	4	6
60	5	5
70	6	4
80	7.5	2.5
90	9	1
100	10	0

anything was missed or done improperly, could it have been improved and if so how, rating their team's performance, steps for improving individual team member's performance and what were the learning points.

■ BEHAVIOR SKILLS

There are important behavior skills that must be there in all healthcare providers trained for neonatal resuscitation. These key skills are summarized here:[7]

- Knowing one's environment (using equipment checklist, aware of where the equipment are, etc.)
- Using available information
- Anticipating problems and planning for it
- Clearly identifying a team leader
- Be able to communicate effectively
- Be able to delegate workload optimally.
- Be able to assess the clinical situation continuously and monitor the skills of personnel to ensure patient safety
- Be able to use available resources effectively
- Call for additional help when needed (know when to call whom to call and how to call)
- Maintain professional behavior.

These skills need constant and frequent reiteration and practice.

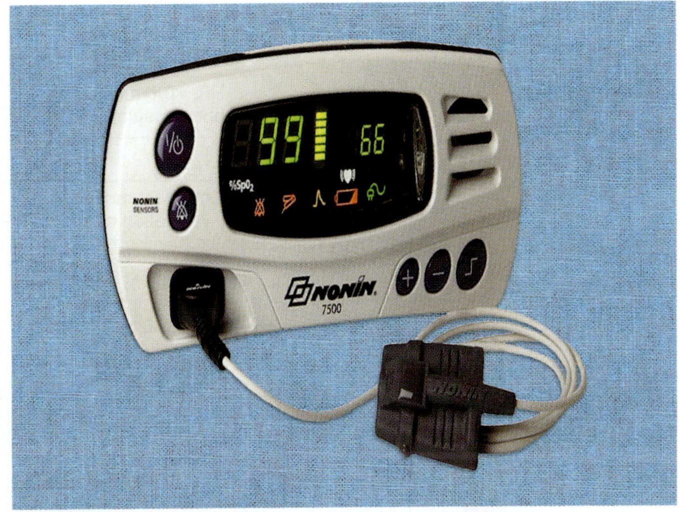

FIG. 2.8 Pulse oximeter with neonatal sensor.

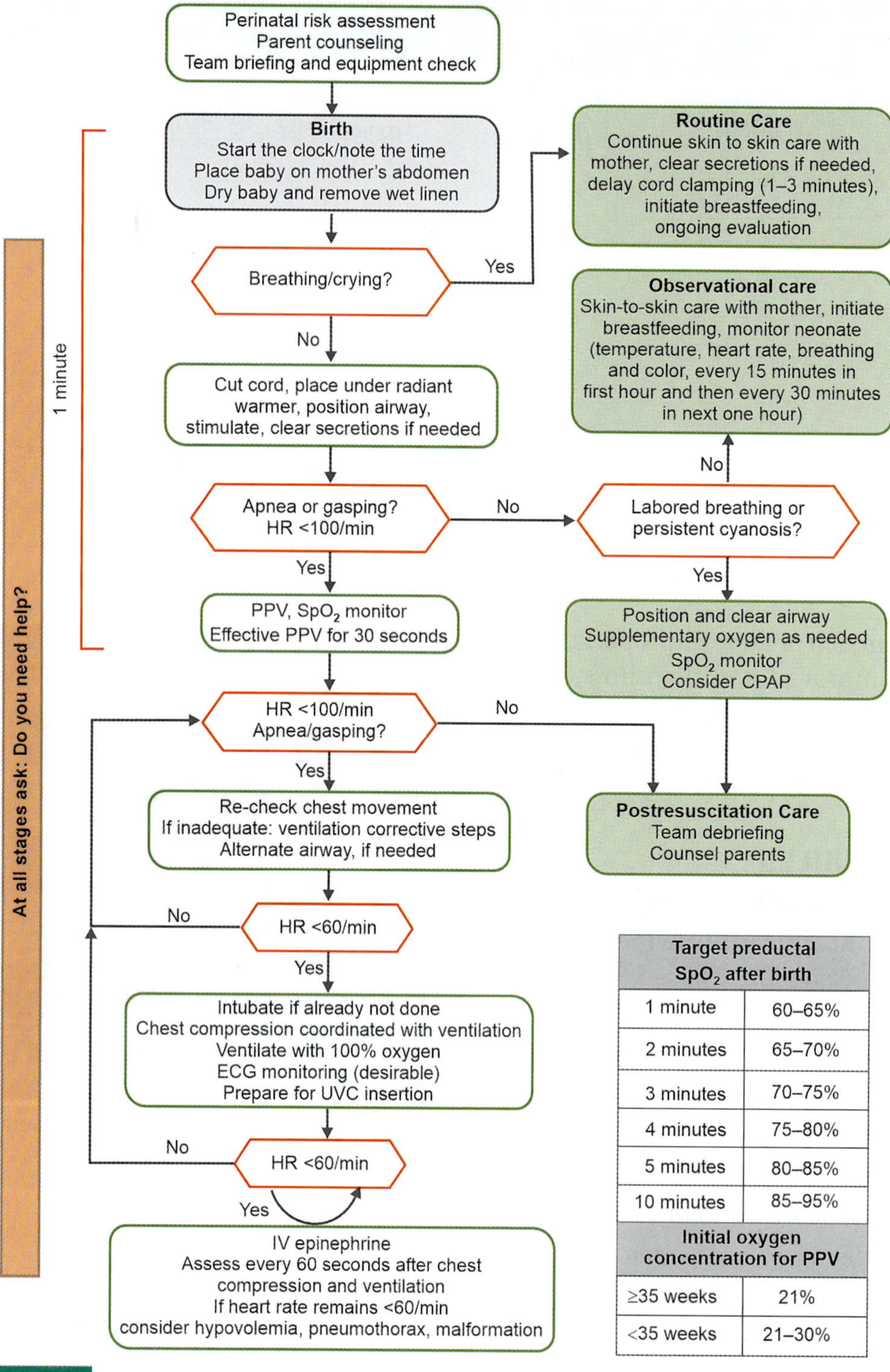

FIG. 2.9 Neonatal resuscitation algorithm.

■ COUNSELING PARENTS

If time permits the healthcare providers should introduce themselves to the parents before birth. They should inform and discuss relevant issues related to the anticipated problems, proposed plan of care and possibility of transfer to neonatal intensive care unit (NICU) if the newborn is high-risk. Parents and/or decision makers in the family should be involved in decision making about extent of resuscitation especially in cases of extreme preterm infants and in those with major malformations.

■ NEONATAL RESUSCITATION ALGORITHM

Figure **2.9** is the flow for the neonatal resuscitation algorithm. All healthcare providers who would be involved in neonatal resuscitation should be familiar with this algorithm. The details of individual sections of the algorithm are being dealt with in subsequent chapters of this book. **Box 2.1** provides an illustrative case of how one prepares for delivery room resuscitation of a newborn infant.

BOX 2.1: ILLUSTRATIVE CASE—PREPARING FOR DELIVERY ROOM NEONATAL RESUSCITATION

A woman is admitted to the delivery room in labor. As the period of pregnancy is 30 weeks, the delivery room informs the neonatal team about the impending delivery. On reaching the delivery room the neonatal team checks with the obstetrician for the number of fetuses and additional risk factors. They are informed that there is a single fetus, and the mother has been leaking per vaginum for over 24 hours and has fever suggesting chorioamnionitis. The team leader ensures that there are at least two members who are trained in advanced neonatal resuscitation. The team leader discusses the anticipated problems and line of action with the team members. Tasks such as receiving the baby and doing initial assessment, performing PPV, intubation, chest compression, administering medication, and documentation are assigned to different persons after confirming their expertise. One team member discusses with the family the possible outcomes and counsels the family about the possible need for resuscitation and subsequent transfer to NICU for care.

*Another team member checks that the windows and fans near the newborn corner are shut, turns on the radiant warmer, and checks it is functioning. Also checks for clean sheets and plastic wrap (as the expected gestation is <32 weeks). They also run a checklist for all the equipment and supplies that may be needed for resuscitation (see **Table 2.4**). The central suction is set to a negative pressure of 80 mm Hg. They assemble and check the function of the self-inflating bag (250 mL). As a T-piece resuscitator is also available, its function is also checked. The flow meter in the central oxygen source is set to 10 L/minute and the oxygen concentration on the blender is set to 30%. The pulse oximeter and its sensor are checked. Equipment for intubation (laryngoscope with straight blades size 0 and 00, endotracheal tubes of 2.5 mm and 3.0 mm ID) are checked. The team also checks for equipment and supplies for umbilical venous cannulation and availability of medication (epinephrine, normal saline).*

All team members have washed their hands following the hand washing protocol, wear gloves and wait for the delivery of the baby.

(NICU: neonatal intensive care unit; PPV: positive pressure ventilation).

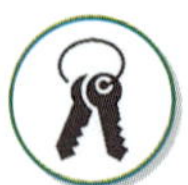

KEY POINTS

1. Majority, but not all newborn, who will require resuscitation can be identified by the presence of perinatal risk factors.

2. Neonatal resuscitation is a team effort, not an individual one.

3. Anticipation and preparation are key to successful resuscitation of newborn.

4. Every delivery room should have a checklist for equipment, supplies and medication required for neonatal resuscitation. All equipment should be functional.

5. All deliveries should be attended by skilled personnel who are solely responsible for the newborn and can perform initial steps, initiate ventilation, and assist in chest compressions.

6. If a high-risk delivery is anticipated, at least two skilled personnel should be present. A team of personnel skilled in advanced resuscitation—intubation, vascular access, and medications, should be readily available if the need arises for all deliveries.

7. Resuscitation is a time bound intervention and demands coordinated teamwork consistently, with high reliability and adaptability.

8. Clear and acknowledged communication is the most basic vital function of a good team and is the one function that fails most frequently.

■ REFERENCES

1. Aziz K, Lee HC, Escobedo MB, Hoover AV, Kamath-Rayne BD, Kapadia VS, et al. Part 5: Neonatal Resuscitation: 2020 American Heart Association Guidelines for Cardiopulmonary Resuscitation and Emergency Cardiovascular Care. Circulation. 2020;142(16_suppl_2):S524-50.

2. Singhal N, Lockyer J, Fidler H, Keenan W, Little G, Bucher S, et al. Helping babies breathe: global neonatal resuscitation program development and formative educational evaluation. Resuscitation. 2012;83(1):90-6.

3. Little GA, Keenan WJ, Niermeyer S, Singhal N, Lawn JE. Neonatal nursing and helping babies breathe: an effective intervention to decrease global neonatal mortality. Newborn Infant Nursin Rev. 2011;11(2):82-7.

4. Shikuku DN, Milimo B, Ayebare E, Gisore P, Nalwadda G. Practice and outcomes of neonatal resuscitation for newborns with birth asphyxia at Kakamega County General Hospital, Kenya: a direct observation study. BMC Pediatr. 2018;18(1):167.

5. Ersdal HL, Mduma E, Svensen E, Perlman J. Birth asphyxia: a major cause of early neonatal mortality in a Tanzanian rural hospital. Pediatrics. 2012;129(5):e1238-e43.

6. World Health Organization. (2012). Guidelines on Basic newborn resuscitation. [online] Available from https://apps.who.int/iris/handle/10665/75157 [Last accessed January, 2023].

7. American Academy of Pediatrics. Textbook of Neonatal Resuscitation, 8th edition. In: Weiner GM, Zaichkin J (Eds). Illinois: American Academy of Pediatrics; 2021.

8. American Academy of Pediatrics and American College of Obstetricians and Gynecologists. Guidelines for Perinatal Care, 8th edition. In: Kilpatrick SJ, Papile LA (Eds). Illinois: American Academy of Pediatrics; 2017.

9. Merchant RM, Topjian AA, Panchal AR, Cheng A, Aziz K, Berg KM, et al. Part 1: Executive Summary: 2020 American Heart Association Guidelines for Cardiopulmonary Resuscitation and Emergency Cardiovascular Care. Circulation. 2020;142(16_suppl_2):S337-57.

10. Ersdal HL, Mduma E, Svensen E, Perlman JM. Early initiation of basic resuscitation interventions including face mask ventilation may reduce birth asphyxia related mortality in low-income countries: a prospective descriptive observational study. Resuscitation. 2012;83(7):869-73.

11. Wyckoff MH, Wyllie J, Aziz K, de Almeida MF, Fabres J, Fawke J, et al. Neonatal Life Support: 2020 International Consensus on Cardiopulmonary Resuscitation and Emergency Cardiovascular Care Science with Treatment Recommendations. Circulation. 2020;142(16_suppl_1):S185-S221.

12. World Health Organization. (2016). WHO Technical Specifications for Neonatal Resuscitation Devices. [online] Available from https://apps.who.int/iris/handle/10665/206540 [Last accessed January, 2023].

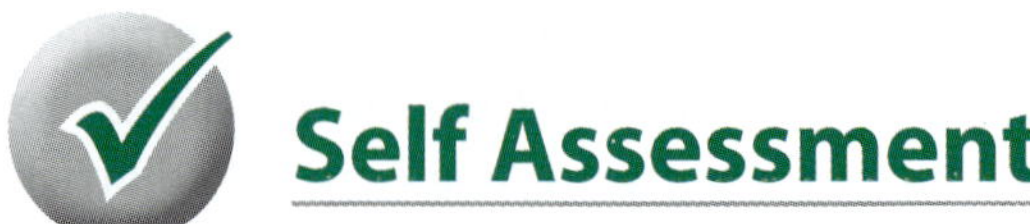

Self Assessment

1. Which of the following statements is not true for preparation at birth?
   a. A person skilled in advanced resuscitation should be available if need arises.
   b. Absence of risk factors suggests no need for skilled person at birth.
   c. All deliveries should be attended by a person skilled in performing initial steps, initiate ventilation, and assist in chest compression.
   d. Resuscitation equipment should be checked before all deliveries.

2. Which of the following is the requirement for a team leader?
   a. Should be the most senior person.
   b. Should be most qualified.
   c. Should be well acquainted with the algorithm, proficient in skills, and demonstrates leadership qualities.
   d. Should be Neonatal Resuscitation Program (NRP) certified.

3. Which of the following is no longer part of essential supplies for newborn resuscitation?
   a. Ringer lactate
   b. Soda bicarbonate
   c. Naloxone
   d. All of the above

4. What happens at a preresuscitation team briefing?
   a. Assess perinatal risk factors.
   b. Identify roles and responsibilities.
   c. Identify anticipated problems and plan of action.
   d. All of the above.

5. Team led resuscitation is advocated in newborns because:
   a. Communication errors are common.
   b. Leads to coordinated efforts.
   c. Leads to better resuscitation outcomes.
   d. All of the above.

6. Which of the following is not a part of essential supplies for newborn resuscitation?
   a. Stylet
   b. End-tidal CO_2
   c. Defibrillator
   d. All of the above.

7. State True/False for the following statements.
   a. With preterm delivery (<37 weeks gestation) special preparations are not required.
   b. The need for resuscitation in newborns can reliably be predicted on risk factors.
   c. A qualified team with full resuscitation skills should be identified and immediately available for every birth where resuscitation is anticipated.
   d. Effective teamwork and communication are optional skills during neonatal resuscitation.

8. What are the questions you should ask obstetrician prior to delivery to identify "risk status"?

9. A primi, 38 weeks' gestation has been admitted in active labor with meconium-stained liquor. You are asked to attend immediately. List how you would prepare for birth of her baby.

Answers

For answers, go to the end of the Book, Page no. 321

SECTION **2**

The Process of Neonatal Resuscitation: Basics

Initial Newborn Care

Somashekhar Nimbalkar

Lessons to Learn

- ○ The immediate steps after birth
- ○ Appropriate timing for umbilical cord clamping after delivery
- ○ Routine care for vigorous newborn babies
- ○ Initial steps for nonvigorous babies
- ○ Assessing the newborn after initial steps
- ○ Observational care for babies responding to initial steps
- ○ Providing free flow oxygen
- ○ Managing babies with difficult breathing

Every newborn infant immediately after birth needs to be assessed to determine if they have normally transitioned from fetal to neonatal life (vigorous at birth) or need assistance to establish adequate spontaneous breathing (delayed transition). Those newborns who are vigorous at birth can be cared for with their mother by providing *"Routine Care"*. Newborns with delayed transition (nonvigorous) would need further assessment and assistance to establish adequate spontaneous breathing. Recent updates to the guidelines for neonatal resuscitation provide the basis for changes in approach to managing the newborn at birth.[1-3] **Box 3.1** provides an illustrative case of a newborn infant who is vigorous at birth, and **Box 3.2** is an illustrative case of a newborn who

---

BOX 3.1: CASE STUDY: NORMAL TRANSITION

A 28-year-old second-gravida woman with an uneventful term pregnancy is admitted to the delivery room in active labor. Her membranes had ruptured 2 hours back on the way to the hospital. A lady companion with the woman said that the amniotic fluid was clear. The labor room nurse carries out a check on equipment and supplies for neonatal resuscitation in case it may be required. The labor progresses normally and after 4 hours a baby girl is delivered vaginally by vertex presentation. As soon as the baby is delivered, "time of birth" is noted. The baby is immediately put on the mother's abdomen and dried using a warm towel and the wet towel is discarded. On assessment, the baby was crying vigorously and had a good tone. The baby is placed prone skin-to-skin on the mother's abdomen and covered with warm linen and noted to be pink. The cord is cut after 1 minute of birth. The baby is then shifted onto the mother's chest in skin-to-skin position and is assessed periodically by the nurse for her breathing, color, temperature, and heart rate. Soon thereafter the mother is assisted to breastfeed the baby.

BOX 3.2: CASE STUDY: DELAYED TRANSITION

A primigravida woman presents at 38 weeks' gestation with active labor and ruptured membranes and noted to have high blood pressure. Cardio-tocograph (CTG) monitoring reveals an indeterminate pattern of fetal heart rate. The neonatal team is informed. The team on arrival enquires from the obstetrician for any additional risk factors and is informed that there are no other risk factors. The team has a briefing session, and then they carry out a check of equipment and supplies. Soon thereafter a male baby is delivered.

Immediately after birth, the time is noted and baby is placed on mother's abdomen and dried. The baby is not crying and appears to have poor tone. The umbilical cord is immediately cut, and baby is brought and placed under a radiant warmer. After positioning the baby in sniffing position, stimulation is provided by gently rubbing his back, and gentle suction of his mouth and nose is done as the baby is noted to have secretions in its mouth. His tone and respiratory effort quickly improve. A team member auscultates to check the heart rate and reports that the baby's heart rate is 140 beats per minute (bpm).

After 3 minutes of birth, the baby's color has not improved and is noted to have central cyanosis. Another team member attaches a pulser oximeter sensor on the baby's right hand and connects it to the pulse oximeter. Oxygen saturation (SpO$_2$) is 66% (which is below the minute-specific target value). The flow meter is set at 10 L/min and the FiO$_2$ on the blender is set at 30% oxygen concentration. Supplemental oxygen is provided by holding the oxygen tubing close to the baby's face. The oxygen concentration is adjusted so that his oxygen saturation remains within the target range. By 10 minutes after birth, the baby has good respiratory efforts with normal target oxygen saturations and supplemental oxygen having been discontinued. Baby is placed in skin-to-skin position on his mother's chest with periodic assessment of breathing, heart rate, color, and temperature. Thereafter the team leader conducts a debriefing session with the team to discuss the resuscitation that had just been carried out.

is nonvigorous at birth and has delayed transition. You can follow these cases as you read through this chapter. *Figure* **3.1** highlights the relevant section in the neonatal resuscitation algorithm.

IMMEDIATE STEPS AFTER THE BIRTH OF BABY

The *time of birth* should be noted as soon as the last fetal part has been delivered and the timer should be started. If no timer is available, the nurse in the delivery room assigned to look after the baby should note the time and record the events observed along with the time. The baby should be placed on the mother's abdomen (*Fig.* **3.2**), dried and wet linen removed and assessed for the following: *Is the newborn breathing or crying?*

If the baby is vigorous (breathing or crying), "**Routine Care**" is provided with the mother. If the baby is nonvigorous, the cord should be clamped and cut, and the baby shifted under the radiant warmer to provide "**Initial Steps.**"

Timing of Cord Clamping

The current recommendations are for delaying cord clamping (DCC). There is no standard definition of delayed cord clamping, and it ranges from 30 seconds to 3 minutes and sometimes even beyond till delivery of the placenta. ***However, the current national guidelines recommend delaying cord clamping for at least 1–3 minutes.*** In preterm infants <34 weeks gestation, DCC marginally improves survival, early cardiovascular stability, and hematological indices; decreases requirement for blood transfusions; and improves iron

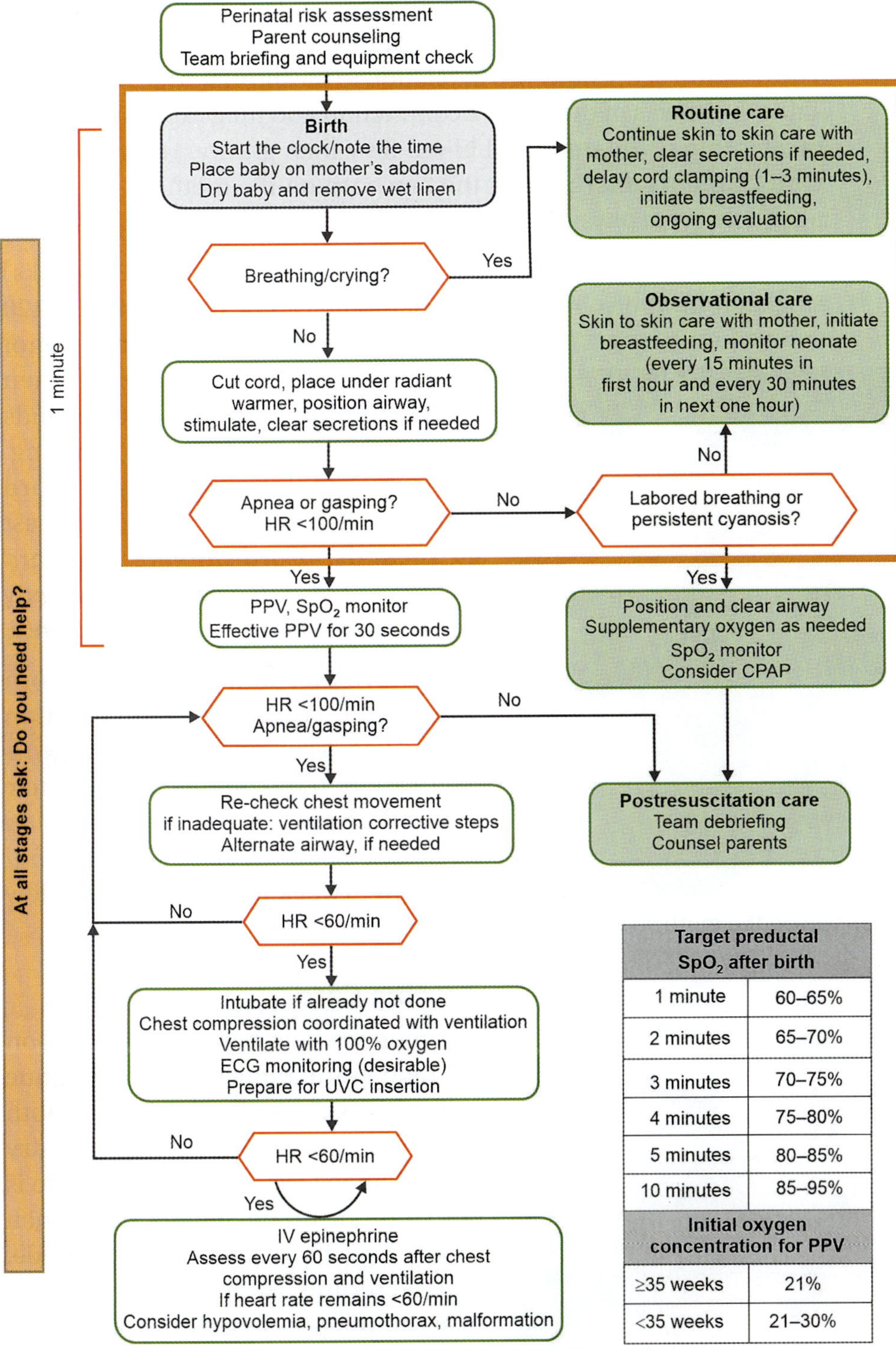

Target preductal SpO2 after birth	
1 minute	60–65%
2 minutes	65–70%
3 minutes	70–75%
4 minutes	75–80%
5 minutes	80–85%
10 minutes	85–95%
Initial oxygen concentration for PPV	
≥35 weeks	21%
<35 weeks	21–30%

FIG. 3.1 Neonatal resuscitation algorithm.
(Boxed area indicates the steps related to providing initial steps).

stores for up to 3–6 months. It also reduces the risk of necrotizing enterocolitis and intraventricular hemorrhage (IVH) in premature infants and improves their developmental outcomes.[4]

In late preterm and term infants, no effect on mortality or need for resuscitation was seen, but circulatory and hematological parameters were better in those neonates who received DCC. A term infant can receive up to 30 mL/kg of additional blood when DCC is performed. The position of the newborn in relation to the introitus does not matter since the effects of the uterine contraction and lung expansion have a greater impact on umbilical blood flow than gravity. Hence delayed cord clamping after placing the newborn on the mother's abdomen after delivery is physiological and evidence based.[5]

In preterm (<37 weeks) and extremely preterm (<28 weeks) singleton newborn infants, cord clamping can be delayed for 60–120 seconds. When cord clamping cannot be delayed for 60–120 seconds, then cord clamping for at least 30 seconds is superior to immediate clamping. In term singletons, delayed cord clamping is recommended for at least 60 seconds.[6] *Cord milking (cut cord or intact cord milking) is not currently recommended due to uncertain evidence.*

However, for nonvigorous newborn infants, the current recommendation state *"For term and preterm infants who require resuscitation at birth, there is insufficient evidence to recommend early cord clamping versus delayed cord clamping"* (weak recommendation, low level evidence).[3]

Routine Care

Vigorous newborn baby who is placed on the mother's abdomen should continue to receive skin-to-skin care with both baby and mother covered with dry (warm) linen (*Fig.* **3.3**). The baby who is placed prone on the mother's abdomen should have its head turned to one side, and secretions (if any) are suctioned using a low-pressure device such as a mucous extractor or bulb suction. While performing all these actions, the care provider should continue to assess the baby for breathing, color, and activity.

The cord is clamped about 1–3 minutes after birth and the baby shifted between the mother's breast and skin-to-skin care continued for at least an hour.

FIG. 3.2 Newborn placed skin-to-skin on the mother's abdomen immediately after delivery.

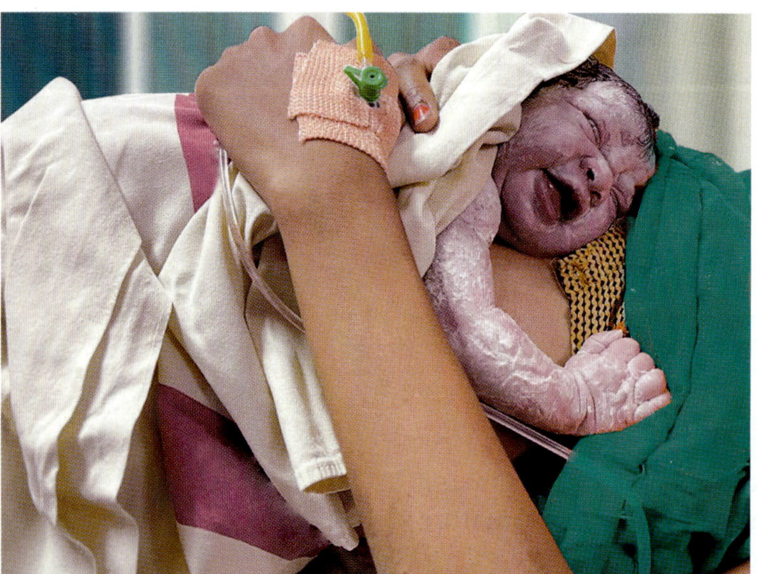

FIG. 3.3 Vigorous newborn receiving skin-to-skin care on mother's abdomen after delivery.

The current recommendation states *"Placing healthy newborn infants who do not require resuscitation skin-to-skin after birth can be effective in improving breastfeeding, temperature control, and blood glucose stability"* (moderate recommendation, moderate level of evidence).[3]

An identification label may be placed on the baby's wrist at this juncture. This should contain the mother's name, sex of baby, date and time of delivery, and the hospital registration number of the mother too. The neonate remains with the mother in skin-to-skin care for an hour. The mother should be encouraged to breastfeed as soon as possible; in most circumstances, this is possible within 30–60 minutes of birth. The accompanying birth companion can help in this process by comforting and supporting the mother.

Procedures such as weighing the newborn, injection of vitamin K, immunization, etc., can be deferred and carried out at the end of the hour. The baby is monitored regularly during the first hour for breathing, color, heart rate, and temperature. The stump should be observed for oozing of blood. The stump is to be left uncovered and allowed to dry, and no medication/substance should be applied to the cord.

■ INITIAL STEPS FOR A NONVIGOROUS BABY

If the baby is nonvigorous, the cord should be cut immediately, and the neonate is placed supine under the radiant warmer (*Fig.* **3.4**). The baby's temperature should be maintained between 36.5°C and 37.4°C. Preterm neonates <32 weeks should be placed in plastic wrap/bag (this can be done even without drying).

Position

The baby's neck is placed in a neutral or slightly extended position (eyes facing the roof) in what may be termed a "sniffing position" (hyperflexion or hyperextension interfere with air flow in the airways) to ensure an open airway. If required to maintain neck position, a shoulder roll (small, rolled towel about 1 inch in height) may be placed under the baby' shoulder. It may also be useful if there is a large caput or the baby is preterm.

Stimulation

If the baby is still not breathing or crying after the above-mentioned steps, provide tactile stimulation by gently rubbing the back. Vigorous stimulation may harm the baby.

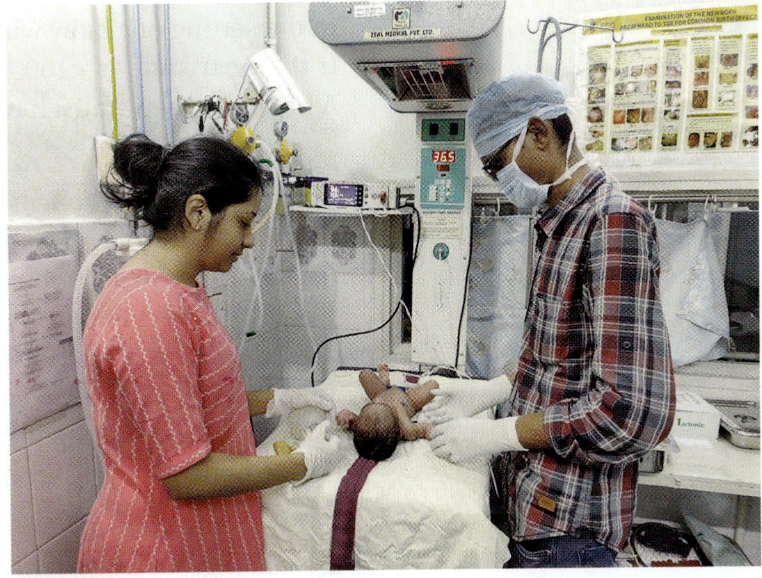

FIG. 3.4 Nonvigorous newborn placed under the radiant warmer.

Clearing Secretions

If the baby is still not breathing, or is gasping or has copious secretions, then clear the airway by suctioning the mouth followed by the nose (depth of insertion of the catheter being not >5 cm in the mouth and 2 cm in the nose—in term neonates). Care should be taken not to suction too deeply as it may cause vagal stimulation leading to bradycardia or apnea. Vigorous suction can damage fragile tissues. For suction, one can either use a mucus extractor or a suction machine (ensure that the suction pressure is between 80 and 100 mm Hg).

The entire process of initial steps should be completed by 30 seconds, and at the end of that period, the healthcare provider assesses the newborn.

◼ ASSESSING NEWBORN RESPONSE TO INITIAL STEPS

A nonvigorous newborn after the initial steps should be assessed for breathing and heart rate. At this stage the following scenarios may be encountered.

Baby not Breathing OR is Gasping

If the baby is not breathing or gasping after initial steps, the baby must be immediately provided positive pressure ventilation (PPV). Prolonging initial steps beyond 1 minute would make the baby more hypoxic. **It must be underscored that ventilation is the most important step during neonatal resuscitation.**

If at this time, there is only one person caring for the baby at the radiant warmer, they must call for additional help immediately.

Newborn is Breathing, but the Heart Rate is <100 bpm

In the setting of a baby who is breathing, heart rate must be assessed. If the heart rate is <100 bpm, PPV must be initiated immediately. A breathing baby must have a heart rate of at least 100 bpm.

Measuring the heart rate: The current recommendations state *"During resuscitation of term and preterm newborns, the use of electrocardiography (ECG) for the rapid and accurate measurement of the newborn's heart rate may be reasonable"* (weak recommendation, low level of evidence).[3] However, ECG may not be available in all delivery rooms. The next best method for assessing heart rate is the auscultation of the precordium with a stethoscope. Heart rate is estimated by counting the beats in 6 seconds and multiplying by 10 (e.g., count of 10 in 6 seconds will provide a heartbeat of 100 bpm).

Cord pulsations for assessing heart rate during newborn resuscitation are no longer recommended as studies have shown that the assessment is unreliable.

Newborn is Breathing, Heart Rate is 100 bpm or more but is Cyanosed

In this scenario, to confirm hypoxia a pulse oximeter sensor must be placed on the baby's right hand to confirm the baby's oxygen saturation level and confirm if there is hypoxia.

Saturation monitor: These are devices used to detect oxygen saturation non-invasively (*Fig.* **3.5**). Appropriate neonatal probes and saturation monitors must be used to detect the newborn's oxygen saturation. The oximeters used during neonatal resuscitation need "minimal averaging time for the SpO_2 values coupled with maximum sensitivity." The oximeter sensors are always placed on the right wrist/palm (*Fig.* **3.6**) as placement at other locations can lead to low saturation readings. It occurs because the recordings are from the post-ductal flow (which has blood leaving the left ventricular chamber) mixing with the poorly oxygenated blood pumped out of the right ventricular chamber via the patent ductus arteriosus, as it has bypassed the lungs. Healthcare providers should familiarize themselves with the workings of saturation monitors as often wrong readings may be noted especially when the perfusion is poor.

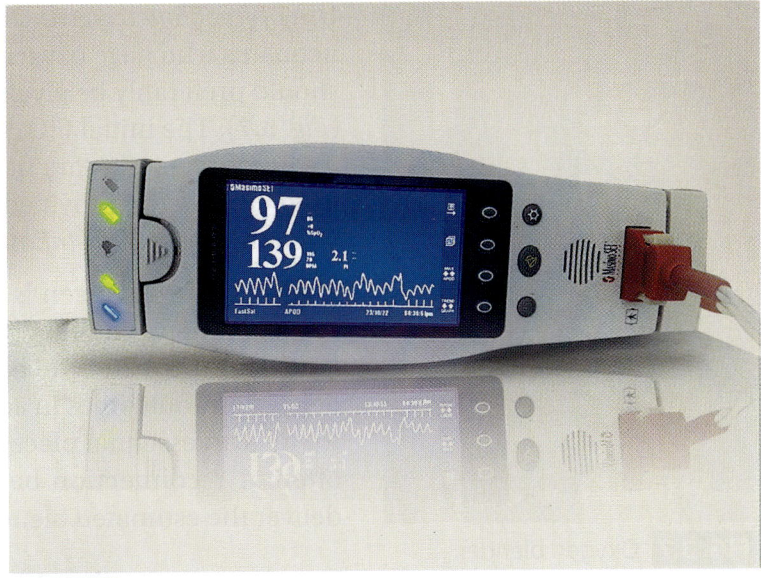

FIG. 3.5 Pulse oximeter displaying the oxygen saturation, heart rate, and the plethysmographic waveforms.

Oxygen saturation targets: In utero, the fetus has a low oxygen saturation of 60%, and it takes some time to achieve normal extrauterine saturation of >90%. Saturation values after birth for normal transitioning term infants have been published and are used in guiding oxygen supplementation during neonatal resuscitation. The pulse oximeter, when connected to the newborn at birth, takes some time to show an appropriate value, and on an average, a stable reading is detected at the end of 1 minute of life. These oxygen saturation targets are evolving, and currently used targets are given in **Table 3.1**. It is also important to remember that saturation readouts are available earlier with vaginal deliveries than cesarean deliveries.[7]

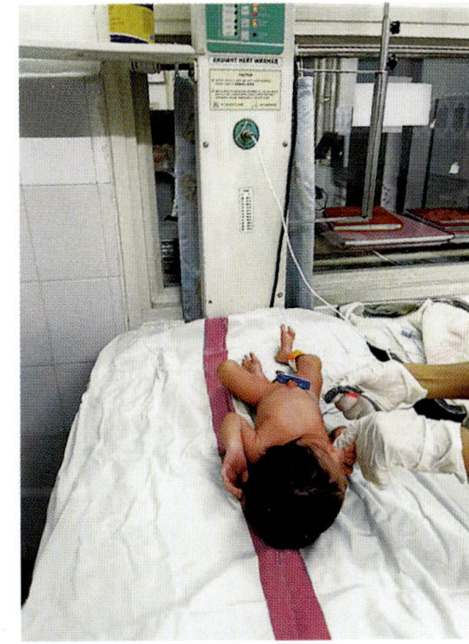

FIG. 3.6 Attaching the probe of pulse oximeter to the right wrist.

TABLE 3.1: TARGET PREDUCTAL OXYGEN SATURATION	
1 minute	60–65%
2 minutes	65–70%
3 minutes	70–75%
4 minutes	75–80%
5 minutes	80–85%
10 minutes	85–95%

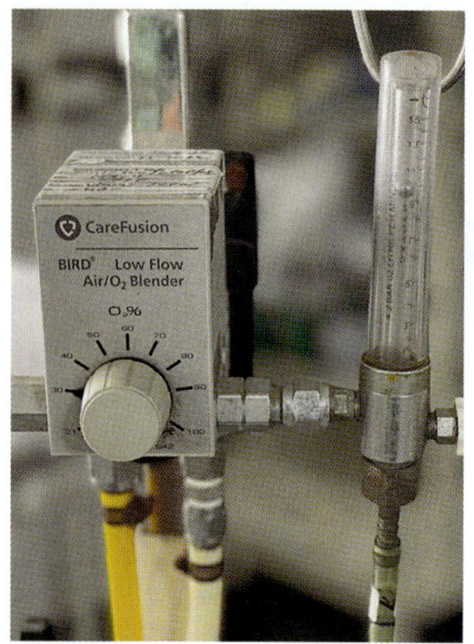

FIG. 3.7 Oxygen blender.

Use of free flow oxygen: Oxygen should be provided to term/preterm neonates who have oxygen saturation below the target levels. Oxygen should preferably be given via a blender at a flow rate of 10 L/minute (*Fig.* **3.7**). The initial FiO_2 should be 30% and can be increased slowly if saturation targets are not being met. Humidified oxygen should be used and can be provided via a mask or via a T-piece device or flow inflating device. *Self-inflating bags cannot provide free flow oxygen.*

Use of 100% oxygen is damaging to the tissues and can result in oxygen radical induced damage to tissues far removed from the lung, and there are studies that link brief oxygen exposure at birth to deleterious outcomes in adolescence. Hence a blender in the delivery room is an essential piece of equipment. In the absence of a blender, often, a Y connection between medical air and oxygen is used to deliver the estimated blended oxygen concentration.

Newborn is having Labored Breathing with Retractions with Heart Rate ≥100 bpm

Neonates who have labored breathing with heart rates ≥100 bpm can benefit from use of CPAP in the delivery room. CPAP can be delivered using a flow-inflating bag or a T-piece resuscitator device, both driven by blended oxygen. T-piece is the preferred device as pressure settings can be easily set. There is lack of studies to back delivery room CPAP for term infants, and hence due to the higher risk of air leak syndromes, it should be given for as short as required. The CPAP pressures should normally be kept at 5–6 cm of H_2O.

*Babies who have cyanosis or labored breathing and are provided free flow oxygen/CPAP in the delivery room should be shifted for "**post-resuscitation care**" to a special care newborn unit or NICU where they can be closely monitored.*

Newborn is Breathing well, Heart Rate ≥100 bpm, and is Pink in Color

Such newborn babies should be provided "**Observational Care**." The baby should be placed back on the mother's abdomen for continued skin-skin-care. Both the newborn and mother should be covered in a warm blankets/linen to maintain warmth and normal body temperature. The mother should be encouraged to breastfeed as soon as possible. The newborn should be checked for breathing, color, heart rate, and temperature at least every 15 minutes in the first hour and every 30 minutes during the next hour.

■ MECONIUM-STAINED AMNIOTIC FLUID

The management of a newborn does not change if the newborn is born through meconium-stained amniotic fluid (MSAF). The current recommendation states *"For nonvigorous newborns (presenting with apnea or ineffective breathing effort) delivered through MSAF, routine laryngoscopy with or without tracheal suctioning is not recommended"* (strong recommendation, low level of evidence due to limited data).

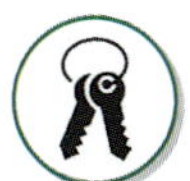

KEY POINTS

1. Most newborn babies transit normally out of the intrauterine environment.
2. About 10% need some assistance in the delivery room after birth to facilitate transition to the extrauterine environment.
3. Delayed cord clamping after 1–3 minutes of birth should be performed for all-term and preterm neonates who are breathing well at birth.
4. All vigorous babies should be provided skin-to-skin care on the mother's abdomen following delivery and supported for breastfeeding during the first hour after birth.
5. Nonvigorous babies should be provided initial steps.
6. Babies not breathing or are gasping or having a heart rate <100 bpm after initial steps should be immediately provided positive pressure ventilation (PPV).
7. Babies after birth who are breathing well with heart rate of 100 bpm or more but cyanosed need to be provided free flow oxygen along with monitoring of their oxygen saturation with an oxygen saturation monitor.
8. Babies with difficult breathing after birth may be considered for continuous positive airway pressure (CPAP) support in the delivery room.

■ REFERENCES

1. Wyckoff MH, Wyllie J, Aziz K, de Almeida MF, Fabres J, Fawke J, et al. Neonatal Life Support: 2020 International Consensus on Cardiopulmonary Resuscitation and Emergency Cardiovascular Care Science with Treatment Recommendations. Circulation. 2020;142(16_suppl_1):S185-221.

2. Madar J, Roehr CC, Ainsworth S, Ersdal H, Morley C, Rüdiger M, et al. European Resuscitation Council Guidelines 2021: Newborn resuscitation and support of transition of infants at birth. Resuscitation. 2021;161:291-326.

3. Aziz K, Lee CHC, Escobedo MB, Hoover AV, Kamath-Rayne BD, Kapadia VS, et al. Part 5: Neonatal Resuscitation 2020 American Heart Association Guidelines for Cardiopulmonary Resuscitation and Emergency Cardiovascular Care. Pediatrics. 2021;147(Suppl 1):e2020038505E.

4. Gomersall J, Berber S, Middleton P, McDonald SJ, Niermeyer S, El-Naggar W, et al. Umbilical cord management at term and late preterm birth: a meta-analysis. Pediatrics. 2021;147(3):e2020015404.

5. Seidler AL, Gyte GML, Rabe H, Díaz-Rossello JL, Duley L, Aziz K, et al. Umbilical cord management for newborns <34 weeks' gestation: a meta-analysis. Pediatrics. 2021;147(3):e20200576.

6. McDonald SD, Narvey M, Ehman W, Jain V, Cassell K. Guideline No. 424: Umbilical Cord Management in Preterm and Term Infants. J Obstet Gynaecol Can. 2022;44(3):313-22.e1.

7. Sankaran D, Lakshminrusimha S, Saugstad OD. Physiology of neonatal resuscitation: Giant strides with small breaths. Semin Perinatol. 2022;46(6):151620.

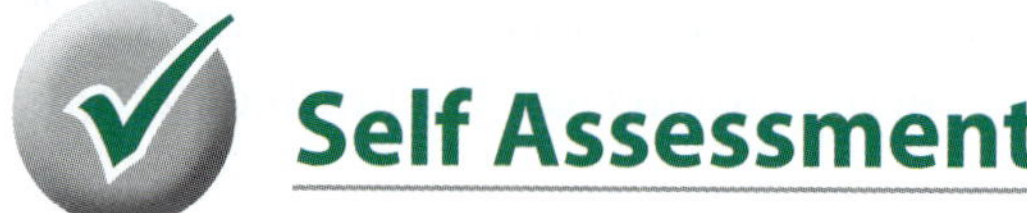

Self Assessment

State TRUE or FALSE

1. During delayed cord clamping, the baby must be held below the level of vaginal introitus till the cord is clamped and cut.

2. The recommended time for skin-to-skin contact on mother's abdomen after birth in a vigorous newborn is at least 60 minutes.

3. There is strong evidence that nonvigorous baby after birth can be resuscitated with intact cord on mother's abdomen.

4. Routine suction in a breathing/crying infant is not recommended.

5. Umbilical cord pulsation is a reliable method to estimate the baby's heart rare after birth.

6. Free flow oxygen can be administered with a self-inflating bag.

7. If an apneic baby does not start breathing after 30 seconds of initial steps, PPV must be immediately initiated.

Fill in the Blanks

8. The correct sequence for initial steps in a nonvigorous baby is __________ ,__________, and__________.

9. Free flow oxygen must be initiated with flow of________L/min and FiO_2 of _____%.

10. What monitoring must be done when the newborn is with the mother during routine care and for how long?

Answers

For answers, go to the end of the Book, Page no. 321

Positive Pressure Ventilation

Rhishikesh Thakre

Lessons to Learn

- ❍ The devices that are used for positive pressure ventilation—self-inflating bag, flow-inflating bag, T-piece resuscitator
- ❍ How to provide positive pressure ventilation (PPV)—when to initiate PPV, how to prepare, providing PPV, oxygen concentration during PPV, evaluating response to PPV
- ❍ Postresuscitation care

About 10% of newborns require some resuscitation at birth. Of those who need assistance for transition at birth, about 40% are estimated to need positive pressure ventilation (PPV) in the delivery room to establish effective ventilation.[1,2] PPV remains the main intervention in neonatal resuscitation, and it is of paramount importance that all healthcare providers who would be assigned the role of caring for the newborn in the delivery room should develop the skills of providing PPV to the newborn infant at birth. Animal studies indicate that in asphyxiated newborn infants, primary apnea leads to secondary apnea and cessation of breathing before occurrence of cardiac arrest. This is different from asphyxiated adults in whom respiratory failure and cardiac arrest occur simultaneously.[2] Hence, it is important that effective ventilation is achieved first before moving further down the resuscitation algorithm to chest compression. **Box 4.1** provides an illustrative case of providing PPV to a baby in the delivery room after birth. You can follow it as you progress through this chapter. *Figure* **4.4** highlights the relevant section in the neonatal resuscitation algorithm that is applicable to PPV.

■ DEVICES USED FOR POSITIVE PRESSURE VENTILATION

There are several devices used for delivering PPV, viz., self-inflating bag, flow-inflating bag, and T-piece resuscitator.[3] It is essential that one is familiar with the equipment available in his/her hospital.

BOX 4.1: ILLUSTRATIVE CASE

A 25-year-old primigravida mother with term gestation is admitted in labor. The progress of labor is slow, and the obstetrician notices a caput on the fetal skull on per vaginal examination and decides to use vacuum extraction for delivering the baby. The neonatal team is informed. The team on arrival enquires from the obstetrician for any additional risk factors and is informed that there are no other risk factors. The team has a briefing session, and they then carry out a check of equipment and supplies. Soon thereafter, a male baby is delivered by vacuum extraction and placed onto the mother's abdomen. The baby is noted to be limp and not breathing. The cord is cut immediately, and baby is handed over to a resuscitation team member who receives the baby in a pre-warmed sheet and places the baby under a radiant warmer in sniffing position to open the airway. The baby is briefly stimulated, by tapping the soles. A quick oropharyngeal and nasal suction is done. As the baby is still not breathing after these initial steps and on auscultation has a heart rate of 80/minute, the resuscitation team decides to initiate positive pressure ventilation.

PPV is initiated with room air (21% oxygen). Another team member reports that the "chest is not rising". Another member of the team places a sensor on the right hand of the baby and connects to a pulse oximeter and begins documenting the events. Ventilation corrective steps are initiated. First the mask is reapplied, and the head and neck of the baby is repositioned. The assistant still reports "no chest rise" with each assisted breath. The mouth and nose are suctioned with a mucus extractor and PPV restarted. Still no chest rise is observed. Then the pressure for PPV is increased at which point the assistant reports "chest is rising". After 15 seconds of PPV, the assistant reports "heart rate is 90/minute". PPV is continued with "squeeze-two-three" mnemonic to provide breaths at 40–60 breaths per minute for next the 15 seconds. At the end of 30 seconds of PPV, the baby has no spontaneous breathing, and the assistant auscultates and reports that the heart rate has increased to 110/minute and the oxygen saturation is 70%. PPV is continued with room air. After 3 minutes of birth, baby is noticed to be breathing spontaneously. The assisted ventilation breaths are decreased and by 4 minutes has good spontaneous breathing, with heart rate of 140/minute with oxygen saturation of 83% and is vigorous. PPV is discontinued. Cord is tied and baby is shown to mother. While part of the team is arranging to transport the baby to the NICU, the team leader explains the subsequent course of action to the mother. Thereafter the team leader conducts a de-briefing session with the team to discuss the resuscitation that was just carried out.

Self-inflating Bag

Self-inflating bag (SIB) (approximately 250 mL) is the most commonly used ventilation device. The bag remains inflated unless it is squeezed. After release, it reinflates on its own due to elastic recoil and draws fresh gas into the bag through the inlet port. If it is not connected to an oxygen source, it draws in 21% oxygen (room air). If it is connected to an oxygen source (with a reservoir bag connected to the bag), the bag is filled with oxygen concentration as the source. The rate of ventilation is determined by how often one squeezes the bag and the inspiratory time (IT) by how quickly one squeezes the bag. The peak inspiratory pressure (PIP) is determined by how much one squeezes the bag. Positive end-expiratory pressure (PEEP) can be given if a PEEP valve is connected to the device.

Parts of the SIB: The parts of an SIB are: (1) Gas outlet, (2) Valve assembly, (3) PEEP valve (optional), (4) Pressure release (pop-off) valve, (5) Gas (oxygen) inlet, (6) Oxygen reservoir (open/closed type), (7) Oxygen tubing, and (8) Manometer (optional). *Figures* **4.1A to E** provide details of the parts of the SIB.

How the self-inflating bag functions: When the bag re-inflates on release from squeeze, gas flows into the bag from the following three sources— air flows in from the holes on rear assembly of the bag, from the oxygen gas inlet (oxygen flows from the blender and flow meter through the oxygen tubing into the inlet) and an oxygen reservoir (where oxygen from the blender accumulates) if there is one attached. When the bag is squeezed, gas from the bag exists via the gas outlet to the patient where an interface such as face mask or endotracheal tube is connected. There is a valve assembly between the bag and gas outlet which has a valve that opens when the bag is squeezed, directing the gas to flow toward the patient and closes when the bag re-expands, thus preventing patient's exhaled gas from entering the bag and prevents rebreathing. There is also a pressure relief valve which is generally designed to open when pressures exceed 30–40 cmH$_2$O; however, one must be cautious as very often they are unreliable. If there is provision for attaching an adjustable PEEP valve, one can use it to deliver PEEP during PPV.

Flow-inflating Bag (Anesthesia Bag)

The bag fills only when a source of compressed gas (oxygen, air, or a mix of the two) flows into the bag, else it remains collapsed. It does not

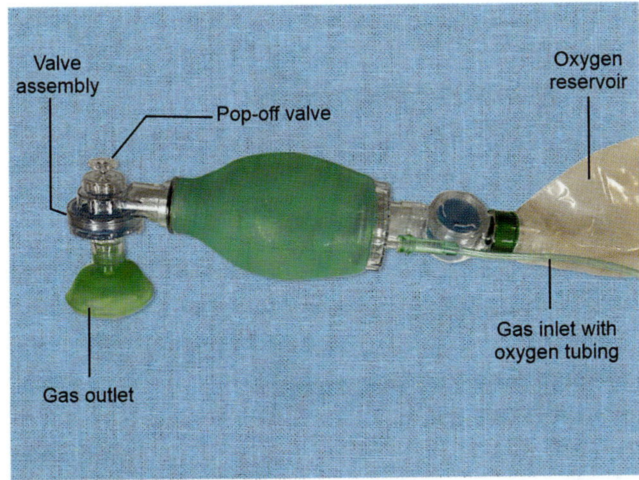

FIG. 4.1A Parts of self-inflating bag.

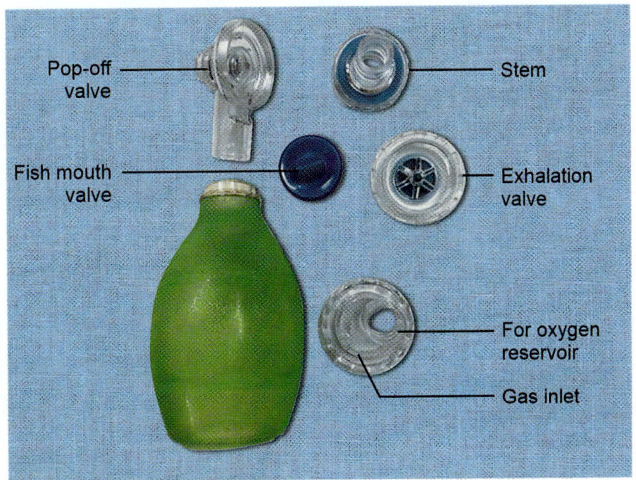

FIG. 4.1B Dissembled self-inflating bag.

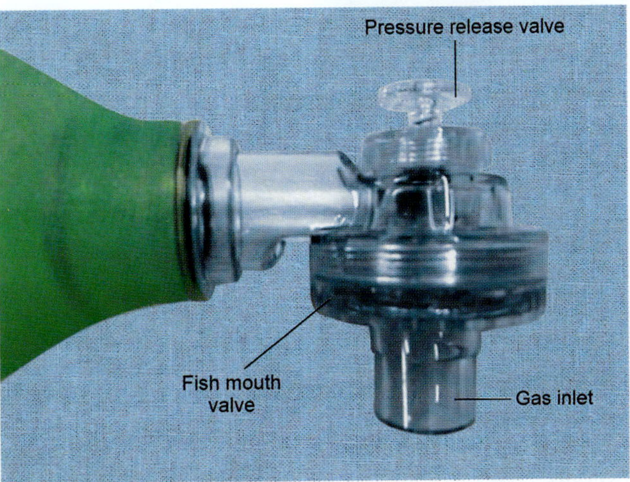

FIG. 4.1C Valves of self-inflating bag.

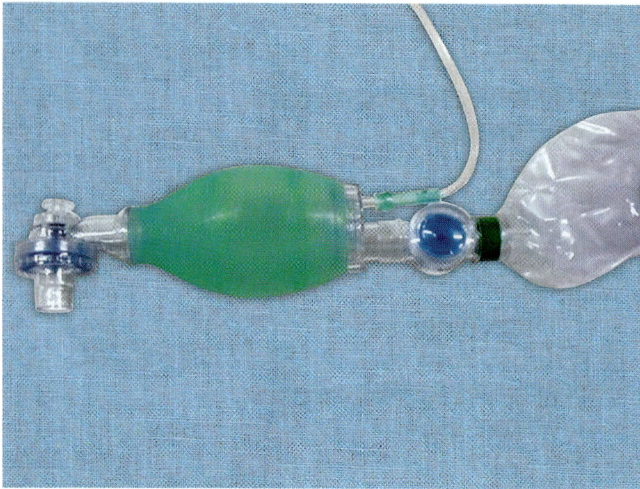
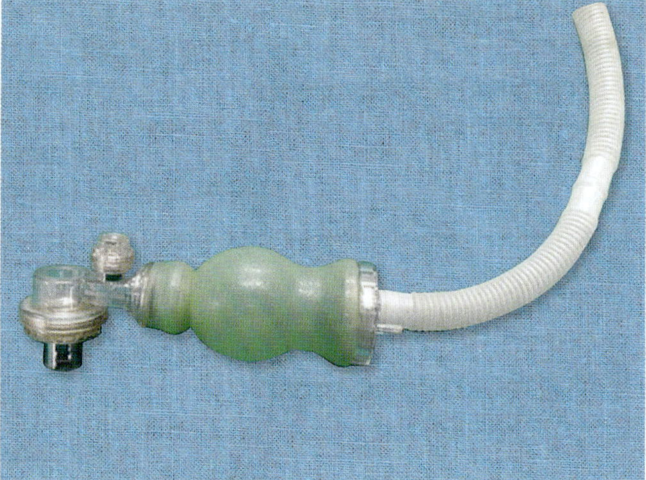

FIG. 4.1D   Self-inflating bag with closed oxygen reservoir (left) and open oxygen reservoir (right).

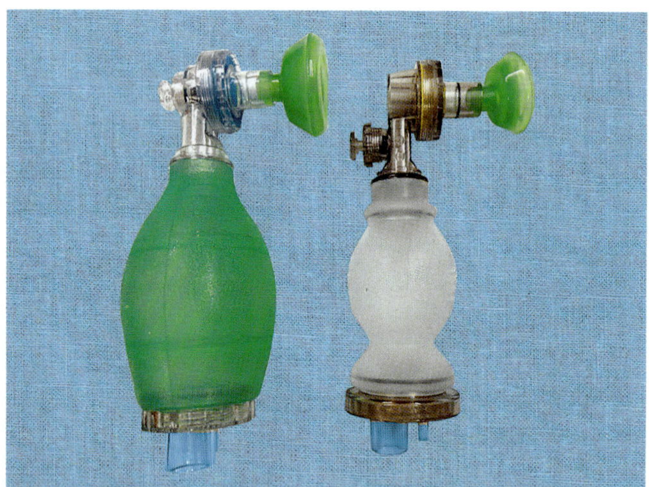

FIG. 4.1E   Term (green) and preterm (white) self-inflating bag.

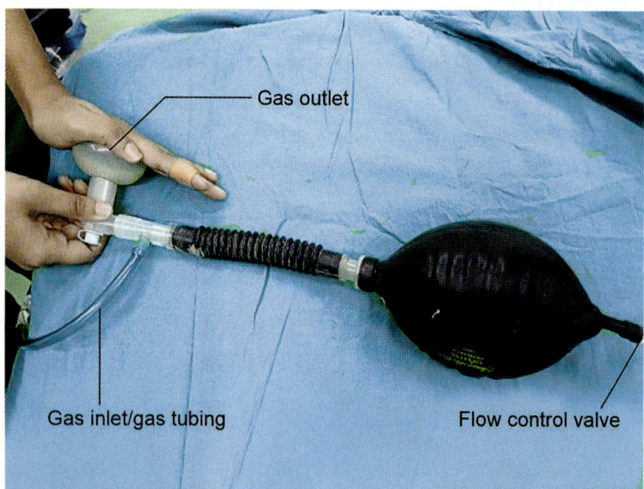

FIG. 4.2   Parts of flow-inflating bag.
Courtesy: Dr Kavita Sreekumar (Goa).

usually have a fixed safety pop-off valve. It may be used with an attached manometer to determine pressure delivery. PEEP can be provided by adjusting the flow of gas out of the bag by the flow control valve.

Parts of flow-inflating bag (Fig. 4.2): The parts of a flow-inflating bag include: (1) Gas inlet, (2) Gas outlet, (3) Flow control valve, (4) Gas tubing, and (5) Manometer (optional).

How the flow-inflating bag functions: The bag expands when compressed gas from the blender flows into the bag through the gas inlet. When the inflated bag is squeezed, gas flows to the neonate through the gas outlet where there is a mask or endotracheal tube as interface. The inflation of the bag is controlled by the balance between the inflow of gas and the outflow from the flow control valve and the gas outlet. If there are large leaks at the face mask, flow is too low, the flow valve is too open or if there is a hole in the bag, it will result in collapse of the bag and inability to deliver any positive pressure breath. The ventilation rate is controlled by how often the bag is squeezed, and the IT by how quickly the bag is squeezed. The PIP is determined by how much one squeezes the bag.

T-piece Resuscitator

It is a flow-controlled pressure limited ventilator device. It requires compressed gas to deliver an inflation. Inflation is achieved by intermittently

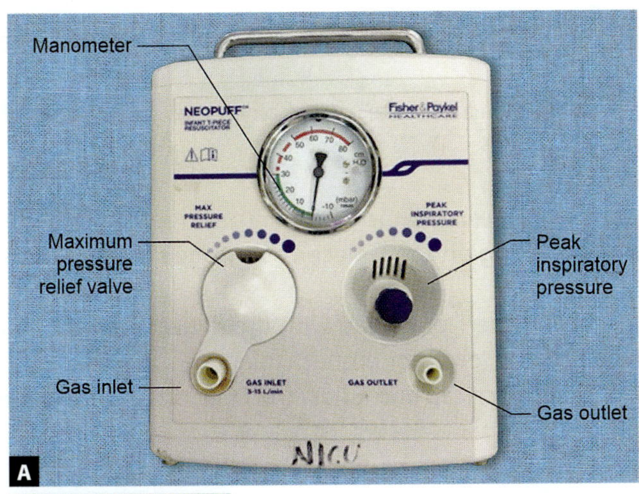

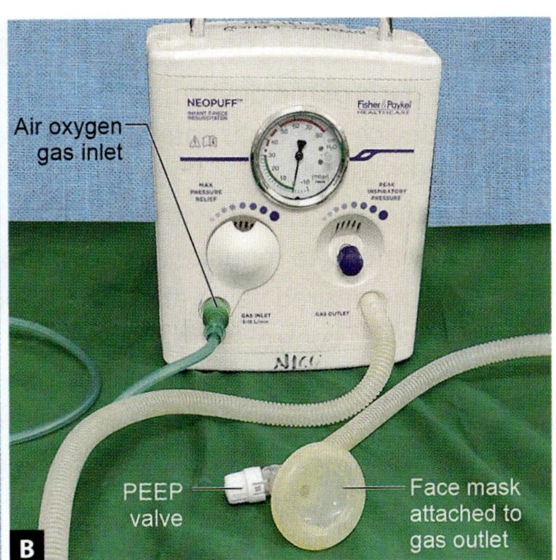

FIGS. 4.3A AND B   Parts of T-piece resuscitator.
Courtesy: Dr Kavita Sreekumar (Goa).

occluding the opening on the cap of the T-piece by a finger by the operator. Rate of ventilation is determined by how often one occludes the opening and IT is determined by how long the opening is occluded. PIP and PEEP can be preset on the device.

Parts of T-piece resuscitator (Figs. 4.3A and B): The parts of the device include: (1) Gas inlet, (2) Proximal gas outlet, (3) T-piece gas outlet, (4) Gas tubing, (5) Manometer, (6) Inspiratory pressure control, (7) Maximum pressure relief valve, (8) T-piece PEEP adjustment dial, and (9) T-piece cap opening.

How the T-piece resuscitator functions: Compressed gas from the blender flows into the device through the gas inlet. The gas then leaves the device through the proximal gas outlet and flows through a corrugated tube to the T-piece gas outlet at the patient end where a mask/endotracheal tube is connected. When the T-piece cap opening is occluded by the operator, the preset inspiratory pressure is delivered to the patient for the duration the opening is occluded. The maximum pressure relief valve (acts like the pop-off valve in a self-inflating bag) controls the maximum pressure delivered and PEEP is adjusted by the valve on the T-piece. The blender controls the concentration of oxygen delivered by the device. **Box 4.2** outlines the steps for setting up a T-piece resuscitator for use.

A self-inflating bag should always be available as a backup to flow-dependent devices in case of failure of compressed gas supply.

Table 4.1 compares the advantages and disadvantages of the above discussed resuscitation devices.

Testing resuscitation devices: **Table 4.2** outlines the steps for testing resuscitation devices before an actual resuscitation takes place as part of equipment checklist for functionality.

BOX 4.2: SETTING UP A T-PIECE RESUSCITATOR

1. Assemble the parts of the device
2. Connect the device to the gas source (it may be delivered via a blender; use of oxygen alone without a blender will deliver 100% oxygen)
3. The patient outlet is occluded with a test lung or finger
4. Adjust the flow meter to regulate gas flow into the T-piece resuscitator (10 L/minute is recommended)
5. Set the PIP to the desired value after occluding the opening on the T-piece cap by one's finger and using the inspiratory pressure control knob
6. The maximum pressure relief control is set by occluding the T-piece cap with the finger using the maximum pressure relief dial. Set to 40 cmH$_2$O for term newborns and lower for preterm infants
7. To set PEEP remove the finger from the opening of the T-piece cap and adjust the PEEP dial to the desired value (recommended is 5 cmH$_2$O).

(PEEP: positive end-expiratory pressure; PIP: peak inspiratory pressure).

TABLE 4.1: COMPARISON OF ADVANTAGES AND DISADVANTAGES OF SELF-INFLATING BAG, FLOW INFLATING BAG, AND T-PIECE RESUSCITATOR

Device	Advantages	Disadvantages
Self-inflating bag	• Easy to use compared to a flow-inflating bag • Pressure limiting valve reduces risk of lung injury • Can be used without a compressed gas supply	• Difficult to deliver consistent inflating pressures • Pop-off valve activates at an inconsistent and wide range of pressures • Dismantling and cleaning is difficult • Cannot deliver free flow oxygen or PEEP • More difficult for the operator to know if he/she has achieved a goodseal • Requires oxygen reservoir to deliver higher concentration of oxygen
Flow-inflating bag	• Can deliver free flow oxygen • Can be used to deliver PEEP • Allows the experienced operator to vary the pressure profile very rapidly in response to the condition of the neonate • Easy to determine when there is a seal on the patient's face	• Needs compressed gas source to work • Requires more training and experience to use • Requires a tight seal between the mask and the patient's face to remain inflated
T-piece resuscitator	• Consistent delivery of PIP and PEEP • Can be used to provide free flow oxygen reliably—21–100% (with blender) • Ability to vary the inspiratory time possible • Provider does not get tired from ventilation	• Costly • Needs compressed gas with a blender • The target pressures cannot be delivered if there are large leaks at the facemask, other leaks in the system, or too low a flow • Requires pressures to be set prior to use • Changing inflation pressure during resuscitation is more difficult

(PEEP: positive end-expiratory pressure; PIP: peak inspiratory pressure).

TABLE 4.2: Testing Resuscitation Devices

Self-inflating bag	<ul><li>Assemble the device correctly</li><li>With a self-inflating bag occlude the face mask against the palm</li><li>Look for following of features as you squeeze the bag:<ul><li>You should feel pressure against the palm</li><li>The fish mouth valve should open and close</li><li>The pop off valve should make a hissing sound or move up and down</li><li>The bag should recoil instantly when pressure is released</li></ul></li><li>If a pressure manometer is attached, it should display the pressure when bag is squeezed.</li><li>Absence of any of the above feature suggests malfunction</li></ul>

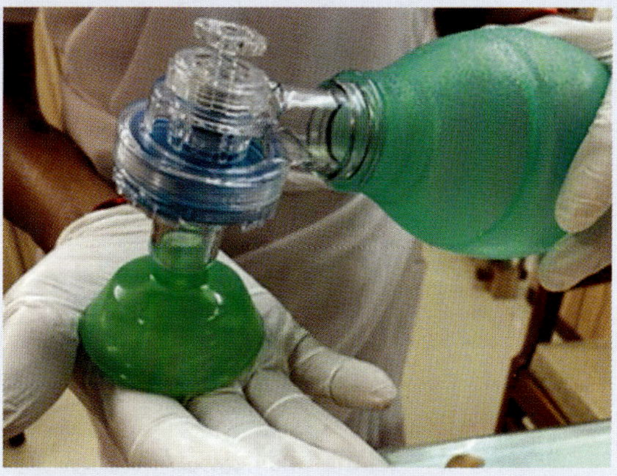

Testing self-inflating bag: Feel for pressure against the palm (above), fish mouthvalve opens and closes with each breath (below)

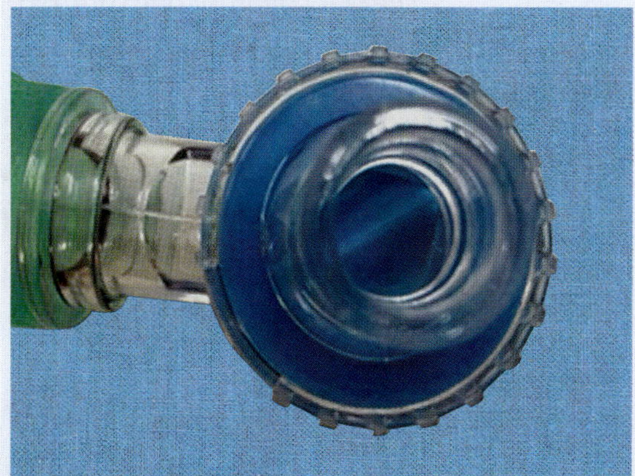

Flow-inflating bag	<ul><li>Block the mask or gas outlet<ul><li>Does the bag fill properly?</li><li>Adjust the flow-control valve to read 5 cmH$_2$O PEEP</li></ul></li><li>Squeeze the bag 40–60 times per minute.<ul><li>Does the bag reinflate quickly when you release your grip?</li><li>Adjust the flow-control valve to read 30–40 cmH$_2$O when squeezed firmly</li><li>Check to be sure that the pressure still reads 5 cmH$_2$O when not being squeezed (PEEP).</li></ul></li><li>If the bag does not fill correctly<ul><li>Is there a crack or hole in the bag?</li><li>Is the flow-control valve open too far?</li><li>Is the manometer attached?</li><li>Is the gas tubing connected securely?</li><li>Is the gas outlet sufficiently blocked?</li></ul></li></ul>

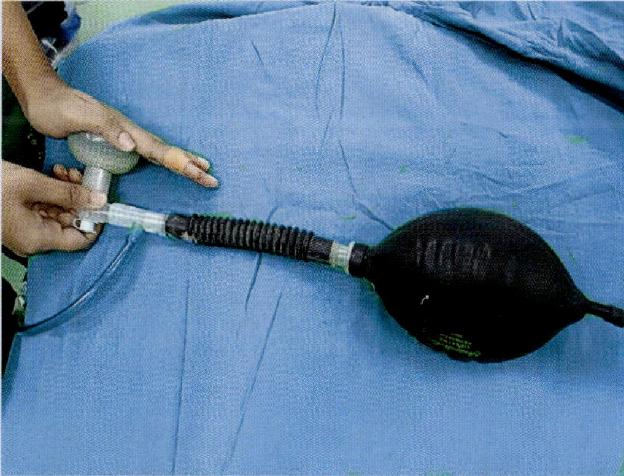

Testing flow resuscitation bag

Contd...

Contd...

T-piece resuscitator	• Block the mask or T-piece gas outlet (patient) without occluding the opening on the T-piece cap
	  – Does the PEEP read 5 cmH_2O?
	• Occlude the opening on the T-piece cap
	  – Does the peak pressure read 20–25 cm H_2O?
	• If the pressure is incorrect,
	  – Is the T-piece gas outlet sealed?
	  – Is the gas tubing connected to the gas inlet?
	  – Is the gas flow sufficient?
	  – Is the gas outlet (proximal) disconnected?
	  – Is the maximum circuit pressure, peak inspiratory pressure, or PEEP incorrectly set?

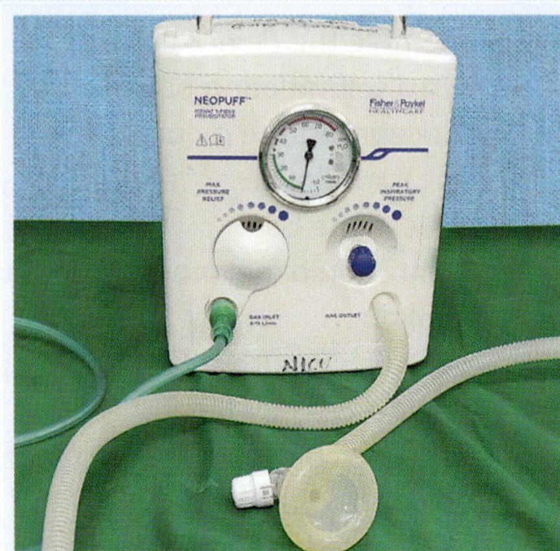

Test T-piece resuscitator by applying the face mask over the palm

(PEEP: positive end-expiratory pressure).

■ PROVIDING POSITIVE PRESSURE VENTILATION

Figure **4.4** indicates the steps in the neonatal resuscitation algorithm that are related to providing PPV.

When to Initiate Positive Pressure Ventilation?

Positive pressure ventilation is indicated, if after initial steps of resuscitation, *(i) the baby is not breathing (apneic) OR (ii) baby is gasping OR (iii) baby has a heart rate <100 bpm.* In newborn infants where it is indicated, PPV should be initiated within 1 minute of birth.

Another relative indication for PPV in the delivery room is in a spontaneously breathing baby with a heart rate ≥100/minute but having an oxygen saturation below the target range despite free flow oxygen or CPAP.

Preparing for Positive Pressure Ventilation

It is advisable to use a standardized sequence before PPV is initiated.

- *Clear secretions:* If secretions have not been cleared earlier from mouth and nose, do so before starting PPV.

- *Position of the care provider:* The team member who would be responsible for providing PPV to the newborn infant should position himself/herself at the head end of the infant. It would be difficult to maintain the position of baby's head, neck, and mask if the provider is standing on the side or the foot end of the baby. The other team members on the side of the baby can help with other procedures and monitoring the progress of resuscitation.

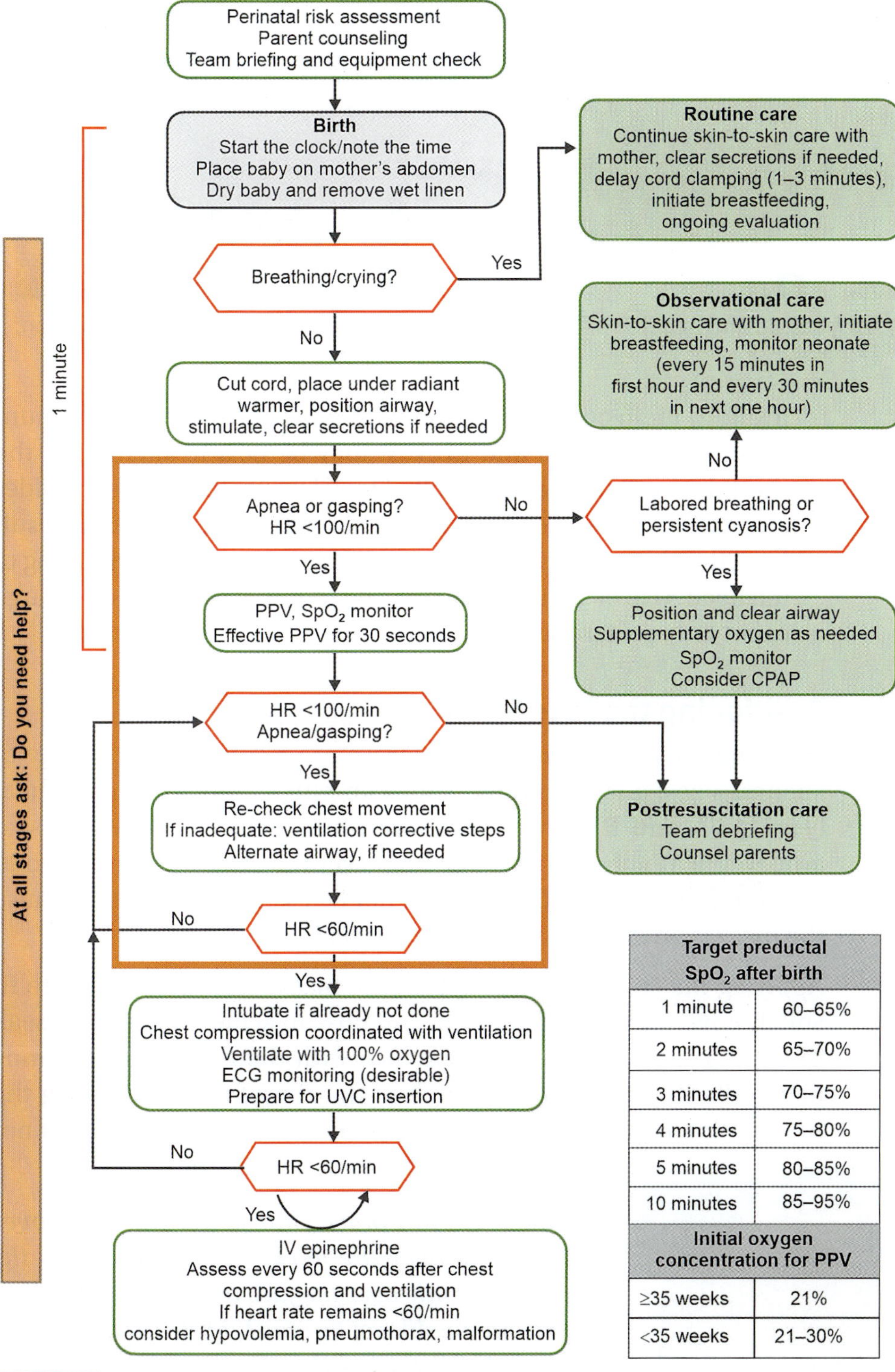

FIG. 4.4 Neonatal resuscitation algorithm *(boxed area indicates the steps related to providing PPV).*

- *Positioning the infant's head and neck:* The baby should be placed on firm, flat, and clean surface. The baby's head and neck should be slightly extended in a "sniffing" position to open the airway (such that the chin and nose face upwards) (*Figs.* **4.5A to C**). Excessive flexion or extension of the neck can obstruct the airway and

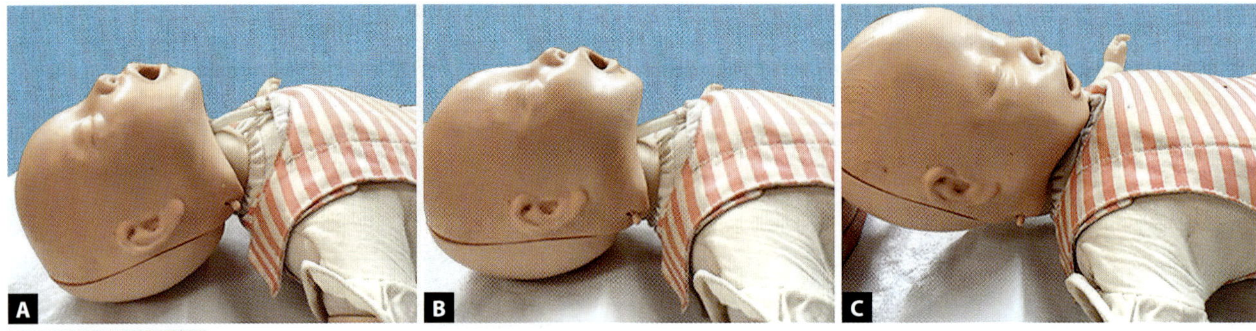

FIGS. 4.5A TO C   Position of baby's head and neck in sniffing position: (A) Extended neck; (B) Sniffing position; (C) Flexed neck.

result in ineffective ventilation with a mask. To get the optimum position of the head and neck, it may be best to slightly lift the shoulder by placing a small rolled towel under the baby's shoulder (*Fig.* **4.6**). Failure to establish normal breathing at birth may result from the absence of a patent airway due to improper positioning of the head. Use of shoulder roll may be required in presence of large caput or in preterm infants.

Positioning the Face Mask

Selecting the correct face mask: Masks are available in a variety of shapes, sizes, and materials. They can either round or anatomical (*Figs.* **4.7A and B**). An appropriately-sized face mask would seal around the mouth and nose but not cover the eyes or extend beyond the chin (*Figs.* **4.8A to C**). It should not be assumed that just because the mask is on the face, there is a good seal.

Applying the face mask: Apply the face mask firmly and gently to fit snugly covering the chin, mouth, and nose to achieve an airtight seal. The mask usually is held on the face with the thumb, index, and/ or middle finger encircling much of the rim of the mask using the nondominant hand (*Figs.* **4.9A to H**). Ensure that the mask does not extend onto the eyes or beyond the chin.

Caution: **Do not place your fingers or hand over the eyes or over the neck.** *Also do not press the mask too firmly over the face as it can cause air to leak from the sides of the mask, obstruct the mask or accidently flex the baby's neck.*

Oxygen Concentration During Ventilation

Studies have shown that normal term newborn infants when they transit from the low oxygen intrauterine environment to the room air (21%) environment show an increase in their oxygenation

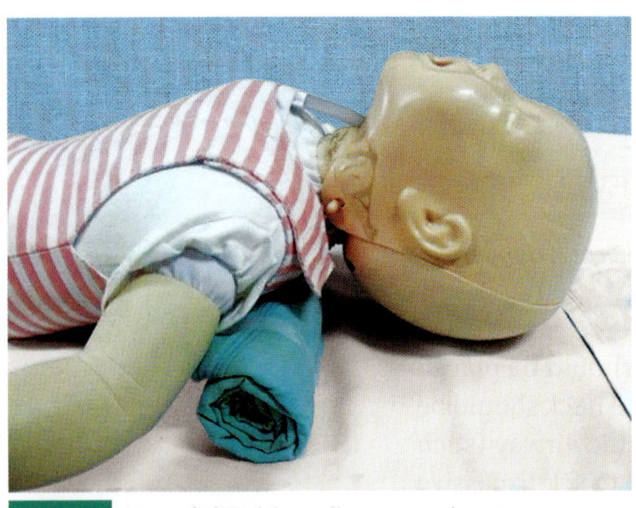

FIG. 4.6   Use of shoulder roll to open the airway.

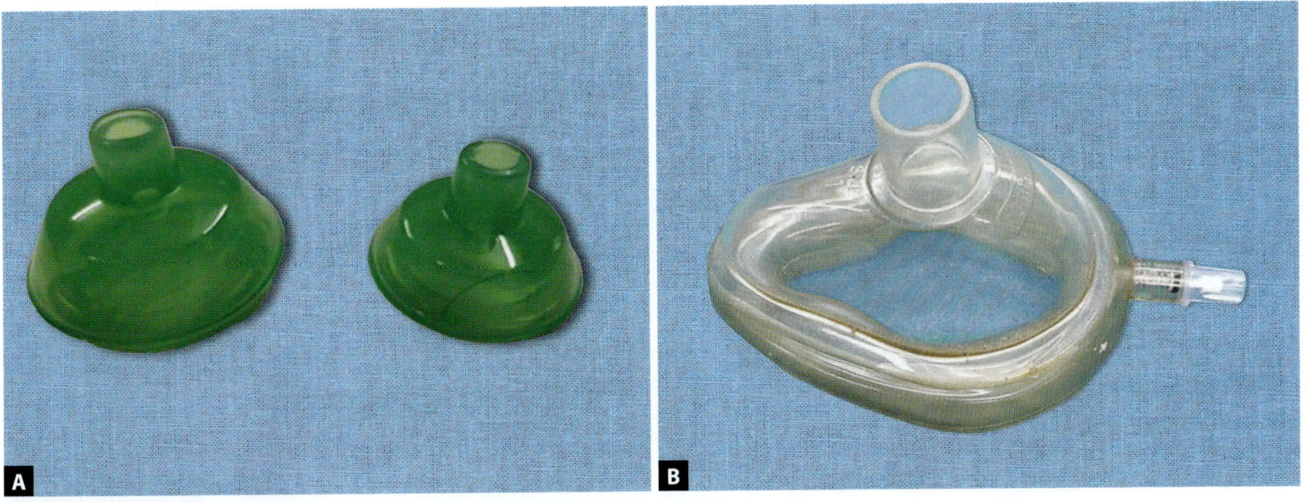

FIGS. 4.7A AND B Face masks—(A) round; (B) anatomic.
Courtesy: Dr Sandeep Kadam (Pune).

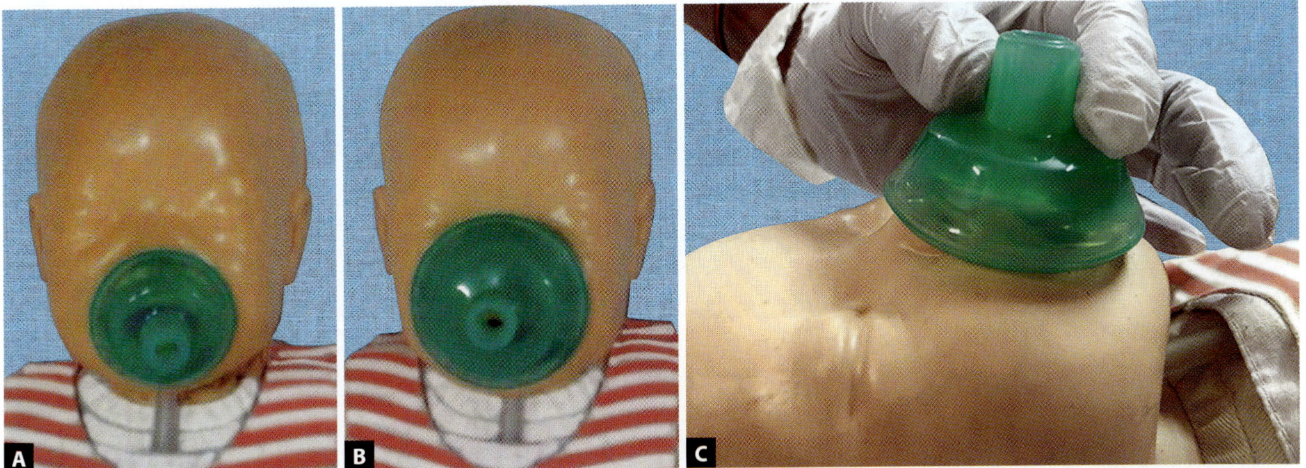

FIGS. 4.8A TO C (A) Appropriate sized mask with correct fit; (B) Mask too large for the face; (C) Mask too small for the face. (B) and (C) are inappropriate sized masks for the baby's face.

over several minutes after birth. Welsford et al.[4] in a systematic review and meta-analysis on the use of room air for initiating newborn resuscitation observed that room air (21% oxygen) was associated with a significant benefit in short-term mortality compared with 100% oxygen [7 RCTs; $n = 1469$; risk ratio (RR) = 0.73; 95% CI: 0.57–0.94]. However, no significant differences were observed in neurodevelopmental impairment or hypoxic-ischemic encephalopathy. In another systematic review and meta-analysis on initial oxygen use for preterm newborn resuscitation,[5] it was noted that there were no significant benefits or harms from starting with lower (50% or less) compared with higher oxygen concentration (>50%) in short-term mortality, long-term mortality, neurodevelopmental impairment, or other key preterm morbidities. Oxygen supplementation may be used during newborn resuscitation to prevent the effects of hypoxia, but the harm

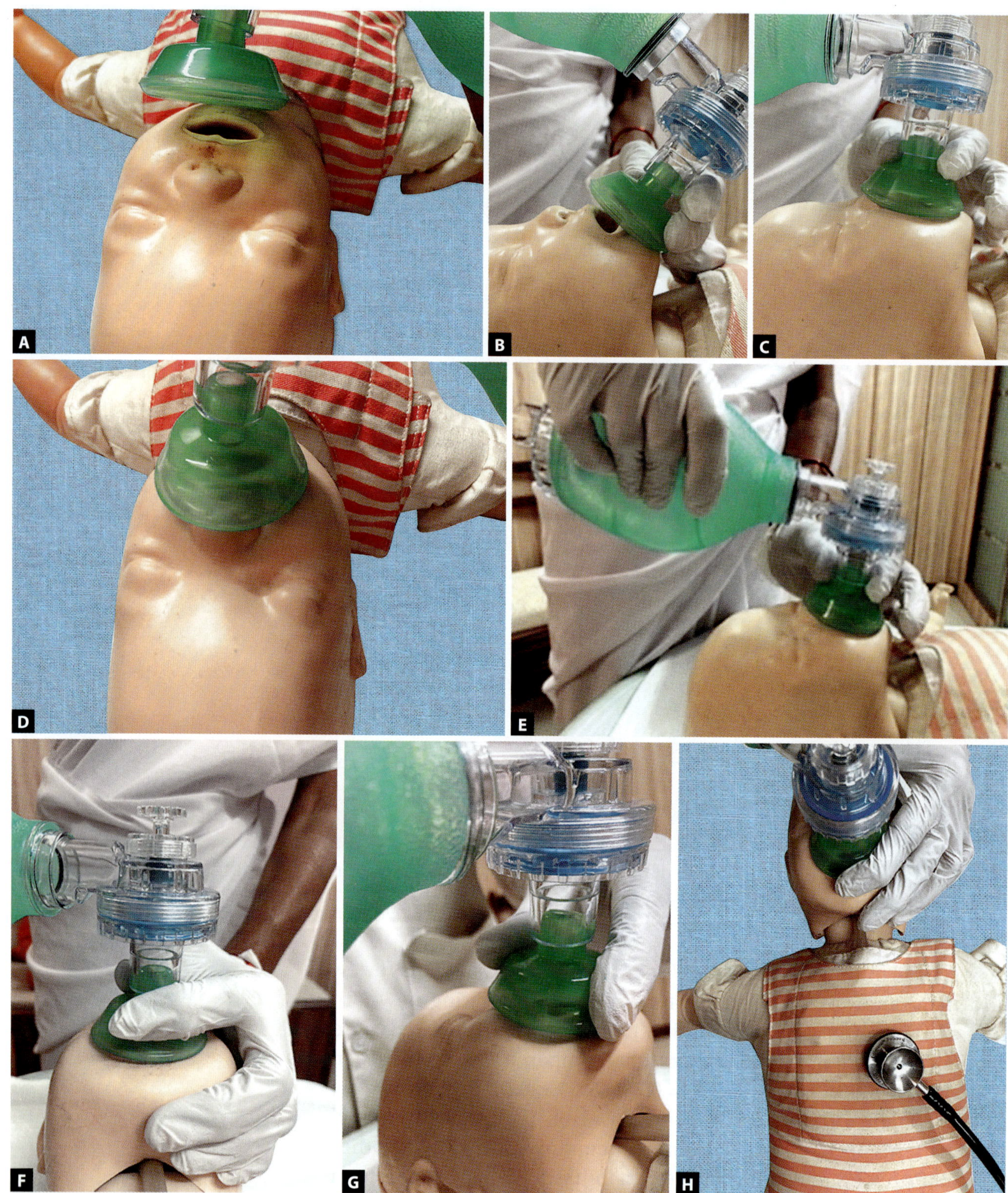

FIGS. 4.9A TO H Steps for placing a face mask and creating an airtight seal.

due to over-exposure to oxygen (hyperoxia) is a matter of serious concern.[6]

Based on the evidence available it has been recommended that for **babies born at term and late preterm neonates (35 weeks gestation or beyond), PPV may be initiated with the oxygen blender set to 21% oxygen** [*Class of recommendation (COR): 2a (moderate), level of evidence (LOE): B-randomized trials*]. **For preterm babies <35 weeks' gestation PPV should be initiated with the blender set to between 21–30% oxygen** [*COR: 2b (weak), LOE: C-limited data*]. Subsequent oxygen delivery should be guided by preductal oxygen saturation targets given in the neonatal resuscitation algorithm in *Figure* **4.4**.

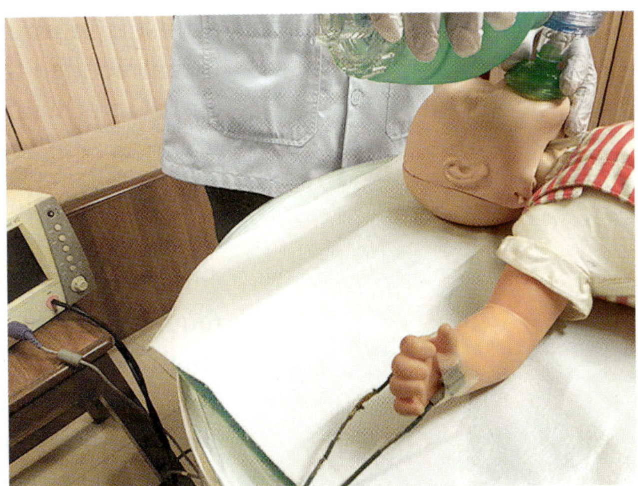

FIG. 4.10 Pulse oximeter sensor on right hand of baby.

The flow meter should be set at 10 L/minute. An assistant should place a pulse oximeter sensor on the right hand/wrist of the newborn infant as soon as PPV is started (*Fig.* **4.10**) to monitor the oxygen saturation of the newborn infant and compare with the recommended oxygen saturation targets to titrate oxygen delivery.

Providing Ventilation

Rate of ventilation: Ventilation should be provided at a rate of 40–60 breaths/minute [*COR: 2a (Moderate); LOE: C-expert opinion*].[2]

Using the rhythm – "**Breathe**, *two, three;* **Breathe**, *two, three;* **Breathe**, *two, three*" will help maintain the required rate. "Breathe" is during squeezing the bag or closing the T-piece resuscitator cap opening while "*two, three*" is during release of the pressure (*Fig.* **4.11**).

Pressure to initiate PPV: In newborns who have not started to breathe after birth, the lung fluid in the alveoli must be cleared to replace it with air. The initial pressure required to ventilate the lungs in such newborn infants is higher. The aim is to inflate the lung sufficient

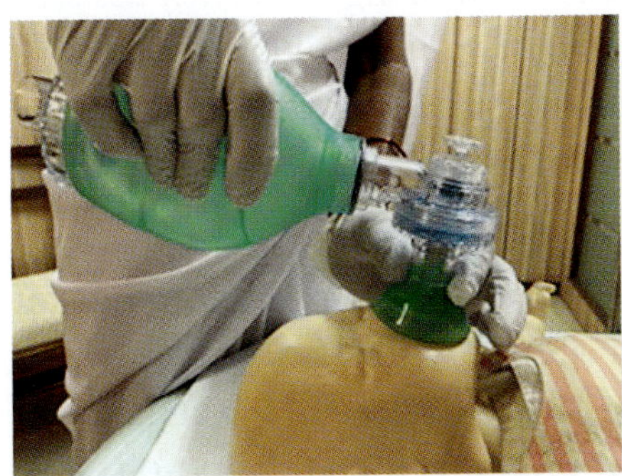

Breathe (squeeze bag)...

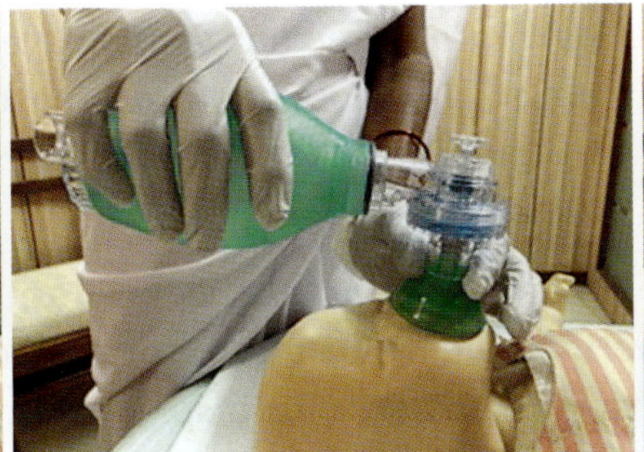

Two (release bag pressure)...

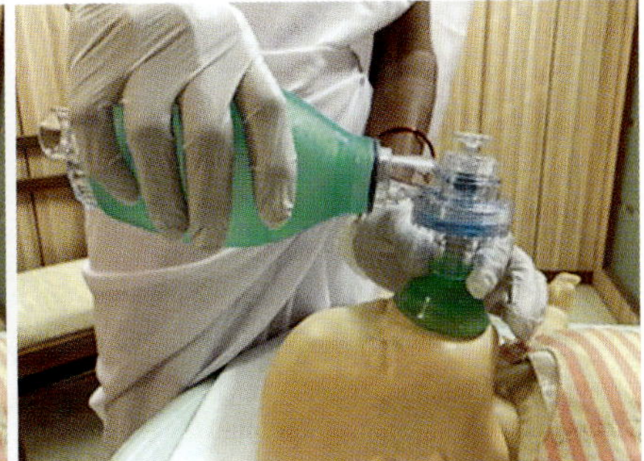

Three (release bag pressure)

FIG. 4.11 Sequence to provide PPV.

to result in an increase in heart rate and oxygen saturation. It is recommended to start PPV with a peak inspiratory pressure of 20–25 cmH$_2$O (term infants may require a higher pressure of 30–40 cmH$_2$O) [*COR: 2a (moderate); LOE: C-limited data*].[2]

Apply sufficient pressure to see a gentle visible rise and fall of the chest with each ventilation provided. One must be aware that the volume in the bag (approximately 250 mL) is larger than the volume required to inflate the lung (4–8 mL/kg; in a 3 kg baby it amounts to about 12–24 mL only) of a newborn infant. Use of excess pressure can injure the lungs and result in a pneumothorax. Hyperinflation can also increase intrathoracic pressure and decrease venous return into the heart and decrease cardiac output.

Use of PEEP with PPV: The evidence for recommending PEEP during PPV for preterm babies is weak with low quality evidence.[7] There is no recommendation for use of PEEP for term newborn infants. If PEEP is used in preterm infants, it should be set at 5 cmH$_2$O.

Evaluating Response to Positive Pressure Ventilation

The most important indicator of effective PPV is a rising heart rate. Heart rate can be measured by auscultation, pulse oximeter, or an ECG monitor. Evaluation of response to PPV is carried out twice—*first is at 15 seconds after initiating PPV* and the next is *at 30 seconds after having noted a chest rise with ventilation.*

(i) Evaluation after 15 seconds: If PPV was initiated for a low heart rate; one expects an increase in heart rate if ventilation is effective.

- *If heart rate is rising,* continue PPV for another 15 seconds and then reassess.

- *If heart rate is not rising,* check for chest movement during each assisted breath. *If heart rate is not rising and chest is moving* with each assisted ventilation—continue PPV and assess after another 15 seconds

- *If heart rate is not rising and chest is not moving with each assisted ventilation,* then one would have to carry out ventilation corrective steps. The most common reasons for chest not rising are leak around the face mask, obstructed airway, or inadequate inflation pressure.

Ventilation corrective steps: **Table 4.3** outlines the sequence of performing ventilation corrective steps; when a manometer is available, increase the inspiratory pressure by 5–10 cmH$_2$O at a time. If one is required to provide >30 cmH$_2$O pressure, then the pop-off valve in the self-inflating bag would have to be occluded; or if one is using a T-piece resuscitator then the PIP dial would have to be adjusted.

TABLE 4.3: SEQUENCE FOR VENTILATION CORRECTIVE STEPS

Problem		Remedial action to be Initiated
Leak around mask	Inadequate seal	Reapply the mask to ensure airtight seal
	Inappropriate position	Reposition the head and neck in sniffing/neutral position
Provide positive pressure ventilation (PPV) and check for chest movement. If not, perform the next steps		
Obstruction of airway		Suction the mouth and nose
		Open baby's mouth and ventilate
Provide PPV and check for chest movement. If not, perform the next steps		
Inadequate pressure	Increase pressure	If using self-inflating bag, squeeze the bag with more pressure till a chest rise is visible, if using T-piece resuscitator adjusts PIP dial
Provide PPV and check for chest movement. If not, perform the next steps		
Consider alternate airway		Insert an endotracheal tube or laryngeal mask airway and continue PPV

At no time should the healthcare provider exceed the recommended limit of 40 cm H_2O pressure. *Increasing the pressure could result in barotrauma and pneumothorax.*[2] If increasing the pressure does not result in chest rise, one must consider use of an alternative airway, i.e., endotracheal intubation or use of laryngeal mask airway (LMA).

(ii) Evaluation after 30 seconds of adequate chest rise: The following situations could be present at this period of evaluation:

- *Heart rate 100 or more beats per minute:* This is an indication that ventilation has been successful. PPV should be continued at the rate of 40–60/minute while monitoring the baby's heart rate and spontaneous breathing effort. If required, oxygen concentration should be adjusted while monitoring the oxygen saturation. If heart rate is consistently 100 or more beats per minute, stimulate the baby to breathe if spontaneous breathing has not been noted by this time.

  Positive pressure ventilation can be gradually tapered and discontinued when heart rate is >100 bpm and baby has regular and adequate spontaneous breathing. After stopping PPV, the baby's oxygen saturation and breathing should be monitored.

- *Heart rate is <100 bpm but at least 60 bpm:* In this situation, PPV should be continued at the rate of 40–60 bpm if the heart rate is improving and reassessed after 30 sec. Oxygen saturation should be monitored and oxygen saturation adjusted to meet oxygen saturation targets already defined. If heart rate is not rising, recheck if ventilation is effective. If there is no chest movement, ventilatory corrective steps should be taken, and strongly consider alternate airway for providing ventilation.

- *Heart rate is <60 bpm:* If heart rate continues to remain <60 bpm even after 30 seconds of adequate ventilation (visible chest rise with each assisted breath), then one must consider use of an alternative airway, e.g., intubation, call for help, increase oxygen concentration to 100% and initiate chest compression to improve circulation of oxygenated blood by improving cardiac contractility and cardiac output.

Baby with Spontaneous Breathing and Heart Rate of 100 bpm or more with Labored Breathing/Low Oxygen Saturation

If a baby has labored breathing or has a low oxygen saturation in spite of free flow oxygen, continuous positive airway pressure (CPAP) may be helpful. CPAP cannot be delivered with a self-inflating bag. It can be delivered with a T-piece resuscitator. The flow should be set to 10 L/minute and the PEEP valve adjusted to start with 5 cmH$_2$O pressure (maximum not exceeding 8 cmH$_2$O pressure). Currently the use of CPAP in the delivery room is recommended for spontaneously breathing preterm babies who need respiratory support (COR-2a; LOE-A).[2,8,9]

Insertion of orogastric tube: During PPV with face mask or CPAP, air enters the stomach through the esophagus. A distended stomach can interfere with ventilation by impeding diaphragmatic movement. During prolonged PPV or CPAP it is recommended that a feeding tube of size 8F be inserted into the stomach to vent the air from the stomach.

■ POSTRESUSCITATION CARE

Newborn infants who have required PPV, CPAP, or free flow oxygen need to be observed and frequently monitored for their breathing, heart rate, oxygen saturation/color, temperature and activity. Those who have required brief PPV (say <1 minute) can be provided care with the mother if they are breathing well, maintaining adequate oxygen saturation on room air, do not have any difficulty in breathing and have good activity. These infants should be monitored for their breathing, heart rate, and oxygen saturation/color every 15 minutes during the first hour and every 30 minutes during the second hour. Newborn infants needing prolonged PPV, needing CPAP, or supplemental oxygen for maintain oxygen saturation and those who needed brief PPV but cannot be monitored with their mother, should be shifted to the NICU for further management and monitoring.

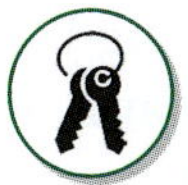

KEY POINTS

1. The most important step of neonatal resuscitation is providing assisted ventilation.
2. Positive pressure ventilation must begin within first minute of birth in infants who are depressed at birth—First Golden Minute.
3. Assisted ventilation must be provided at a rate of 40–60 breaths per minute.
4. In infants who are term gestation or late preterms (35 weeks gestation or more), ventilation may be initiated with room air (21%) and with 21–30% oxygen in infants <35 weeks gestation.
5. Rise in heart rate is the most objective parameter to assess response to assisted ventilation.
6. The most frequent reasons for ineffective-assisted ventilation are leaks around face mask seal, obstructed airway, or need for higher inspiratory pressure.
7. Free flow oxygen cannot be delivered through the face mask of a self-inflating bag.
8. In spontaneously breathing preterm neonates with labored breathing in the delivery room, CPAP can be considered for initial stabilization.

▮ REFERENCES

1. Zanardo V, Weiner G, Micaglio M, Doglioni N, Buzzacchero R, Trevisanuto D. Delivery room resuscitation of near-term infants: role of the laryngeal mask airway. Resuscitation. 2010;81(3): 327-30.

2. Aziz K, Lee CHC, Escobedo MB, Hoover AV, Kamath-Rayne BD, Kapadia VS, et al. Part 5: Neonatal Resuscitation 2020 American Heart Association Guidelines for Cardiopulmonary Resuscitation and Emergency Cardiovascular Care. Pediatrics. 2021;147(Suppl 1):e2020038505E.

3. Trevisanuto D, Roehr CC, Davis PG, Schmölzer GM, Wyckoff MH, Liley HG, et al. International Liaison Committee on Resuscitation neonatal life support task force. Devices for Administering Ventilation at Birth: a systematic review. Pediatrics. 2021;148(1):e2021050174.

4. Welsford M, Nishiyama C, Shortt C, Isayama T, Dawson JA, Weiner G, et al. Room air for initiating term newborn resuscitation: a systematic review with meta-analysis. Pediatrics. 2019;143(1):e20181825.

5. Welsford M, Nishiyama C, Shortt C, Weiner G, Roehr CC, Isayama T, et al. Initial oxygen use for preterm newborn resuscitation: a systematic review with meta-analysis. Pediatrics. 2019;143(1):e20181828.

6. Saugstad OD. Hyperoxia in the term newborn: more evidence is still needed for optimal oxygen therapy. Acta Paediatr. 2012;101(464): 34-8.

7. Wyckoff MH, Wyllie J, Aziz K, de Almeida MF, Fabres J, Fawke J, et al. Neonatal Life Support Collaborators. Neonatal Life Support: 2020 International Consensus on Cardiopulmonary Resuscitation and Emergency Cardiovascular Care Science With Treatment Recommendations. Circulation. 2020;142(16_suppl_1):S185-221.

8. Schmölzer GM, Kumar M, Pichler G, Aziz K, O'Reilly M, Cheung PY. Noninvasive versus invasive respiratory support in preterm infants at birth: systematic review and meta-analysis. BMJ. 2013;347:f5980.

9. Ramaswamy VV, Abiramalatha T, Bandyopadhyay T, Shaik NB, Pullattayil S AK, Cavallin F, et al. Delivery room CPAP in improving outcomes of preterm neonates in low- and middle-income countries: a systematic review and network meta-analysis. Resuscitation. 2022;170: 250-63.

Self Assessment

1. The most appropriate size of self-inflating bag (SIB) for newborn resuscitation is:
   a. 125 mL
   b. 250 mL
   c. 650 mL
   d. 750 mL

2. Regarding use of mask during PPV, all the following are TRUE except:
   a. Different sizes of masks should be available at every delivery.
   b. The mask should cover the chin, mouth, and nose, but not the eyes.
   c. Effective ventilation of a preterm baby with a term-infant size mask is possible.
   d. Round, cushioned mask, or anatomical-shaped face masks are preferred during newborn resuscitation.

3. Once positive pressure ventilation administration is begun, assessment should consist of:
   a. Respiration, heart rate, and color
   b. Respiration, heart rate, and blood pressure
   c. Respiration, heart rate, and tone
   d. Heart rate, respiratory rate, and if possible, evaluation of the state of oxygenation (pulse oximetry)

4. Which is the correct method to hold the mask over the face?

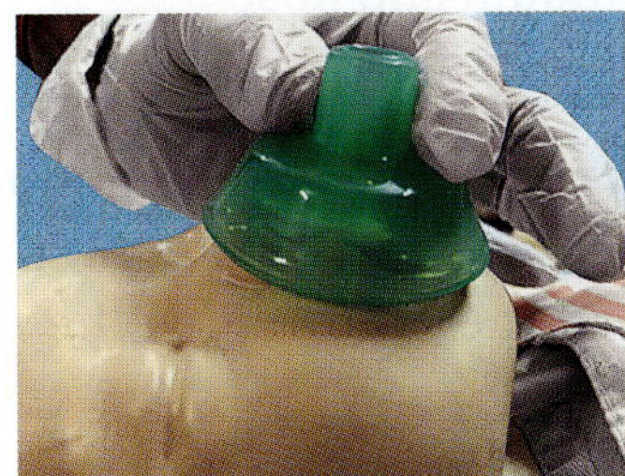 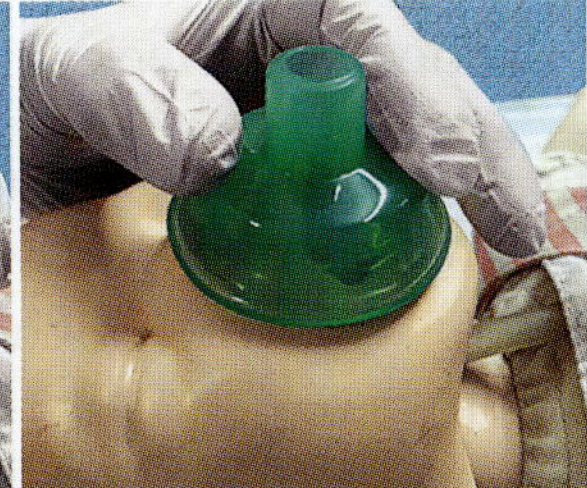 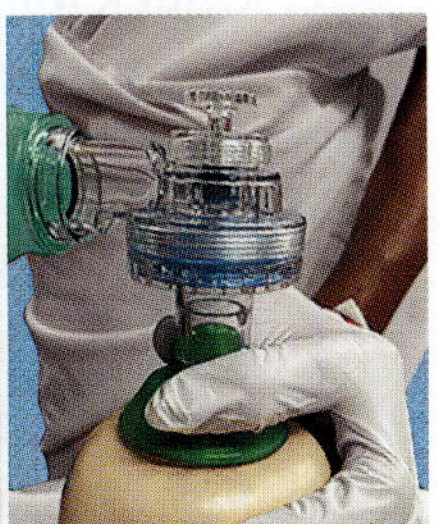

   a. Stem hold   b. Top hold   c. Rim hold

5. The concept of "First Golden minute" at birth means:
   a. Initial steps be completed within 1 minute
   b. Positive pressure ventilation (PPV) should be completed in 1 minute
   c. PPV should be initiated within 1 minute of birth
   d. Baby should establish cry within 1 minute

6. The best indication that the mask has formed a good seal and the lungs are being adequately inflated is:
   a. Rise in heart rate
   b. Improvement in tone
   c. Improvement in color
   d. Bilateral equal air entry

7. If the chest does not move adequately it may be due to:
   a. The seal is inadequate.
   b. The airway is blocked.
   c. Not enough pressure is being given.
   d. All of the above

8. If PPV with a mask is to be continued for more than several minutes, you should consider:
   a. Assess heart rate periodically every 30 seconds
   b. Putting an orogastric tube
   c. Consider intubation
   d. All of the above

9. Ventilation should be provided at a rate of:
   a. 30–40/minute
   b. 40–60/minute
   c. 30–60/minute
   d. All of the above

10. You are attempting to ventilate a term newborn with bag and mask. There is no improvement in heart rate and no perceptible chest movement. Which of the following would be an inappropriate action?
    a. Reapply the mask to the baby's face and lift the jaw forward
    b. Apply continuous positive airway pressure (CPAP)
    c. Check for secretions; suction the mouth and nose
    d. Reposition the head and neck

11. As you initiate bag and mask resuscitation you find the baby becoming blue. You take corrective actions for ventilation, but baby continues to worsen. Which of the following is the next appropriate action?
    a. Insert a laryngeal mask airway
    b. Intubate and ventilate with bag to tube
    c. Give 10 mL/kg of normal saline push
    d. Insert an oral airway

Answers

For answers, go to the end of the Book, Page no. 321

Laryngeal Mask Airway

Ashish Mehta

Lessons to Learn

- Indications for use of laryngeal mask airway (LMA) in neonatal resuscitation
- Types of LMA devices for neonates
- Technique of inserting LMA and ascertain its correct placement
- The benefits and limitations of using LMA in neonatal resuscitation

The use of face mask and endotracheal intubation for providing positive pressure ventilation in neonates needing resuscitation has been considered a challenge for resuscitators in spite of the training provided to them. There has, therefore, been a felt need for devices that can be used for positive pressure ventilation (PPV) that require less training than for endotracheal intubation. Over the years, it has been suggested that laryngeal mask airway (LMA) could be the possible effective alternate device for providing PPV. LMA was first made available for clinical use in adults and children in the late 1980s. In the last decade of the 20th century and the early 21st century its feasibility in neonatal resuscitation was reported.[1,2]

LARYNGEAL MASK AIRWAY IN NEONATES

A Cochrane review[3] concluded LMA to be more effective than face mask in terms of shorter resuscitation, ventilation times, and need for endotracheal intubation. When compared with bag and mask resuscitation, supraglottic airway decreased need of endotracheal intubation [risk ratio (RR) 0.24, 95% CI 0.12–0.47 and risk difference (RD) –0.14, 95% CI –0.14 to –0.06] (moderate quality evidence).[1] In a more recent systematic review, Yamada et al.[4] observed that use of LMA as compared to face mask for providing PPV in neonates reduced the probability of failure to improve and the need for intubation. But they also concluded that the quality of evidence for most outcomes was low to very low certainty.

In a recent clinical trial, Pejovic et al.[5] observed that in neonates ≥34 week and birth weights ≥2000 g who needed resuscitation, there was no difference in death or neonatal intensive care unit (NICU) admission due to moderate-severe encephalopathy when resuscitated by midwives using face mask or LMA.

IN WHOM TO USE

Currently, it is recommended that its use should be considered in infants of ≥34 weeks gestation (whose weight is expected to be about 2,000 g, although some devices have been used successfully in infants weighing as low as 1,500 g)[6] in the following situations:

- If there are problems with establishing effective ventilation with a facemask.

- Where it is difficult to achieve a good seal for facemask ventilation because of orofacial congenital anomalies, and/or where intubation is not possible due to lack of equipment or provider skill.

- As an alternative to tracheal intubation as a secondary airway— however, current literature also supports its use as a primary interface to provide PPV, but it would require structured training as a part of neonatal resuscitation program and LMA should be easily available.

When not to use LMA: In situations where pulmonary compliance is expected to be low and high pressures are required to inflate the lung, it is not advisable to use LMA for PPV as the device provides a low pressure seal.

LARYNGEAL MASK AIRWAY DEVICES

Since its first use, laryngeal mask airway has undergone several modifications. First generation LMA was a simple device with an elliptical mask-shaped inflatable cuff, 15 mm universal connector, and ventilatory pathway with internal diameter of 5.3 mm. To inflate the cuff, it had an inflating line with a one-way pilot valve. Two aperture bars in the middle of mask lumen, prevented the epiglottis from herniating into the airway (*Figs.* **5.1 to 5.3**).

Second generation LMAs have an esophageal drain tube through which gastric tube can be inserted to vent the stomach (*Fig.* **5.4**).

The newer LMA devices which have been evaluated in neonates have a soft gel, noninflating preshaped sealing device (*Fig.* **5.5A and B**). The modifications from the original design have found it to be more effective and have also reduced its potential complications. **The recommended size for use during neonatal resuscitation is LMA size 1.**

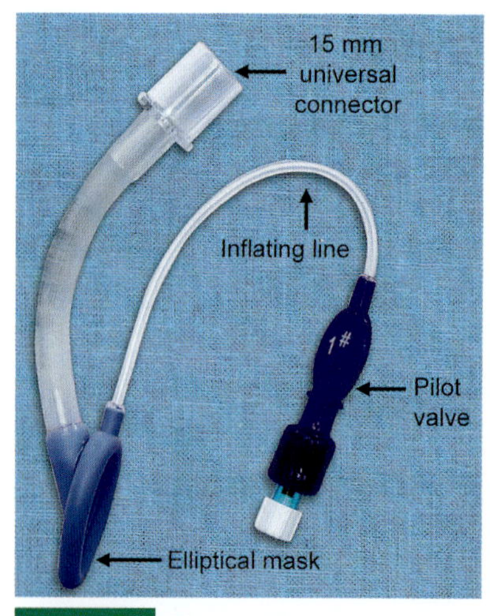

FIG. 5.1 First generation LMA and its parts.

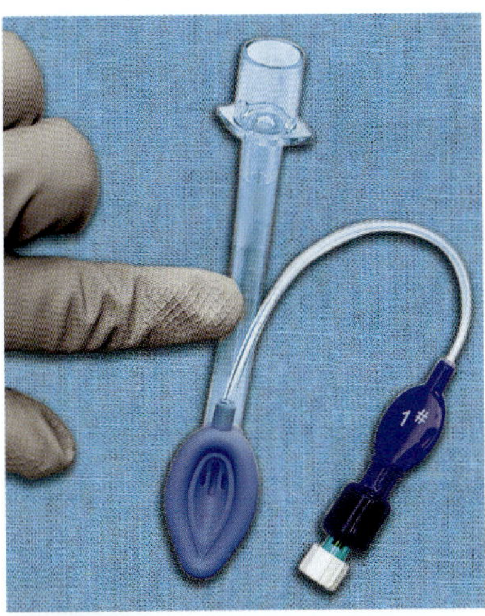

FIG. 5.2 Ventilatory tube in an LMA.

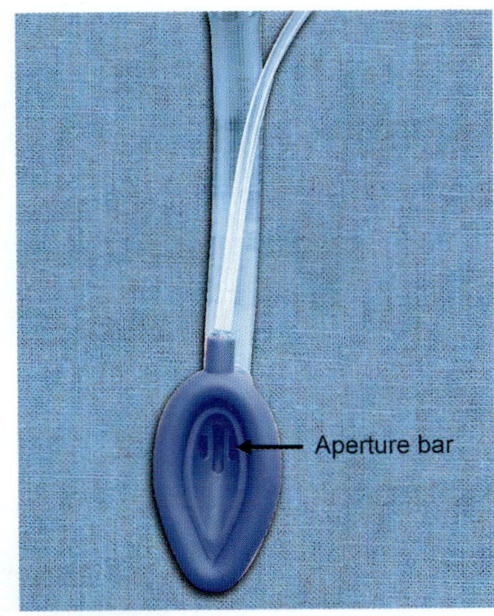

FIG. 5.3 Aperture bars in the mask lumen of LMA.

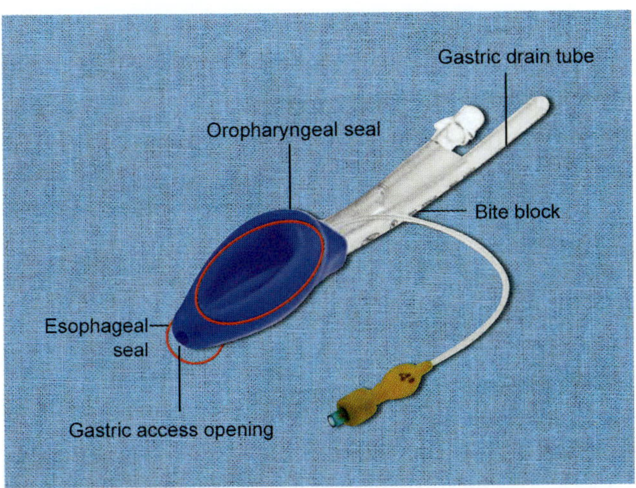

FIG. 5.4 Parts of second generation LMA.

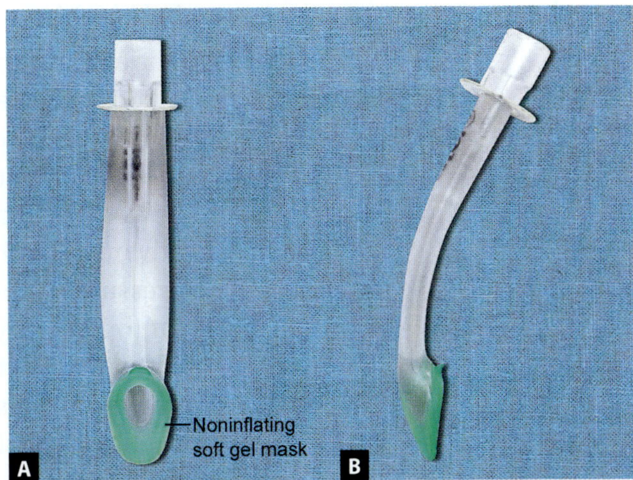

FIGS. 5.5A AND B LMA with no inflating mask: (A) Front view; (B) Side view.

TECHNIQUE OF INSERTION OF LARYNGEAL MASK AIRWAY

Since direct visualization of the glottis is not required to insert a laryngeal mask airway, a laryngoscope is not required. One is expected to adhere to all aseptic precautions required during any procedures performed on the neonate.

- For inserting a LMA for neonatal resuscitation in the delivery room lubrication is generally not required as oral and pharyngeal secretions of the infant would provide the lubrication. If lubrication is required it should be a water-based lubricant.

- If one is using an LMA with inflatable mask, the cuff should first be fully deflated prior to its insertion.

- The healthcare provider stands at the head end of the baby. The baby's neck is extended slightly as if in sniffing position. The baby's

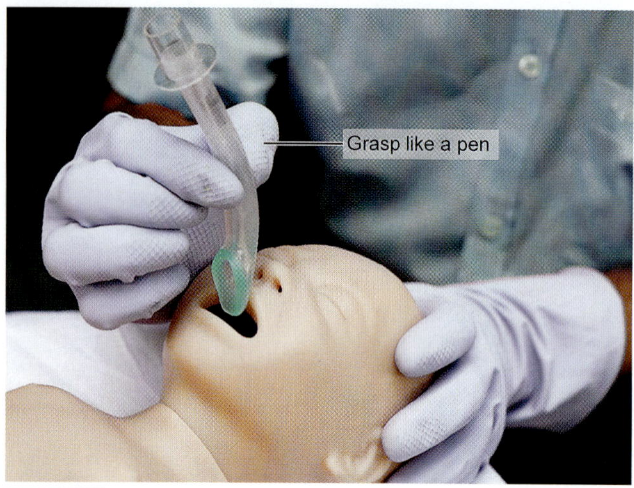

FIG. 5.6 The technique of holding an LMA for insertion.

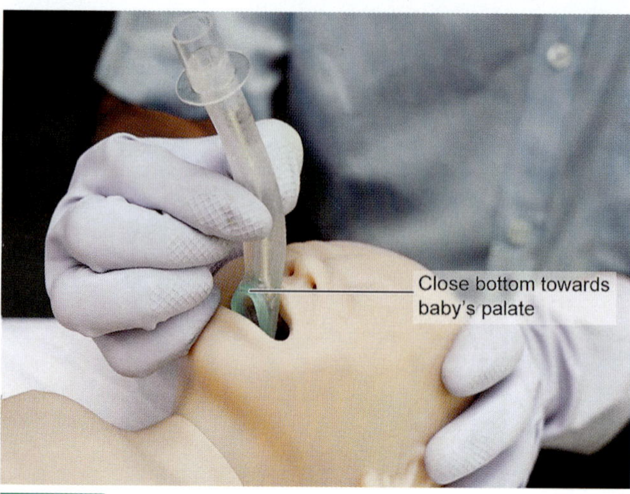

FIG. 5.7 Technique of inserting the LMA.

mouth is opened by gentle jaw thrust, pressing gently downward on baby's chin.

- The airway tube part of LMA is grasped in one's right or left hand like a pen with the index finger at the junction between the mask and the distal end of the airway tube (*Fig.* **5.6**). Hold it in such a way that the closed bottom of the mask faces the baby's palate, and the open bowl of the mask faces the baby's chin (*Fig.* **5.7**). The LMA is gently advanced with one single movement, while applying continuous pressure on the palate and following the contour of the hard palate on top of baby's tongue. One continues pushing the LMA against soft palate so that the cuff passes along posterior pharyngeal wall and tip locates itself in the hypopharynx until resistance is felt—it cannot be pushed further inward (*Fig.* **5.8**).

- If one is using an LMA device with inflatable mask, inflate it with minimal volume of air volume necessary to establish an adequate seal. One can see the ventilation tubing shaft moving outward during cuff inflation, so one must not hold the shaft of LMA at the time of cuff inflation.

- *Confirming correct placement of LMA:* Once the LMA is in place it can be connected to a device for providing PPV. Correct insertion of LMA would be indicated by a visible chest rise and breath sounds on both side of the chest on auscultation during PPV. If there is a sound of air leak from the baby's mouth or a visible bulge in the baby's neck, it is indicative of malposition of the airway or inadequate seal.

- If there is no leak during PPV, the LMA can be secured with a tape. Effective PPV via a LMA should be accompanied by rising heart rate and oxygen saturation.

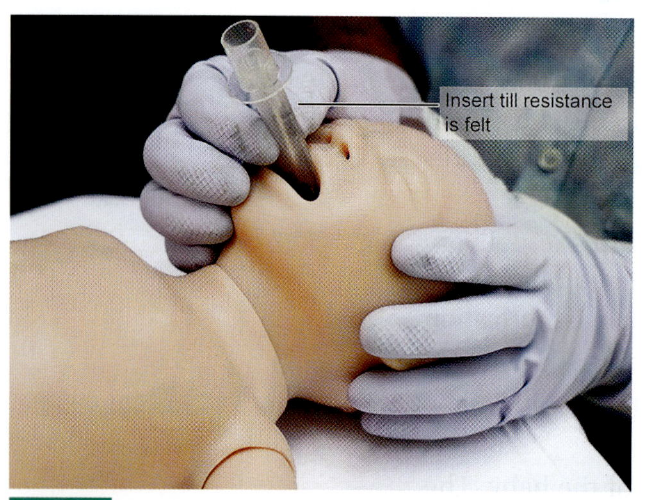

FIG. 5.8 How far to insert the LMA?

- One can hear the baby crying when baby starts breathing spontaneously, as the vocal cords can still adduct despite LMA being in place.

Pros and Cons of LMA

Advantages of LMA: There are several potential benefits that have been cited for the use of a LMA in neonatal resuscitation. These include its ability to provide more effective positive pressure ventilation in comparison to face mask, less skill being required to maintain effective PPV in comparison to face mask and endotracheal tube, easier placement by less experienced personnel and lesser time required to place it in position compared to endotracheal intubation.[7]

Limitations: There are greater chances of gastric insufflation when LMA without gastric vent is used. It may not provide effective ventilation when pressure needed is high as LMA provides only a low-pressure seal. It is not possible to suction airway through the LMA. Also, administration of medication is difficult and since placing a LMA is a blind procedure, medication given through LMA may leak into stomach. Hence, the use of LMA for medication is currently not recommended.

Complications: Complications are not frequent but those documented include tissue trauma, gastric distension, and laryngospasm.

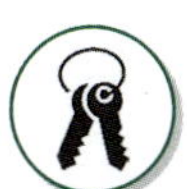 **KEY POINTS**

1. Laryngeal mask airway (LMA) also known as supraglottic airway is meant to provide positive pressure ventilation in neonates.
2. Laryngoscopy or direct visualization of glottis is not required while placing an LMA, hence it is an effective alternative compared to endotracheal intubation when face mask ventilation is unsuccessful.
3. Many designs of LMA are available commercially, but technique to place it remains same. For neonates, LMA size 1 is recommended.
4. It is currently recommended for use in babies ≥34 weeks gestation and/or birth weight >2,000 g. But it has also been used successfully in infants with birth weight >1,500 g.
5. Laryngeal mask airway is not currently recommended for intratracheal administration of medications.

REFERENCES

1. Brimacombe J, Gandini D. The laryngeal mask airway: potential applications in neonatal health care. J Obstet Gynecol Neonatal Nurs. 1997;26:171-8.
2. Trevisanuto D, Micaglio M, Ferrarese P, Zanardo V. The laryngeal mask airway: potential applications in neonates. Arch Dis Child Fetal Neonatal Ed. 2004;89:F485-9.

3. Qureshi MJ, Kumar M. Laryngeal mask airway versus bag-mask ventilation or endotracheal intubation for neonatal resuscitation. Cochrane Database Syst Rev. 2018;3(3):CD003314.

4. Yamada NK, McKinlay CJ, Quek BH, Schmölzer GM, Wyckoff MH, Liley HG, et al. Supraglottic airways compared with face masks for neonatal resuscitation: a systematic review. Pediatrics. 2022;150(3):e2022056568.

5. Pejovic NJ, Myrnerts Höök S, Byamugisha J, Alfvén T, Lubulwa C, Cavallin F, et al. A randomized trial of laryngeal mask airway in neonatal resuscitation. N Engl J Med. 2020;383(22):2138-47.

6. Madar J, Roehr CC, Ainsworth S, Ersdal H, Morley C, Rüdiger M, et al. European Resuscitation Council Guidelines 2021: Newborn Resuscitation and Support of Transition of Infants at Birth. Resuscitation. 2021;161:291-326.

7. Mani S, Pinheiro JMB, Rawat M. Laryngeal Masks in Neonatal Resuscitation: a Narrative Review of Updates 2022. Children (Basel). 2022;9(5):733.

 # Self Assessment

1. The following statement(s) are TRUE regarding laryngeal mask airway:
   a. It is known as supraglottic airway.
   b. Size 1 mask is for neonates.
   c. Aperture bars in the middle of mask are to increase air flow.
   d. It can be placed by anyone who deals with neonatal resuscitation.

2. Laryngeal mask is used in neonates when:
   a. With face mask ventilation SpO_2 is not increasing.
   b. If no improvement after 5 minutes of resuscitation.
   c. When face mask ventilation is not effective and attempts at endotracheal intubation were unsuccessful.
   d. When medical staff is not available.

3. Rearrange steps to introduce LMA in neonates:
   a. Attach device to provide positive pressure ventilation (PPV) to LMA.
   b. Progress LMA in the mouth till resistance is felt.
   c. Inflate the mask with minimum air volume.
   d. Hold mask like pen with index finger.

4. State True/False.
   a. LMA can be used in neonates >28 weeks.
   b. It should be placed in front of glottis with the help of laryngoscope.
   c. LMA is safe and more effective than face mask as primary interface.
   d. It also can be used for suctioning and for intratracheal delivery of medications.

Answers

For answers, go to the end of the Book, Page no. 321

The Process of Neonatal Resuscitation: Advanced

6 Endotracheal Intubation

Suman Rao PN

Lessons to Learn

- Indications for endotracheal intubation
- What are the supplies required for the procedure?
- Procedure of endotracheal intubation
- Confirming the position of the endotracheal tube
- How to secure the endotracheal tube?
- Role of the assistant during endotracheal intubation
- What are the complications of intubation and how to improve patient safety?

Endotracheal intubation is placement of a tube into the trachea by passing it through the glottis between the vocal cords. It is done under direct visualization of the vocal cords using a laryngoscope. It is the gold standard for securing the airway during neonatal resuscitation when the provider is unable to ventilate adequately with mask ventilation. *Figure* **6.1** is the NRP flow diagram where the steps related to endotracheal intubation is highlighted by an outlined area. **Box 6.1** provides an illustrative case of a neonate who required endotracheal intubation as part of resuscitation. You can follow the case and the flow diagram as you read through this chapter. The chapter also includes the newer aspects of the procedure such as video-laryngoscopy, cuffed endotracheal tube and methods to improve the safety of the procedure.

■ WHEN SHOULD THE BABY BE INTUBATED?

Table 6.1 lists the indications for endotracheal intubation.

Personnel and Supplies

When endotracheal intubation is needed, it should be immediately inserted with aseptic precautions. Hence a provider with intubation skills must always be available during a high-risk delivery. The team member assisting in endotracheal intubation has several roles to play and must be trained. At least one complete set of the supplies indicated

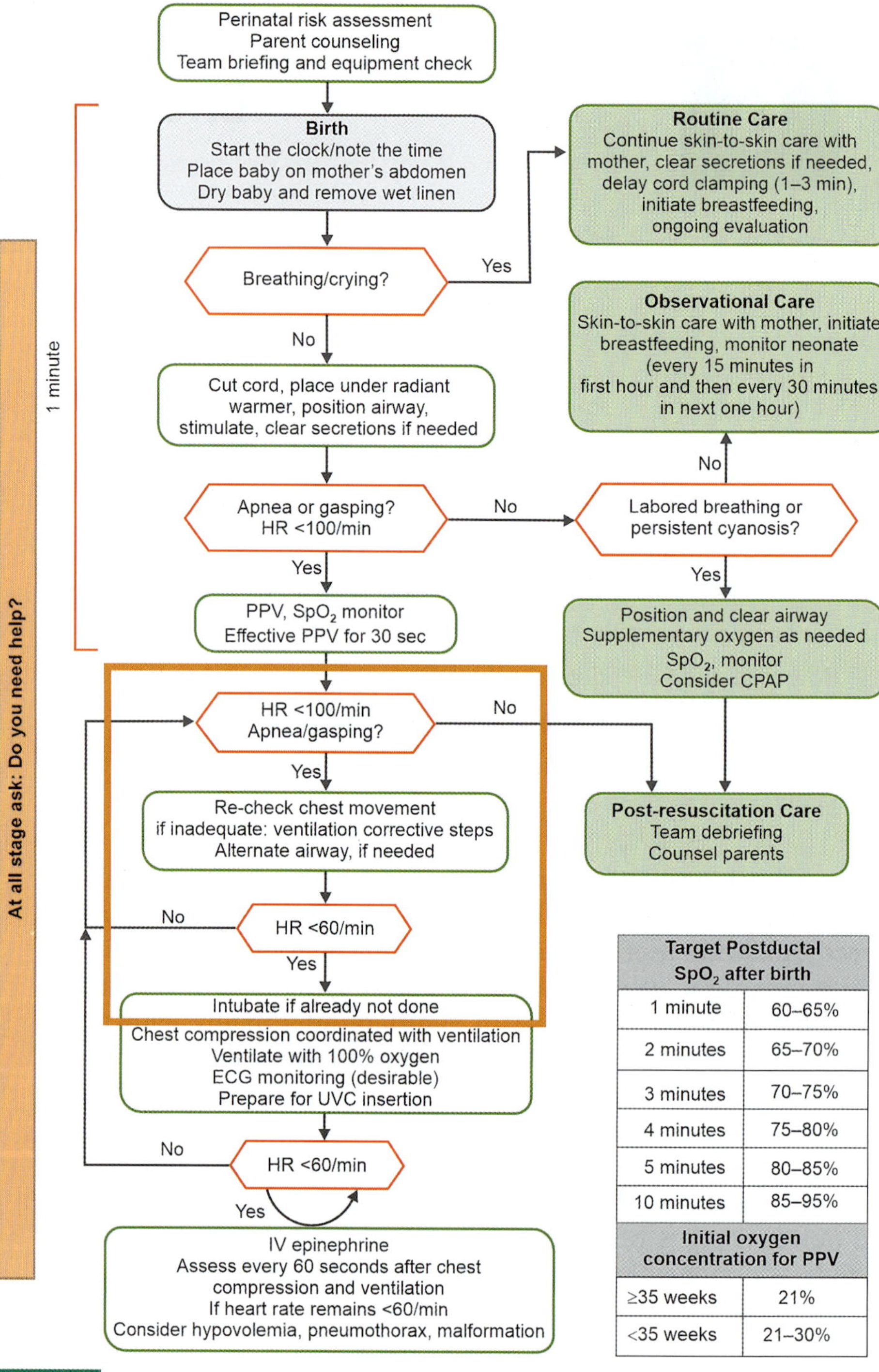

Target Postductal SpO2 after birth	
1 minute	60–65%
2 minutes	65–70%
3 minutes	70–75%
4 minutes	75–80%
5 minutes	80–85%
10 minutes	85–95%
Initial oxygen concentration for PPV	
≥35 weeks	21%
<35 weeks	21–30%

FIG. 6.1   Neonatal resuscitation flow diagram *(boxed area indicates the steps related to endotracheal intubation).*

in **Table 6.2** must be assembled and must be easily accessible in each newborn care corner (NBCC) (*Fig.* **6.2**).

Endotracheal Tube

The endotracheal tube (ET) used in neonatal resuscitation is a non-cuffed tube with uniform diameter throughout the length of the tube.

BOX 6.1: ILLUSTRATIVE CASE

A woman is admitted in preterm labor at 35 weeks with fetal distress. She is taken up for emergency cesarean section. The neonatal resuscitation team is informed. The physician and the nurse complete a pre-resuscitation briefing, check the equipment, and switch on the radiant warmer. The baby is limp and apneic at birth. The obstetrician immediately clamps and cuts the cord and hands over the baby to the nurse, who brings the infant to a radiant warmer for resuscitation.

The baby is positioned, dried, provided tactile stimulus and mouth and nose suctioned to clear secretions. As the baby is still not breathing, positive pressure ventilation (PPV) with room air is initiated. The nurse auscultates the heart. Heart rate is 70 bpm and the nurse notes that there is no chest rise. With readjustment of the mask, there is chest rise and the heart rate improves to >100 bpm and PPV is continued. A pulse oximeter probe is placed on the baby's right hand and connected to the oximeter. The oxygen saturation is 70% at 2 minutes and 80% at 3 minutes. But as there is no spontaneous respiratory effort even after 3 minutes, the team decides to intubate the baby.

The nurse provides a laryngoscope with blade 0 and a 3.5 mm endotracheal tube. She keeps the suction ready, steadies the head of the baby. The physician intubates the baby and the tube's adaptor is connected to the PPV device. Auscultation of the chest confirms that the breath sounds are heard equally in the axillae and not over the stomach. The baby's chest is moving well, and the heart rate remains >100 bpm. PPV is continued at 40 breaths/minute. The saturations remain 90–92%. The team updates the family on the baby's status and prepares to shift the baby to the neonatal intensive care unit. Thereafter the team has a debriefing to evaluate the management of the baby.

TABLE 6.1: INDICATIONS FOR ENDOTRACHEAL INTUBATION

Indication	Additional comments
For effective positive pressure ventilation (PPV)	When heart rate remains <100 and is not increasing despite PPV or when there is no chest rise on PPV despite ventilatory corrective steps (after mask adjustment, repositioning, suctioning of airway, opening of mouth, and increased pressure), endotracheal intubation is indicated to facilitate effective PPV
Prolonged PPV	If PPV is prolonged (lasts for a few minutes or more), endotracheal intubation improves the efficacy of ventilation and allows for transport of the infant
Before chest compression	Endotracheal intubation is strongly recommended before chest compression. PPV for 30 seconds after intubation could avert the need for chest compression. It aids in coordinating with compressions. It also allows the person providing chest compression to stand at the head end to provide chest compression. If heart rate is <60 despite PPV and chest compression for 1 minute, the endotracheal tube (ET) can be used to provide adrenaline, while IV access is being established
For tracheal suction	In an infant born through meconium-stained amniotic fluid, if the airway is obstructed and chest rise cannot be achieved with PPV, endotracheal intubation followed by suction as the tube is withdrawn should be considered
If there is a suspicion of congenital diaphragmatic hernia (CDH)	In a baby with antenatally diagnosed diaphragmatic hernia or if there is a suspicion of CDH (scaphoid abdomen with displaced heart sounds), endotracheal intubation should be done to provide PPV. Mask ventilation will further compress the lungs and is contraindicated
For administration of surfactant	Endotracheal intubation is one method of administration of surfactant though it is not routinely indicated in the labor room. Noninvasive methods of surfactant administration such as less invasive surfactant administration (LISA) are currently preferred[32]

TABLE 6.2: SUPPLIES REQUIRED FOR INTUBATION

Supplies	Remarks
Endotracheal tubes with internal diameters (ID) of 2.5, 3.0, and 3.5 mm	
Laryngoscope handle with batteries and bulb	An extra set of batteries and bulbs should be available. A video laryngoscope is a recent option for a difficult airway
Laryngoscope blades: No.1 (term babies) No. 0 (preterm babies) No. 00 (extremely preterm optional)	The laryngoscope blades for newborns are straight (Miller)
Stylet (optional)	Routine use of stylet is discouraged but it may be considered in difficult airways
Adhesive tapes	½ or ¾ inch tapes to secure the tube must be pre-cut and available. Skin protective adhesives for extreme preterm babies are preferred
Measuring tape	For determining the nasal-tragus length
Scissors to cut tape	
Tracheal aspirator	A tracheal aspirator (meconium aspirator) is rarely required to suction the trachea
Stethoscope	These are required for earlier steps of resuscitation and are essential during endotracheal intubation
Self-inflating bag/T-piece resuscitator	
Pulse oximeter or cardiac monitor	
Gloves	

Most commonly the endotracheal tube needed ranges from 2.5–3.5 mm. Size 2.0 mm and size 4.0 mm are routinely not required but may be considered in special situations. Choice of the size of the ET is based on birth weight or gestation age **(Table 6.3)**. Too large a tube will be difficult to insert and can injure the airway, too small a tube will increase the resistance and work of breathing. In special situations such as a difficult airway, a smaller size tube may be chosen.

The tube should have markings in centimeters throughout the length of the tube. At the tip of the tube, there is usually another marking which is the vocal cord guide (this part of the tube indicates the depth the tube should be below the vocal cords, but this is only an approximation). The tube also has another line that is radiopaque and indicates the tube on X-ray. The tube is connected to an adapter that connects the ET to the positive pressure ventilation (PPV) device. This adapter is size specific. The ET has a side hole at the tip (*Fig.* **6.3**).

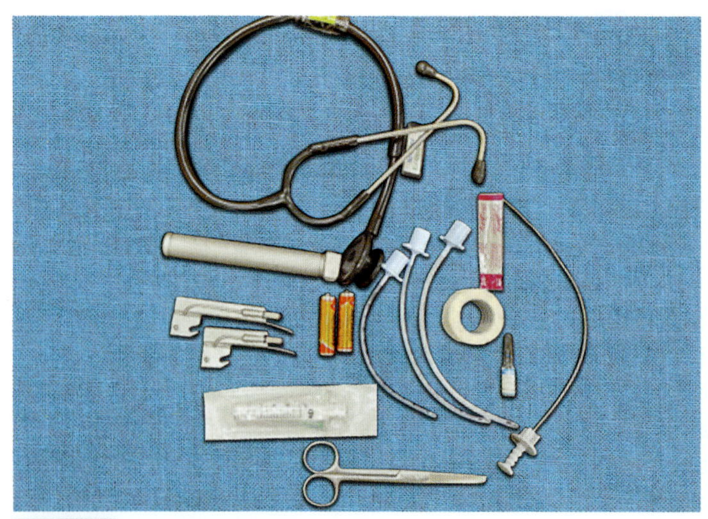

FIG. 6.2 Supplies for neonatal resuscitation.

TABLE 6.3: Selecting the Size of Endotracheal Tube

Weight	Gestational age	ET size
<1 kg	<28 weeks	2.5 mm ID
1–2 kg	28–34 weeks	3.0 mm ID
>2 kg	>34 weeks	3.5 mm ID

(ET: endotracheal tube; ID: internal diameter).

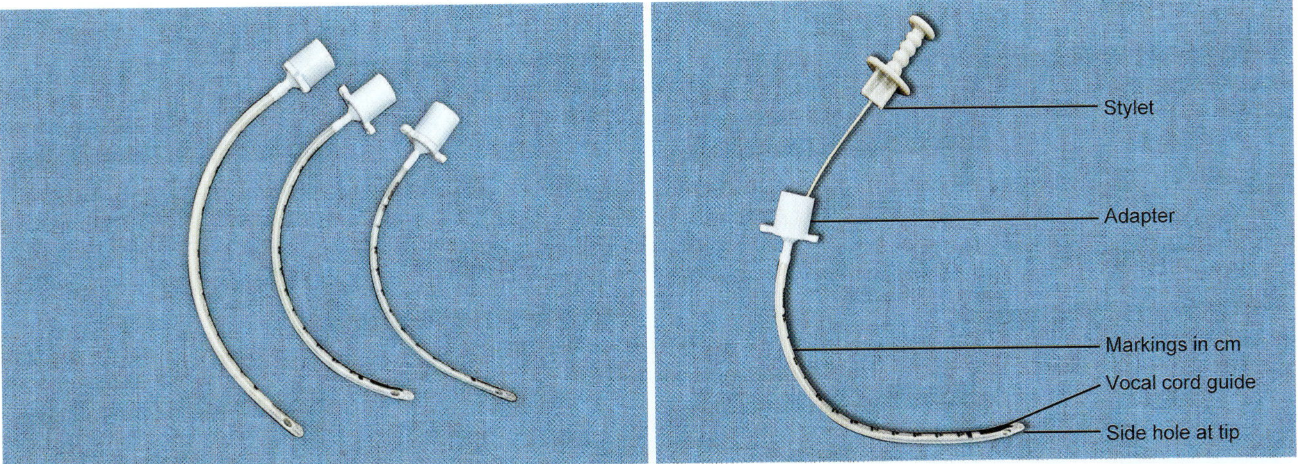

FIG. 6.3 Endotracheal tube and its components.

The neonatal airway is similar to the adult airway and is more cylindrical rather than funnel shaped with the narrowest part of the larynx being the glottic region.[1] This has led to reconsideration on use of cuffed ET. The advantages of cuffed ET include decreased reintubation rate, decreased ET leak, decreased aspiration, and ventilator-associated pneumonia and potentially less airway damage. However, limited evidence precludes routine recommendation for use of cuffed ET.

Stylet

The use of a stylet in newborn endotracheal intubation is optional. If it is used, it should be secured (either with a plug or bent at the top) such that the tip of the stylet does not protrude beyond the tip of the ET or through the side hole as this may cause injury to the airway. It should not fit snuggly into the tube and should be easily removable once inserted without displacing the tube. *Figures* **6.4A and B** show how a stylet can be used with the ET tube.

Though it is considered optional, majority of neonatal airway providers reported using stylet in a survey with the belief that it improves the success of intubation.[2] However, the evidence from a Cochrane meta-analysis found no difference in success with the use of stylet among pediatric trainees.[3] In a review of 5,292 primary oral intubations from 16 centers, 73% used stylets. Success of first attempt intubation, adverse events, and severe desaturations were similar with and without use of stylet.[4]

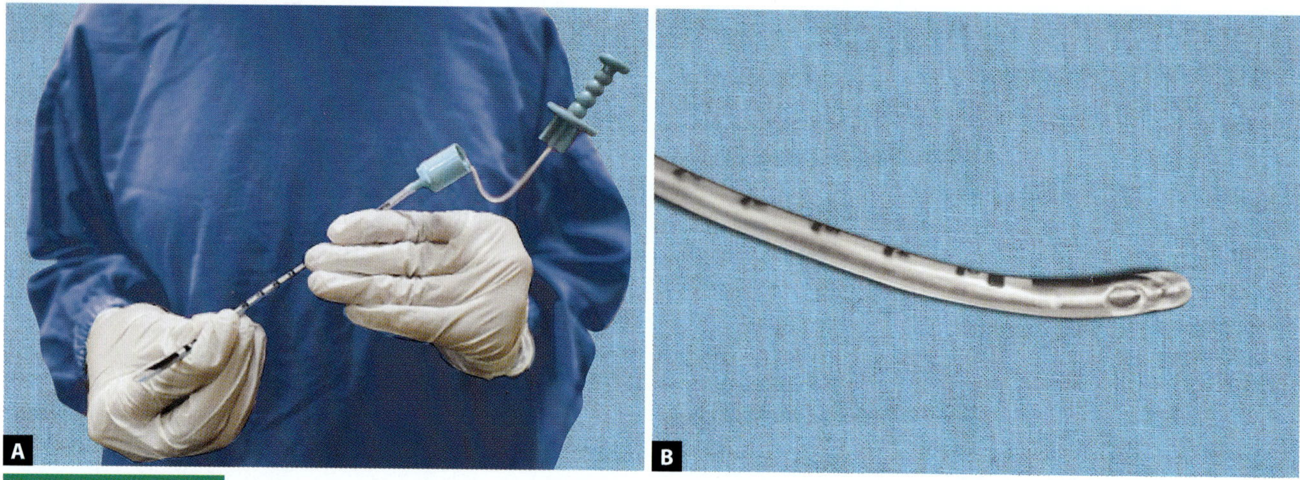

FIGS. 6.4A AND B Using a stylet with the endotracheal tube: (A) The stylet has to be bent at the top; (B) The tip of stylet should not protrude beyond the tip of the ET.

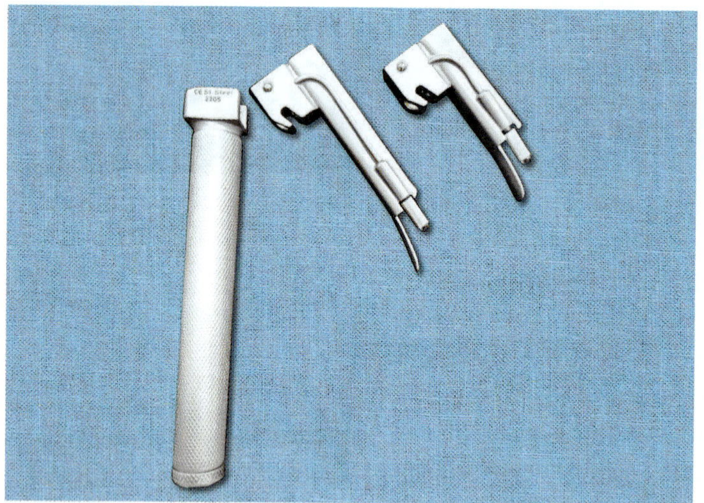

FIG. 6.5 Laryngoscope handle with size '0' and size '1' blades.

Laryngoscope

One must choose the appropriately sized laryngoscope blade. Blade No. 1 is used for term babies and No. 0 for preterm babies (*Fig.* **6.5**). Consider use of 00 size for extremely preterm infants. The Miller straight blade laryngoscope is superior for visualization of the laryngeal inlet in the newborn due to the unique upper airway anatomy of infants and the large posteriorly angled epiglottis. The light of the laryngoscope must always be checked and if it is dim or flickers, tighten the bulb and change the batteries, if needed. The laryngoscope should be kept closed till it is needed to avoid overheating of the bulb and blade.

Video-laryngoscopes with a camera that show the magnified images of the airway on the screen are available and particularly useful in a difficult airway. Studies have shown that learning endotracheal intubation using the video-laryngoscope improved success rates of endotracheal intubation and reduced esophageal intubations.[5,6] Data from the National Emergency Airway Registry for Neonates have shown that video-laryngoscope use was associated with higher first attempt success and lower adverse events but there was no difference in severe desaturation.[7]

Positive Pressure Ventilation Device

Positive pressure ventilation devices (self-inflating bag or T-piece resuscitator) are essential for endotracheal intubation not only to confirm the position of the tube but to continue PPV after intubation.

Suction Device with Suction Catheters

For suctioning obstructed ET, suction catheters of size 5F or 6F are recommended. Tracheal aspirator (meconium aspirator) should be part of the endotracheal intubation procedure kit. In the presence of obstruction with meconium that prevents chest rise, the tracheal aspirator can be directly connected to the ET to suction thick secretions or meconium as one withdraws the tube while applying continuous suction.

Supplies to Fix the Endotracheal Tube

Adhesive tapes (½ or ¾ inch width) pre-cut as "H" or "pantaloon" should be kept ready to fix the ET. A pair of scissors and a tape to measure the nasal-tragus length are also essential.

Monitoring Devices

The baby should be monitored with a pulse oximeter during the procedure. A cardiac monitor may more reliably provide the heart rate. A CO_2 detector that changes color on successful intubation is useful but not mandatory.

■ PROCEDURE OF ENDOTRACHEAL INTUBATION

Preparation for Intubation

The following steps help in preparing for endotracheal intubation:

1. Select the appropriate size of ET based on gestational age or approximate birth weight
2. Select appropriate size blade and attach it to the handle
3. Check the light, if the light is dim or flickering change the batteries.
4. Keep suction apparatus ready
5. Keep PPV device ready

Technique of Endotracheal Intubation

The provider performing endotracheal intubation should be familiar with the anatomic landmarks in the neonatal airway. *Figure* **6.6** provides a view of vocal cords and surrounding structures as seen during laryngoscopy. **Box 6.2** and *Figures* **6.7 to 6.10** provide the steps of endotracheal intubation.

Confirming the Position of the Endotracheal Tube in the Trachea

A rapidly increasing heart rate is the primary method of confirming that the ET is in the

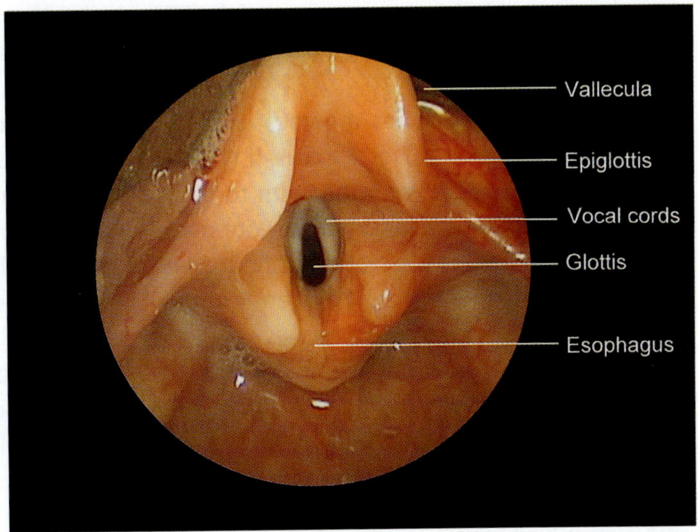

FIG. 6.6 Laryngoscopic view of the vocal cords and surrounding structures.

trachea. There are several other signs given in **Box 6.3** that indicate successful placement of the ET in the trachea.

It is important to note that breath sounds in babies are easily transmitted across the chest. Hence, a small stethoscope should be placed in the axillae as sounds from the esophagus or stomach may easily be heard by a large stethoscope placed on the center of the chest.

If the tube is not placed in the trachea, it is best to withdraw the tube, provide ventilation with PPV device and mask, stabilize the

---

BOX 6.2: STEPS OF ENDOTRACHEAL INTUBATION

1. Position the baby with the head in the "sniffing" position, slightly extended such that the airway is open (*Fig.* **6.7**). A shoulder roll may aid in positioning the baby
2. Stand at the head end of the baby. Adjust the height of the warmer bed such that the baby's head is at the level of your lower chest or upper abdomen
3. Stabilize the head of the baby with your right hand or this can be done by the assistant, who ensures that the baby's body is straight and head is in "sniffing" position
4. Always hold the laryngoscope blade in your **LEFT** hand (even if you are a left-handed person) (*Fig.* **6.7**)
5. Gently open the mouth with your right thumb and index finger. Insert the laryngoscope in the midline, over the tongue till the tip lies in the vallecula (the space between the base of the tongue and the epiglottis)
6. Lift the laryngoscope in the direction of the handle to expose the glottis. Do not bend your wrist and "rock" the laryngoscope toward yourself (*Fig.* **6.8**) as this will injure the baby's gums and lips
7. At times, the tip of the blade may need to be placed directly under the epiglottis to move it out gently away from the laryngeal inlet. The vocal cords appear as an inverted "V"
8. If the vocal cords are not seen, it may be because the blade is not inserted far enough, and you see only the base of the tongue. The laryngoscope then needs to be inserted further. If the blade is too far in, you see the esophagus and you need to withdraw the tube. You may also need to ask the assistant to apply downward pressure on the cricoid toward the baby's right ear to bring the glottis into view (*Fig.* **6.9**). If secretions are blocking the view, remove the secretions with a 10 F or 12 F suction catheter. You should attempt to put in the ET *only after* visualization of the vocal cords
9. Hold the laryngoscope steadily while the assistant places the appropriate-sized ET in your right hand. Hold the tube with the concave curve of the ET in the horizontal plane and insert the tube into the right side of the baby's mouth toward the vocal cords. Do not pass the tube through the groove in the laryngoscope as this will block your view
10. As the tip approaches the vocal cords, rotate the tube such that the tip is directed upward. Gently pass between the open vocal cords. If the vocal cords remain closed, do not touch the cords with the tube or laryngoscope but wait for them to open. If cords do not open in 30 seconds, remove the laryngoscope, continue PPV with mask before your make another attempt
11. Once the tube is inserted into the trachea, securely hold the tube against the baby's hard palate with your right index finger (*Fig.* **6.10**). Gently remove the laryngoscope. If stylet is used, it should be carefully removed without dislodging the tube
12. With the help of the assistant, connect the PPV device to the ET to provide ventilation
13. The procedure of intubation is an emergency intervention and should take not more than 30 seconds. If you are unable to insert the ET in 30 seconds, remove the laryngoscope and provide mask ventilation. Do not make more than three attempts, as repeated attempts can cause soft tissue trauma
14. If intubation is unsuccessful, consider calling for help from an expert (more experienced neonatologist, anesthetist). Continue PPV with mask till help arrives. Use of laryngeal mask airway is an alternative as it needs lesser skill and experience

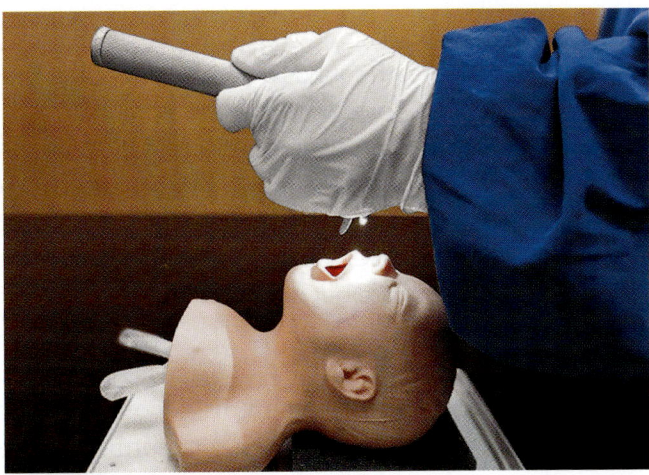

FIG. 6.7 Position the baby in the sniffing position and hold the laryngoscope in left hand.

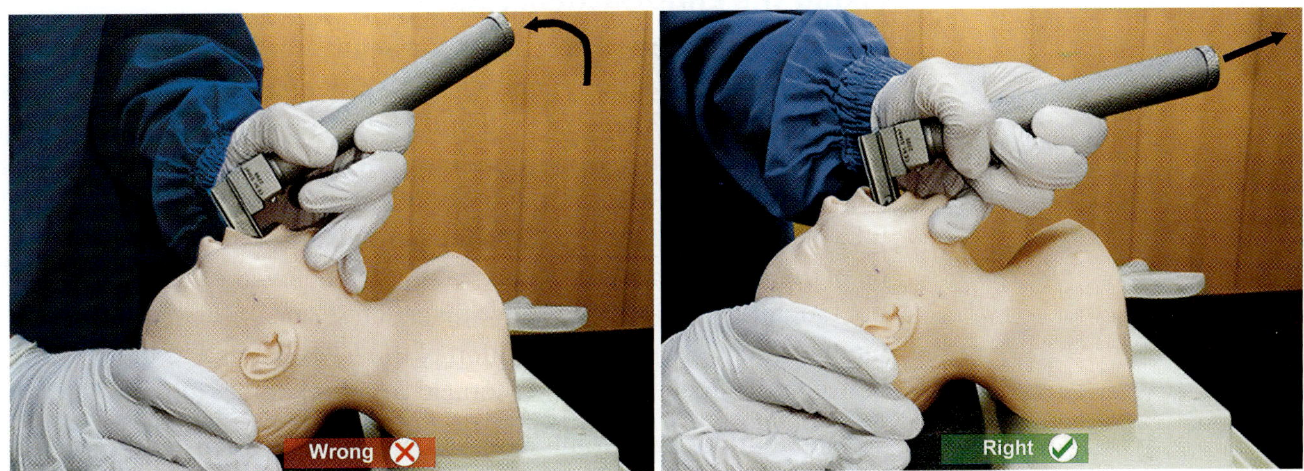

FIG. 6.8 Lift the laryngoscope in the direction of the handle and avoid rocking motion.

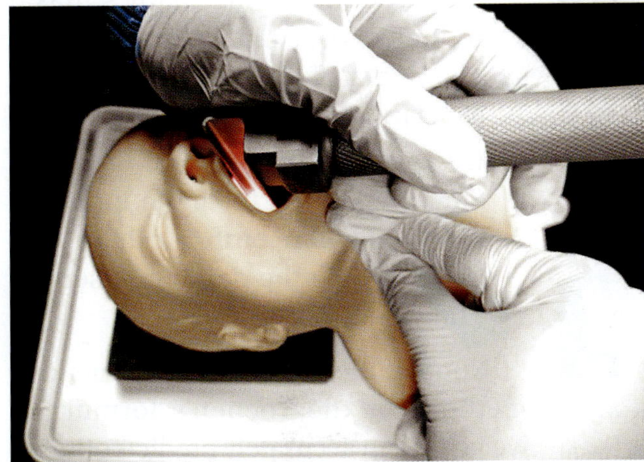

FIG. 6.9 Application of cricoid pressure.

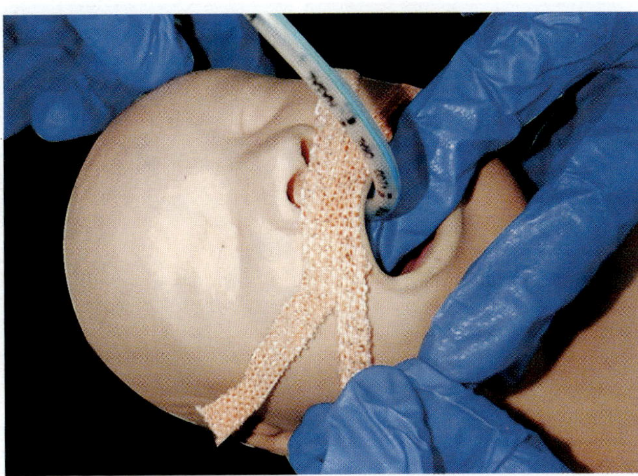

FIG. 6.10 Stabilizing the ET while the laryngoscope is withdrawn.

> **BOX 6.3: CONFIRMING THE POSITION OF THE ENDOTRACHEAL TUBE IN THE TRACHEA**
> 1. Equal breath sounds on both sides of the chest near the axillae, but decreased or absent over the stomach
> 2. Adequate and symmetrical chest movements with each breath
> 3. No gastric distention with ventilation
> 4. Presence of mist in the tube
> 5. Detection of CO_2 in the exhaled gas by colorimetric CO_2 detectors is also a gold standard but not frequently available at all health facilities

baby and then try again. A "second look" procedure reinserting the laryngoscope and checking to confirm if the tube is inserted between the vocal cords can be considered if one is sure of intubation despite the absence of signs. X-ray is the gold standard to confirm the position of the ET.

Fixing the Endotracheal Tube

Optimal depth of insertion of the ET is essential, for too high a placement (above T1 vertebral body) may cause accidental extubation, and too low a placement (below T4 vertebral body) may cause intubation of a main stem bronchus, usually on the right side. Optimal placement is vital to allow for the flexion and extension of neck without significant tube displacement during these movements. Aim the tip of the ET to be in the middle part of the trachea, 1–2 cm below the vocal cords and not touching the carina (usually adjacent to T3 or T4) or entering into a main bronchus. Optimum position of the ET is defined as the tip lying between the first and second thoracic vertebral bodies (T1 and T2).[8]

The depth of insertion is assessed by the tip to lip distance, i.e., the marking on the tube adjacent to the baby's lip. This can be determined by several methods:

- *Nasal-tragus length (NTL):* The distance from the baby's nasal septum to the ear tragus is measured. The depth of insertion is calculated as NTL+1 cm (*Fig.* **6.11**).

- *Gestational age-based method*[9]: Since very often the gestational age is known before birth, it can be used to determine the depth of insertion **(Table 6.4)**.

None of the currently recommended methods or the Tochen's formula of weight +6 cm accurately predicts optimal ET length in Indian neonates.[10] There could be variations across ethnic groups.

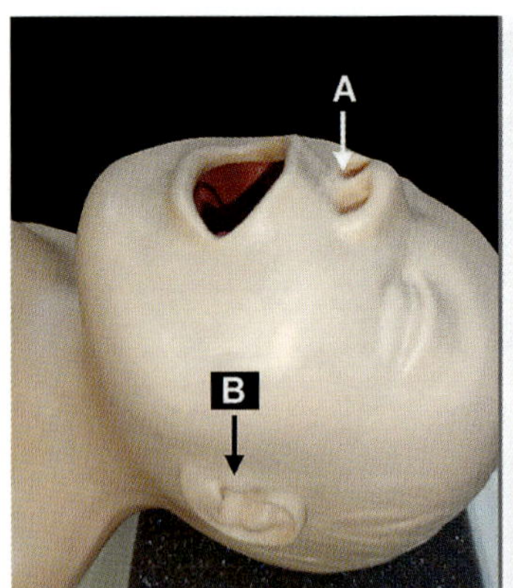
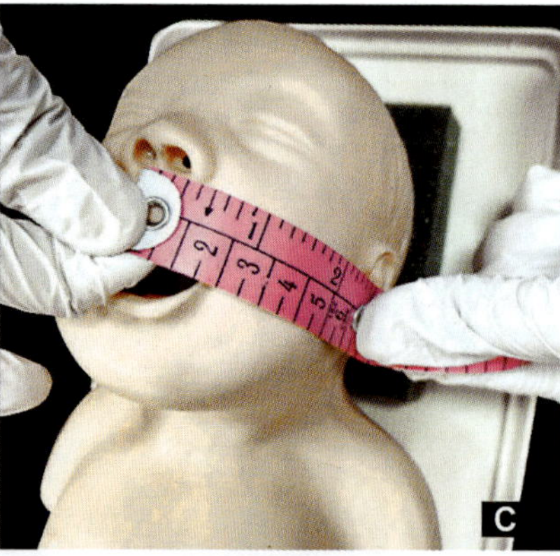

FIG. 6.11 Nasal-tragus length to determine the depth of insertion of the endotracheal tube. Measure from the middle of the nasal septum (A) to the tragus of the ear (B). Measure this length as shown in (C).

TABLE 6.4: GESTATIONAL AGE-BASED ESTIMATION OF THE DEPTH OF INSERTION OF THE ENDOTRACHEAL TUBE

Gestation	Endotracheal tube insertion depth at lips	Baby's weight
23–24 weeks	5.5 cm	0.5–0.6 kg
25–26 weeks	6.0 cm	0.7–0.8 kg
27–29 weeks	6.5 cm	0.9–1 kg
30–32 weeks	7.0 cm	1.1–1.4 kg
33–34 weeks	7.5 cm	1.5–1.8 kg
35–37 weeks	8.0 cm	1.9–2.4 kg
38–40 weeks	8.5 cm	2.5–3.1 kg
41–43 weeks	9.0 cm	3.3–4.2 kg

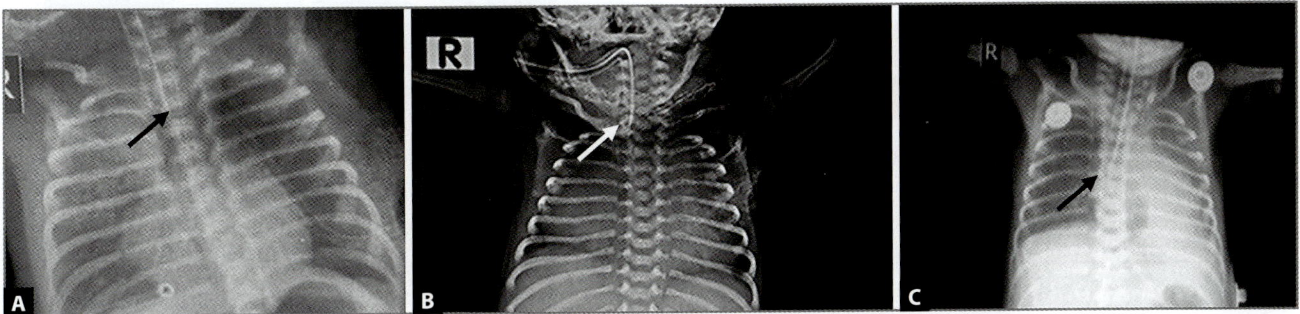

FIGS. 6.12A TO C X-ray confirmation of ET position. (A) Correct position; (B) ET is high up; (C) ET is too far in.

In LBW babies, modified Tochen's formula (weight +5 cm) may enable more optimum placement of ET.[11]

These formulae are only estimates. It is, therefore, important to auscultate for breath sounds in both axillae and over stomach after inserting the tube to determine the correct placement. When correctly placed, breath sounds should be equally heard in both the axillae and not on the stomach. X-ray is the gold standard to confirm the correct position of the ET (*Figs.* **6.12A to C**). Point-of-care ultrasound is emerging as a rapid, reliable alternative.[12,13]

Securing the Endotracheal Tube

It is essential to secure the ET tube if it is planned to keep it beyond the initial resuscitation. Cut sufficient length of the ½ or ¾ inch tape so that it can extend from one side of the baby's mouth, cross the upper lip and extend about 2 cm onto the opposite cheek of the baby. In the pantaloon method, the tape is split along half its length, mimicking two legs of a pant. The uncut section should be at the corner of the baby's mouth, one leg of the pant should be across the upper lip and the other carefully wound around the ET. The other way of securing the ET is by the "H" method (*Figs.* **6.13A and B**). Here the tape is split along its length from both ends so that it appears as an "H". One limb of the "H" should be across the upper lip and the two sections of the other limb of the H are wound around the ET.

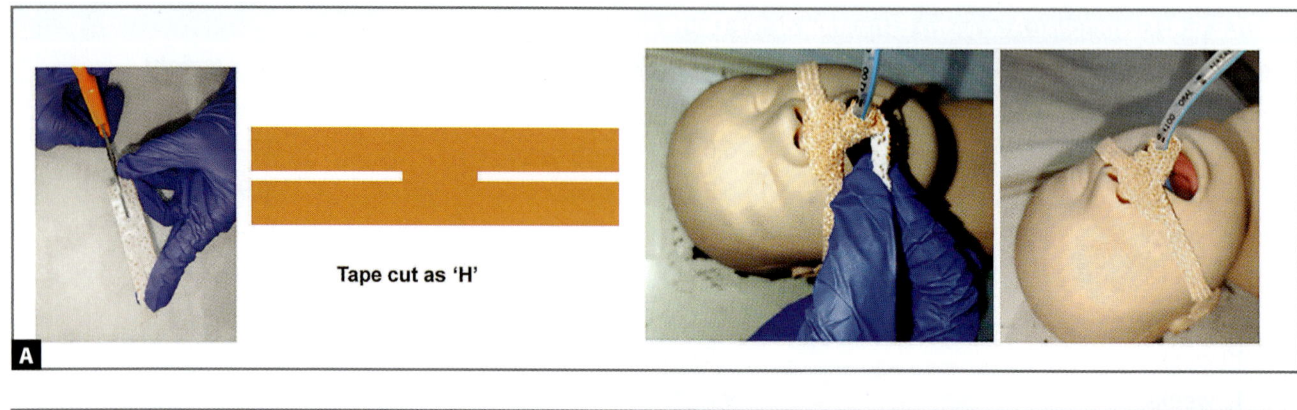

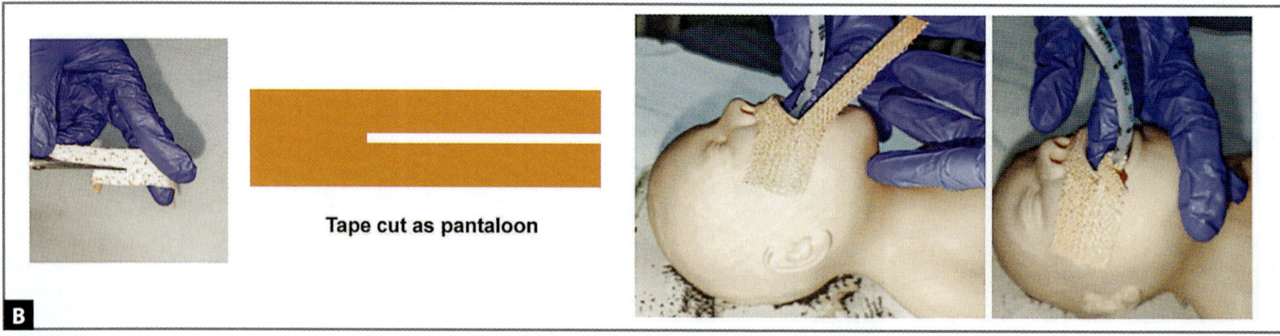

FIGS. 6.13A AND B Techniques for fixing endotracheal tube. (A) Using the 'H'-shaped tape; (B) Using the pantaloon-shaped tape.

It is advisable that the adhesive tapes are not directly applied on the skin. Skin friendly adhesives should first be applied on the skin and the tapes secured over them to prevent skin injury especially in the very preterm babies. Ensure that the desired centimeter mark on the ET is against the upper lip while fixing, as often the tube slips deeper in during securing of the ET. The most effective and safe method to stabilize the endotracheal tube in the ventilated neonate is not clear and well-designed studies are needed.[14]

Role of the Assistant

The team member assisting the procedure of endotracheal intubation has several tasks to perform which are listed in **Box 6.4**. Effective team work aids in successful and timely intubation.

■ SUCTIONING WITH AN ENDOTRACHEAL TUBE

The goal of neonatal resuscitation is to establish effective positive pressure ventilation. If it is not possible to get adequate chest movements despite endotracheal intubation, one must consider thick secretions blocking the tube especially in babies born through meconium-stained liquor. These secretions can be removed either by passing a suction catheter inserted through the ET or by using a tracheal (meconium) aspirator. In the first method, the suction should be protected. The tip of the suction catheter should be just beyond the tip of the ET and should not touch the carina. A tracheal aspirator

BOX 6.4: ROLE OF THE ASSISTANT IN ENDOTRACHEAL INTUBATION

1. Ensures the baby is correctly positioned. Stabilizes the head throughout the procedure
2. Holds equipment and passes them as directed. Helps in suction so that the provider need not look away from the anatomic landmarks
3. Monitors the baby's heart rate. Calls out if the attempt is >30 seconds
4. Provides cricoid pressure as needed
5. After intubation helps to remove the stylet, if used and connects ET to the positive pressure device
6. Auscultates for heart rate and for breath sounds in the baby's axilla and over stomach to confirm the position
7. Assesses the tip-to-lip insertion depth
8. Secures the tube

TABLE 6.5: OCCASIONAL COMPLICATIONS ASSOCIATED WITH ENDOTRACHEAL INTUBATION

Complication	Possible causes	Prevention or corrective action to be considered
Hypoxia, bradycardia/apnea	• Taking too long to intubate • Incorrect placement of tube	• Halt intubation attempt after 30 seconds • Monitor saturations on pulse oximeter • Reposition tube
Pneumothorax	• Over ventilation of one lung due to tube in right main bronchus • Excessive ventilation pressures	• Place tube correctly • Use appropriate ventilating pressures
Contusions or lacerations of tongue, gums, or airway	• Rough handling of laryngoscope or tube • Inappropriate "rocking" rather than lifting of laryngoscope • Laryngoscope blade too long or too short	• Obtain additional practice/skill • Select appropriate equipment
Perforation of trachea or esophagus	• Too vigorous insertion • Stylet protrudes beyond end of tube	• Handle tube gently • Place stylet properly
Obstructed endotracheal tube	Kink in tube or tube obstructed with secretions	Try to suction tube with catheter or with tracheal aspirator
Infection	Introduction of organisms via hands or equipment	Take all aseptic precautions during the procedure

directly connected to the ET is a better option in the presence of thick secretions, as the larger diameter ET is used as the suction catheter. The ET is withdrawn while applying suction pressure (not to exceed 80–100 mm Hg) by occluding the suction port of the tracheal aspirator. If needed, this procedure can be repeated.

■ COMPLICATIONS OF ENDOTRACHEAL INTUBATION

In skilled hands, the complications are few. Significant hypoxemia and bradycardia are common occurrences during endotracheal intubation. In addition, there may occasionally be other complications (**Table 6.5**). *If the baby suddenly deteriorates after endotracheal intubation* it may be because the tube has got displaced, is obstructed with secretions or the baby has developed a pneumothorax. The procedure also has the potential for adverse physiological changes such as systemic and intracranial hypertension that can cause intraventricular hemorrhage in preterm neonates.[15]

In a prospective study of 162 infants, 35% intubations were associated with non-severe events such as esophageal intubation and 8% with severe adverse events such as hypotension requiring treatment. Emergency intubations and increased number of attempts were predictors of adverse events.[16] One of the long-term effects of neonatal intubation is the enamel defect in primary dentition of children in the region of the incisors which corresponds to the area affected by the laryngoscope toggle.[17]

■ IMPROVING SAFETY OF ENDOTRACHEAL INTUBATION

Premedication for Neonatal Intubation

To ameliorate the adverse physiological changes during endotracheal intubation, premedication is advised for elective/semi-elective intubations.[18] This commonly includes an analgesic or anesthetic dose of a hypnotic drug, muscle relaxant, and anticholinergic drug. A sedative or a muscle relaxant should not be used alone. Premedication results in more optimal intubation with fewer attempts and shorter time and adverse events are reduced.[19]

Though the common drug regimens (morphine, atropine, and suxamethonium) often have hemodynamic effects, the use of premedication has improved over the past decade.[15] An intubation readiness score (IRS) of 3–4 by evaluating the response to a firm stimulus (1 = spontaneous movement; 2 = movement on slight touch; 3 = movement on firm stimulus; 4 = no movement) has been suggested to predict optimal conditions for intubation after premedication.[20]

In the delivery room, where endotracheal intubation is an emergency procedure, premedication use is low. It was only seen in 5.1% of premature infants in the EPIPAGE 2 cohort.[21] Premedication in delivery room has been attempted with nasal medication.[22] Nasal midazolam was found more efficient than nasal ketamine to sedate neonates; the hemodynamic and respiratory effects of both the drugs were comparable.[23]

High Flow Nasal Therapy

High flow nasal therapy has been shown to extend time to desaturation among children and adults. A recent randomized controlled trial in 202 infants with 251 intubations showed that use of nasal high flow therapy during the procedure improved the likelihood of first attempt success (68.5% vs. 54.3%) without physiological instability.[24]

Quality Improvement Approach to Improve Safety

Improving the success of endotracheal intubation and reducing adverse events is an important goal for a neonatal intensive care unit (NICU). A quality improvement approach of sequentially implementing three interventions—standardized checklist for intubation, premedication algorithm, and computerized provider order entry set for intubation resulted in 10% absolute reduction in adverse events.[25]

Competency in Endotracheal Intubation

First attempt success in neonatal intubation is the goal of training providers in this skill. First attempt success is not only associated with fewer adverse effects but also reduced intraventricular hemorrhage and improved neurodevelopmental outcomes among extremely low birth weight infants.[26,27] Physician training level has been shown to be associated with first attempt success. A report from National Emergency Airway Registry for Neonates (NEAR4NEOS) found first attempt success was 23% among residents, 53% among fellows, and 60% among consultants.[28] The suboptimal success among trainees likely reflects their limited experience. While it is mentioned that about 100 intubations are needed for proficiency, a pediatric resident may have a median of three intubation opportunities during training.[29] This calls for developing alternate methods to ensure competency such as use of simulation and video-advanced resuscitation laryngoscopy.[6] In a randomized controlled trial of coaching using video, higher success rate in intubation was seen in the video group (57%) than the traditional group (33%).[30] Tools to provide formative and summative assessments to improve competency have been developed and validated.[31]

 **KEY POINTS**

1. Endotracheal intubation is a "must learn" skill for healthcare providers involved in providing advanced neonatal resuscitation.

2. It is recommended at several steps in the neonatal resuscitation flow diagram to provide effective positive pressure ventilation, prior to chest compression.

3. The size of the endotracheal tube and the laryngoscope blade is based on gestational age.

4. The endotracheal tube must be placed such that the tip is in the middle of the trachea. The position of the tube in the trachea can be confirmed by several methods but the gold standard is an X-ray. Each attempt should be limited to 30 seconds.

5. The procedure could be associated with several complications, but these can be minimized with care and expertise.

▣ REFERENCES

1. Thomas R, Rao S, Minutillo C. Cuffed endotracheal tubes for neonates and young infants: a comprehensive review. Arch Dis Child Fetal Neonatal Ed. 2015;0:F1-F7.

2. Gray MM, Umoren RA, Harris S, Strandjord TP, Sawyer T. Use and perceived safety of stylets for neonatal endotracheal intubation: a national survey. J Perinatol. 2018;38(10):1331-6.

3. O'Shea JE, O'Gorman J, Gupta A, Sinhai S, Foster JP, O'Connell LAF, et al. Orotracheal intubation in infants performed with a stylet versus without a stylet. Cochrane Database Syst Rev. 2017;6:CD011791.

4. Gray MM, Rumpel JA, Brei BK, Krick JA, Sawyer T, Glass K, et al; National Emergency Airway Registry for Neonates: NEAR4NEOS Investigators. Associations of Stylet Use during Neonatal Intubation with Intubation Success, Adverse Events, and Severe Desaturation: A Report from NEAR4NEOS. Neonatology. 2021;118(4):470-8.

5. Assaad MA, Lachance C, Moussa A. Learning neonatal intubation using the videolaryngoscope: a randomized trial on mannequins. Sim Healthcare. 2016;11:190-3.

6. O'Shea JE, Thio M, Kamlin O, McGrory L, Wong C, John J, et al. Videolaryngoscopy to teach neonatal intubation: a randomized trial. Pediatrics. 2015;136:912-9.

7. Mousa A, Sawyer T, Puia-Dumitrescu M, Foglia EE, Ades A, Napolitano N, et al. Does videolaryngoscopy improve tracheal intubation first attempt success in NICUs? A report from the NEAR4 NEOS. J Perinatol. 2022;42:1210-5.

8. Tochen ML. Orotracheal intubation in the newborn infant: a method for determining depth of tube insertion. J Pediatr. 1979;95(6):1050-1.

9. Kempley ST, Moreiras JW, Petrone FL. Endotracheal tube length for neonatal intubation. Resuscitation. 2008;77(3):369-73.

10. Priyadarshi M, Thukral A, Sankar MJ, Verma A, Jana M, Agarwal R, et al. 'Lip-to-Tip' study: comparison of three methods to determine optimal insertion length of endotracheal tube in neonates. Eur J Pediatr. 2021;180(5):1459-66.

11. Tatwavedi D, Nesargi SV, Shankar N, Mathias P, Rao Pn S. Efficacy of modified Tochen's formula for optimum endotracheal tube placement in low birth weight neonates: an RCT. J Perinatol. 2018;38(5):512-6.

12. Salvadori S, Nardo D, Frigo AC, Oss M, Mercante I, Moschino L, et al. Ultrasound for endotracheal tube tip position in term and preterm infants. Neonatology. 2021;118(5):569-77.

13. Jaeel P, Sheth M, Nguyen J. Ultrasonography for endotracheal tube position in infants and children. Eur J Pediatr. 2017;176(3):293-300.

14. Lai M, Inglis GDT, Hose K, Jardine LA, Davies MW. Methods for securing endotracheal tubes in newborn infants. Cochrane Database Syst Rev. 2014;7:CD007805.

15. Maheshwari R, Tracy M, Badawi N, Hinder M. Neonatal endotracheal intubation: how to make it more baby friendly. J Pediatr Child Health. 2016;52:480-6.

16. Hatch LD, Grubb PH, Lea AS, Walsh WF, Markham MH, Whitney GM, et al. Endotracheal intubation in neonates: a prospective study of adverse safety events in 162 infants. J Pediatr. 2016;168:62-6.

17. Melo NSF, Da Silva PGVC, de Lima AAS. The neonatal intubation causes defects in primary teeth of premature infants. Biomed Pap Med Fac Univ Palacky Olomouc Czech Repub. 2014;158(4):605-12.

18. Kumar P, Densor SE, Mancuso TJ. Clinical report: premedication for nonemergency endotracheal intubation. Pediatrics. 2010;125:608-15.

19. Ozawa Y, Ades A, Foglia EE, DeMeo S, Barry J, Sawyer T, et al. Premedication with neuromuscular blockade and sedation during neonatal intubation is associated with fewer adverse events. J Perinatol. 2019;39(6):848-56.

20. de Kort EHM, Andriessen P, Reiss IKH, van Dijk M, Simons SHP. Evaluation of an intubation readiness score to assess neonatal sedation before intubation. Neonatology. 2019;115:43-8.

21. Walter-Nicolet E, Courtois E, Milesi C, Ancel PY, Beuchee A, Tourneux P, et al. Premedication practices for delivery room intubations in premature infants in France: results from the EPIPAGE 2 cohort study. PLoS ONE. 2019;14 (4):e0215150.

22. Baleine J, Milesi C, Mesnage R, Novais ARB, Combes C, Durand S, et al. Intubation in the delivery room: experience with nasal midazolam. Early Hum Dev. 2014;90:39-43.

23. Milesi C, Baleine J, Mura T, Benito-Castro F, Ferragu F, Thiriez G, et al. Nasal midazolam vs ketamine for neonatal intubation in the delivery room: a randomized trial. Arch Dis Child Fetal Neonatal Ed. 2018;103(3):F221-6.

24. Hodgson KA, Owen LS, Kamlin COF, Roberts CT, Newman SE, Francis KL, et al. Nasal high-flow therapy during neonatal endotracheal intubation. N Engl J Med. 2022;386(17):1627-37.

25. Hatch LD, Grubb PH, Lea AS, Walsh WF, Markham MH, Maynord PO, et al. Interventions to improve patient safety during intubation in the neonatal intensive care unit. Pediatrics 2016;138 (4):e20160069.

26. Sauer CW, Kong JY, Baleine J, Milesi C, Mesnage R, Novais ARB, et al. Intubation in the delivery room: experience with nasal midazolam. Early Hum Dev. 2014;90(1):39-43.

27. Wallenstein MB, Birnie KL, Arain YH, Yang W, Yamada NK, Huffman LC, et al. Failed endotracheal intubation and adverse outcomes among extremely low birth weight infants. J Perinatol. 2016;36(2):112-5.

28. Johnston L, Sawyer T, Ades A, Moussa A, Zenge J, Jung P, et al. Impact of physician training level on neonatal tracheal intubation success rates and adverse events: a report from National Emergency Airway Registry for Neonates (NEAR4NEOS). Neonatology. 2021;118:434-42.

29. Sawyer T, Foglia E, Hatch LD, Moussa A, Ades A, Johnston L, et al. Improving neonatal intubation safety: a journey of a thousand miles. J Neonatal Perinatal Med. 2017;10(2):125-31.

30. Volz S, Stevens TP, Dadiz R. A randomized controlled trial: does coaching using video during direct laryngoscopy improve residents' success in neonatal intubations? J Perinatol. 2018;38(8):1074-80.

31. Johnston L, Sawyer T, Nishisaki A, Whitfill T, Ades A, French H, et al. Neonatal intubation competency assessment tool: development and validation. Acta Pediatr. 2019;19(2):157-64.

32. Abdel-Latif ME, Davis PG, Wheeler KI, De Paoli AG, Dargaville PA. Surfactant therapy via thin catheter in preterm infants with or at risk of respiratory distress syndrome. Cochrane Database Syst Rev. 2021;10;5(5):CD011672.

Self Assessment

1. Endotracheal intubation should be performed prior to chest compression. True/False

2. Premedications are essential prior to endotracheal intubation in the delivery room. True/False

3. What is the recommended size of the endotracheal tube for babies <28 weeks?

4. List two methods of determining the tip to lip distance prior to securing the tube.

5. List four indications for endotracheal intubation during resuscitation.

6. Which of the following is a correct statement:
   a. The tip of the stylet should protrude just beyond the tip of the ET.
   b. It improves the success of endotracheal intubation.
   c. It should snuggly fit into the ET.
   d. Use of stylet is optional.

7. Despite endotracheal intubation in a baby born through meconium-stained liquor, positive pressure ventilation does not achieve chest rise. All are potential next steps except:
   a. Suction the tube with a catheter inserted into the tube.
   b. Use a meconium aspirator and suction the tube.
   c. Confirm that the tube is positioned in the trachea.
   d. Initiate chest compression and give adrenaline through umbilical route.

8. Name the structure indicated in the figure:

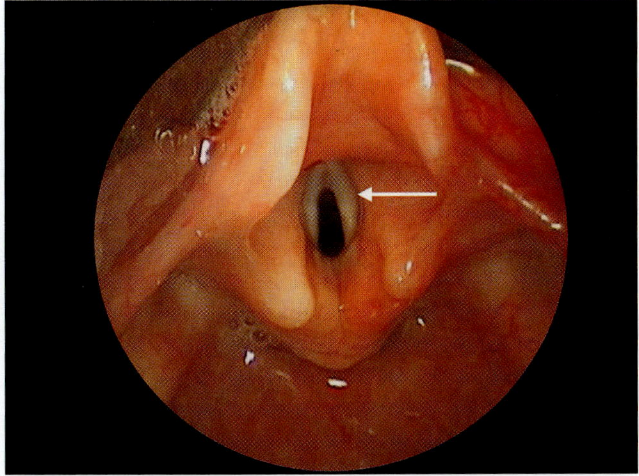

9. All are known complications of endotracheal intubation EXCEPT
   a. Hypoxia
   b. Trauma
   c. Shock
   d. Air leak

10. The assistant should limit the duration of intubation to
   _____________seconds.

Answers

For answers, go to the end of the Book, Page no. 321–322

Chest Compressions

Abiramalatha T

Lessons to Learn

- ○ *When to initiate chest compressions:* In this section, the reader will understand when to initiate chest compressions, and that one should never attempt to initiate chest compressions before achieving effective ventilation.

- ○ *Measures to be taken before initiating chest compressions:* This section will describe the important steps (and their rationale) that should be performed before initiating chest compressions.

- ○ *Technique of providing chest compression:* This section will describe the recommended technique to provide chest compressions and its basis.

- ○ *Coordinating chest compressions with positive pressure ventilation:* This section will describe the sequence used to provide coordinated chest compressions and ventilation.

- ○ *Stopping chest compressions:* This section will describe when to stop chest compressions and when to proceed to providing medication.

Most of the newborn infants who need assistance at birth respond to initial steps and positive pressure ventilation (PPV). The need for chest compressions is infrequent and is estimated to be around 1–2 per 1,000 live births in term neonates and around 5–6% in very preterm neonates.[1-3]

Neonates who do not respond to effective PPV are likely to have significant hypoxemia, acidemia, and severely impaired myocardial function. Enabling flow of oxygenated blood into the coronary arteries is essential to restore cardiac function in such neonates. This requires the steps in the neonatal resuscitation algorithm related to chest compressions and use of medications such as epinephrine (*Fig.* **7.1**). **Box 7.1** depicts an illustrative case of an asphyxiated newborn who needed chest compressions. You may follow it as you read through this chapter.

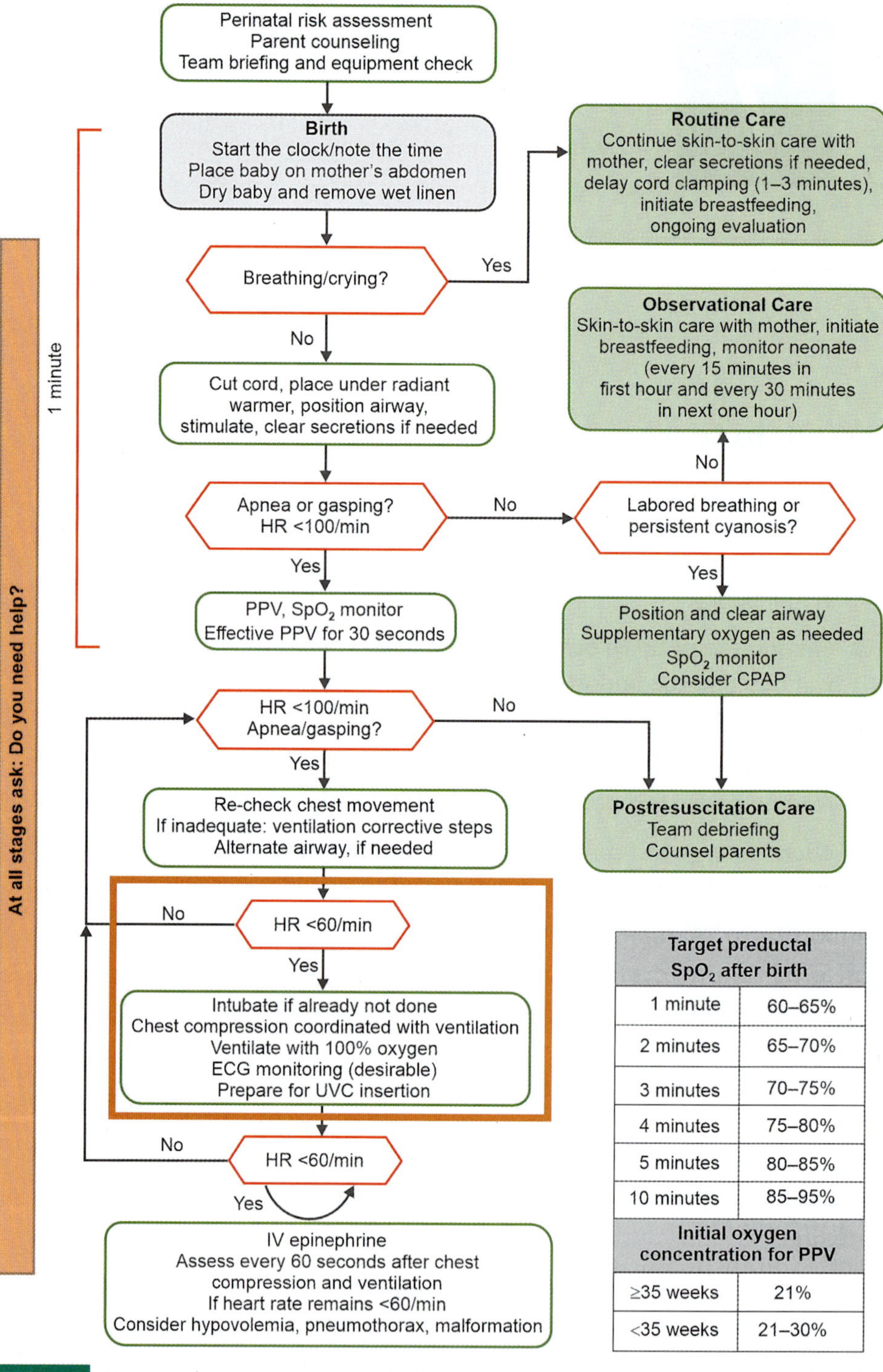

Target preductal SpO2 after birth	
1 minute	60–65%
2 minutes	65–70%
3 minutes	70–75%
4 minutes	75–80%
5 minutes	80–85%
10 minutes	85–95%
Initial oxygen concentration for PPV	
≥35 weeks	21%
<35 weeks	21–30%

FIG. 7.1 Neonatal resuscitation algorithm *(boxed area indicates the steps related to providing chest compression).*

PHYSIOLOGY OF CHEST COMPRESSIONS

Chest compressions are rhythmic compressions delivered on the chest wall with the aim of manually generating a cardiac output. The two theories postulated regarding the mechanism of blood flow during chest compressions are "cardiac compression" theory and "thoracic

BOX 7.1: ILLUSTRATIVE CASE

A 30-year third gravida who has gestational diabetes and is on insulin therapy, is admitted at 36 weeks' gestation with history of reduced fetal movements for 12 hours. Nonstress test was nonreactive. Hence, the obstetric team decides to deliver her by emergency cesarean section. The neonatal team is informed. The team has a briefing session, and they then carry out a check of equipment and supplies.

A baby girl is delivered who is not breathing and is limp. The umbilical cord is clamped immediately, and baby is shifted to a prewarmed radiant warmer. The baby is positioned in sniffing position with a shoulder roll, dried, tactile stimulation is provided by gently rubbing the back and the airway is cleared by suctioning the mouth and then the nose. As the baby is not breathing and heart rate is 50 beats per minute (bpm) after initial steps, the team decides to initiate positive pressure ventilation.

Positive pressure ventilation (PPV) is initiated with room air at the rate of 40 bpm. Another team member applies the pulse-oximeter sensor on the right hand of the baby and connects it to a pulse oximeter. Another team member announces that "there is chest rise". After 30 sec of effective PPV, the heart rate is counted for 6 sec by auscultation over the precordium. The heart rate is reported as 50 bpm, the pulse oximeter has no reliable signal and the baby is still not breathing. The team decides to initiate chest compressions.

Before initiating chest compressions, the team decides to intubate the baby. After intubation, PPV is continued with ventilation through the endotracheal tube, the FiO_2 is increased to 100%, coordinated chest compression and ventilation is initiated and a call is made for additional help. After 60 sec of coordinated chest compressions and PPV, baby's heart rate improves to 80 bpm. Chest compressions are discontinued and PPV alone is continued. After another 30 sec of PPV, heart rate rises to 110 bpm and baby is noted to have intermittent breathing efforts. Pulse oximeter signal is reliable and baby's oxygen saturation was improving. FiO_2 is gradually reduced titrating with the target saturations. The baby's heart rate rises to 150 bpm, the respiratory efforts and tone improve. The parents are counseled, and the baby is shifted to NICU for post-resuscitation care. Thereafter the team members have a de-briefing session to review their management of the baby.

pump" theory.[4,5] According to "cardiac compression" theory, the heart is directly squeezed between the sternum and spine during chest compression and this pushes blood from the heart into the aorta and blood vessels. When pressure on the sternum is released, oxygenated blood from the lungs refills the cardiac chambers. According to "thoracic pump" theory, pressing the sternum downward increases the intrathoracic pressure. The increase in intrathoracic pressure pushes blood from the heart and intrathoracic blood vessels into peripheral vessels generating a forward blood flow.

The major mechanism by which chest compressions help is by improving blood flow to the myocardium. During coordinated PPV and chest compressions, PPV helps to oxygenate the blood in the lungs, and chest compressions help in the flow of oxygenated blood into coronary arteries. This improves oxygen delivery to the myocardium, to make the heart pump effectively.

Unlike older children and adults, providing chest compressions without PPV is futile in neonates. There are two major reasons for this: (1) Perinatal asphyxia is almost always due to respiratory failure causing impaired gas exchange, unlike the cardiac etiology (typically ventricular fibrillation) for cardiorespiratory collapse in older children and adults; and (2) In children and adults, immediately after cardiac arrest, the aortic blood has normal pH and oxygen concentration close to the pre-arrest state; the major problem is the lack of flow rather than the oxygen content of blood. Hence, when chest compressions are initiated, blood with adequate oxygen content flows into the coronary arteries. On the contrary, the neonate has hypoxemia, hypercarbia, and acidemia following perinatal asphyxia. Hence, PPV to reverse the hypoxemia and hypercarbia is critical in asphyxiated neonates.

■ WHEN TO INITIATE CHEST COMPRESSIONS?

In neonatal resuscitation, chest compressions are initiated *if the heart rate (HR) remains <60 beats per minute (bpm) after 30 seconds of effective PPV.* It is important to note that even if the first assessed HR (the HR checked after "initial steps") is <60 bpm, we must initiate PPV alone. Chest compressions are to be initiated only if the HR is persistently <60 bpm after effective PPV.

Effective PPV is one that produces a visible chest rise. If the chest is not moving with PPV, it means the lungs are not yet getting inflated. We should focus on steps to achieve effective ventilation and carry out ventilation corrective steps, rather than initiating chest compressions. For all practical purposes, it is prudent to provide 30 seconds of *PPV via a properly placed endotracheal tube* before considering chest compressions.

Important Steps that Should Accompany Chest Compressions

The following measures should be addressed as we prepare for/initiate chest compressions.

- *Intubate the baby if not done earlier:* It will ensure a secure airway for ventilation during chest compressions. It will also facilitate insertion of umbilical venous catheter during chest compressions.

- *The FiO₂ should be increased to 100%:* The reasons for this are many. Hypoxemia reduces oxygen delivery to the myocardium, which in turn worsens myocardial function. Hence, it is essential to provide adequate FiO_2 to ensure that the blood flowing to the coronaries is adequately oxygenated. Also, pulse oximeter readings are unreliable when HR is <60 bpm and hence one may not be able to titrate FiO_2 to achieve the target oxygen saturations.

- *Position of resuscitation team members:* Neonates who require chest compressions have a high probability of requiring epinephrine administration as well. To facilitate insertion of umbilical venous catheter, the resuscitation team members may have to switch positions. The person providing PPV (with a secure endotracheal tube) would need to move to the side of the baby and the person providing chest compressions would need to move to the head end of the neonate. This creates space for a third member of the team to be able to insert an umbilical venous catheter (*Fig.* **7.2**).

- *ECG leads to monitor HR:* It is currently recommended that in neonates requiring resuscitation, especially during chest compressions, ECG can be used to provide rapid and accurate estimation of heart rate. However, this recommendation is a weak one based on low certainty of evidence and largely on expert opinion.[6,7] One might consider using multiparameter monitors where the facility is available.

PROVIDING CHEST COMPRESSIONS

Box 7.2 summarizes the key aspects of providing chest compressions.

Site for compression: Anatomically, the left ventricle of the heart is placed behind the lower one-third of sternum. Hence, chest compressions are provided in the midline at the lower third of the sternum below the nipple line and above the xiphoid process (*Fig.* **7.3**). Nipple line is an imaginary line joining the two nipples. The correct position should be identified by running a finger along the lower margin of the rib cage to locate the xiphoid, then placing the thumbs above the xiphoid process.

Technique of chest compression: Two-thumb technique with hands and fingers encircling the chest is the recommended method to provide chest compressions (weak recommendation with low certainty of evidence)[6] (*Fig.* **7.3**). The thumbs are placed on the lower third of sternum with slight flexion at the distal interphalangeal joints. The thumbs should either meet in midline or be placed one over the other. The hands and the remaining four fingers should encircle the chest and reach the back to provide a firm support to deliver effective chest compressions.

Two-finger technique is using the tips of index and middle fingers or middle and ring fingers to provide compressions while the other hand is placed behind the baby's back to provide a firm support. This technique is not recommended, since the two-thumb technique has the following advantages: (1) it generates greater blood pressure and coronary perfusion pressure, (2) there is less variability of the compression depth, (3) it enables consistent correct position on the chest, and (4) there is less fatigue to the provider.[8]

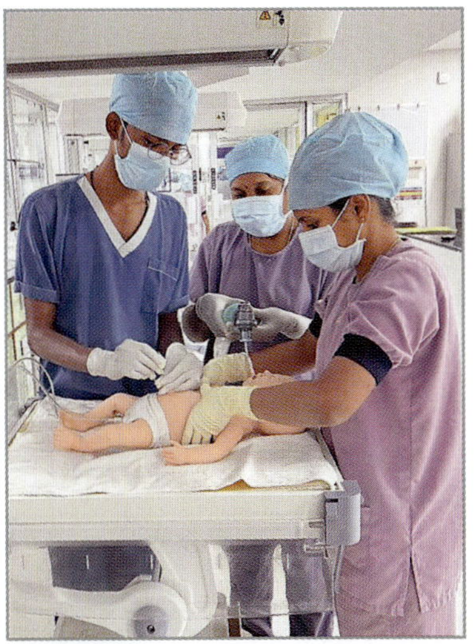

FIG. 7.2 Positions of the team members performing PPV (via endotracheal tube), chest compressions, and umbilical venous access.

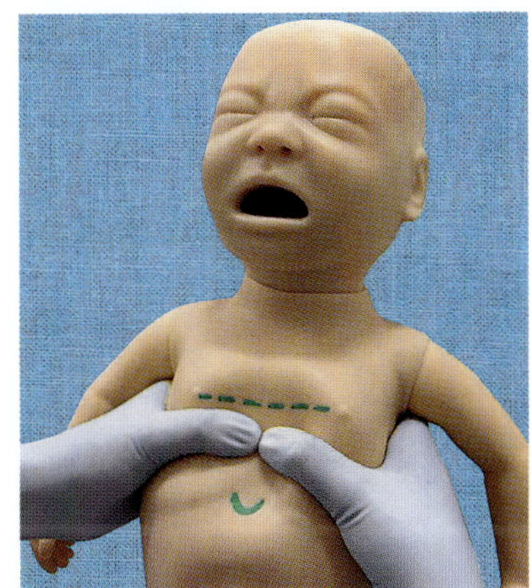

FIG. 7.3 Figure depicting the landmarks for chest compressions (below the nipple line and above the xiphisternum) and the two-thumb technique with hands and fingers encircling the chest.

BOX 7.2: HOW TO PROVIDE CHEST COMPRESSIONS?

Technique: 2-thumb with hands and fingers encircling the chest.
Site: Lower one-third of sternum below the nipple line and above the xiphoid process.
Depth: One-third of the anteroposterior diameter of the chest.
Sequence: "One-and-two-and-three-and-breathe-and".
Rate: 120 events per minute (90 chest compressions and 30 breaths).
Duration of each cycle: 60 s.

However, the two-finger technique may be used in exceptional circumstances such as (1) single resuscitator, where only one person is available to provide both PPV and chest compressions, and (2) where there is space constraint, for a short duration when the umbilical catheter is being inserted.

Many other techniques such as pinched finger technique using thumb, middle, and index/ring finger, flexed two fingers technique and a new two-thumb technique are being evaluated.[9-11] None of these have been confirmed to being superior to the currently recommended two-thumb technique.

Depth of compression: The sternum should be depressed up to one-third of the anteroposterior diameter of the chest. The actual depth varies with the size of the baby. Pressing to the correct depth is critical, as more superficial compressions will not generate adequate stroke volume and deeper compressions may cause complications such as cardiac contusion or rib fracture.

It is imperative to release the pressure completely after each compression and allow the chest wall to recoil back to its position. This is to ensure venous return and refilling of cardiac chambers. More importantly, blood flow into the coronary arteries occurs exclusively in diastole during chest compressions. Hence, adequate release after compression is critical.

The thumbs should remain in contact with the chest during both the compression and release. The reasons being placing the thumbs back in the correct position for each compression will result in wastage of time, and the thumbs may be placed back in improper position resulting in ineffective chest compressions and other complications.

Sequence of chest compressions and PPV: Coordinated chest compressions and PPV should be provided in 3:1 ratio. The sequence is *"one-and-two-and-three-and-breathe-and.........".* The "one", "two", and "three" indicate the timing of compressions and the "and" in between indicate the timing of release of the compressions. The "breathe-and" is the timing for inhalation, while exhalation happens during the next compression.

Each sequence should be completed in 2 seconds. There should be a total of 120 events in 1 minute (90 chest compressions and 30 PPV). The compressor should say the rhythm loudly, so that the person ventilating can perform PPV coordinating with chest compressions. It is essential to ensure coordination and avoid delivering both chest compressions and PPV simultaneously.

When compared to the greater chest compressions to PPV ratio in older children (15:2) and adults (30:2), we aim to provide more

PPV in neonates, as PPV is more important in neonates than chest compressions, for reasons discussed above. Other chest compressions to ventilation ratios such as 15:2, 9:3, 2:1, 4:1, etc., that are being evaluated in animal studies showed no advantage over 3:1 ratio for outcomes such as time to return of spontaneous circulation (ROSC) and mortality.[12]

Cycle: Each cycle of coordinated chest compressions and PPV should be provided for 60 seconds. One of the critical components of high-quality cardiopulmonary resuscitation (CPR) is to minimize interruptions.[13] Interruption of chest compressions to assess HR decreases coronary perfusion pressure, which takes time to improve again when chest compressions are resumed. Thus, frequent or prolonged interruption of chest compressions impairs coronary blood flow and should be avoided. In circumstances where ECG is unavailable and pulse oximeter is not picking a reliable signal, brief pauses for 6 seconds to assess HR (HR counted for 6 seconds multiplied by 10 gives the HR in beats per minute) is recommended.

Ergonomics

Surface: A hard surface with an elevated platform such as a radiant warmer or a resuscitation table [with other source(s) of heat] is the most suitable to provide chest compressions to neonates.

Compressor position: The depth and quality of chest compressions delivered from the head end are as good as those from the side of the neonate. The head end position has the added advantage of less compressor fatigue. Further, it creates space for umbilical venous access as discussed above. It is also suitable for single rescuer managing both the airway and chest compressions.

Switch roles if required: If the compressor becomes tired, the team members should switch roles and another member of the team should take over chest compressions.

Potential Complications

Direct pressure on the xiphoid process during chest compressions should be avoided as it may cause fracture of xiphoid resulting in hepatic laceration or laceration of the heart and cardiac tamponade. Positioning the thumbs centrally over the sternum is also critical to reduce the risk of rib fracture, which in turn may cause flail chest or pneumothorax, both of which will impair ventilation of the lungs.

Monitoring HR during Chest Compressions

Monitoring HR during chest compressions may be performed by auscultation of precordium, pulse oximetry, or ECG **(Box 7.3)**.

BOX 7.3: MONITORING HEART RATE DURING CHEST COMPRESSIONS

- HR monitoring during chest compressions is routinely performed by auscultation of precordium (HR counted for 6 seconds and multiplied by 10)
- In centers where multipara monitors are available, one might use ECG leads to monitor HR.
- Pulse oximeter may not give a reliable signal when HR is <60 bpm
- *Palpation of umbilical pulse is prone to errors and is no longer recommended as a method to assess HR during neonatal resuscitation.*

Available limited evidence suggests that ECG may be faster and more reliable than pulse oximetry for the determination of HR when there is bradycardia and poor perfusion.[14] Auscultation of precordium may be less reliable than ECG.[15] Further, it requires interruption of chest compressions and/or PPV, which would compromise the efficiency of resuscitation.

The major barrier for ECG use in neonatal resuscitation is that it is not available in the delivery room in many health facilities. The other disadvantage of using ECG for HR assessment is that pulseless electrical activity (PEA) may be mistaken as normal HR and chest compressions may be stopped.[16,17] PEA is diagnosed when the ECG displays electrical rhythm while the heart is in asystole. PEA should be treated as asystole and cardiac compressions and other resuscitation measures should be continued.

NONIMPROVING HEART RATE WITH CHEST COMPRESSIONS AND PPV

If HR is not improving despite 60 seconds of chest compressions and PPV, it is prudent to recheck the quality of various steps of resuscitation while the venous access is being established. The checklist is provided in **Box 7.4**.[18]

If HR remains persistently <60 bpm despite adequate chest compressions and PPV for 60 seconds, it is an indication that one needs to secure umbilical venous access and administer epinephrine.

BOX 7.4: REVIEW CHECKLIST IF HR IS NOT IMPROVING WITH CHEST COMPRESSIONS AND PPV

1. Chest movement. Is the chest moving with PPV?
2. Airway. Is the airway secured with a properly placed endotracheal tube?
3. Rate. Is the CPR provided at the correct rate of three chest compressions and one PPV every 2 s?
4. Depth. Is the depth of chest compressions adequate?
5. Inspired oxygen. Is the FiO_2 100%?

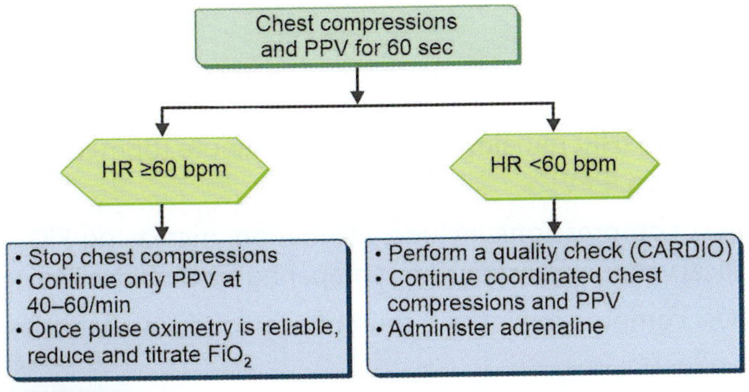

FIG. 7.4 Next steps after chest compressions and PPV.

DISCONTINUATION OF CHEST COMPRESSIONS

If HR improves to >60 bpm, chest compressions are stopped and PPV alone is continued at the rate of 40–60 breaths/minute (*Fig.* **7.4**). As soon as the pulse oximeter signals become reliable, one should reduce and titrate the FiO_2 to maintain oxygen saturations within the target range. This is critical to avoid oxidative stress and its harmful effects on various organ systems.

COORDINATION AND TEAMWORK

Chest compressions is a situation that requires multiple team members to work seamlessly to ensure all steps and procedures of resuscitation are carried out in the correct sequence along with timely support from all team members. The team needs to have a team leader who can delegate responsibilities to various team members based on their competence and skills. They need to anticipate and plan the next steps, be familiar with the environment where they are performing resuscitation and be able to effectively communicate with one another during the entire procedure of resuscitation.

FUTURE RESEARCH

Clinical research studies on chest compressions in neonates are a challenge, as it is a rare event. Most of the data on chest compressions come from animal studies and mathematical modelling. The following are some of the aspects of chest compressions that need further research:

- The need of different management approaches for asystole versus bradycardia.
- Efficacy of asynchronous chest compressions and ventilation to achieve a greater number of breaths per minute.
- The ideal FiO_2 that should be administered during chest compressions.
- Abrupt versus gradual weaning of FiO_2 once heart rate improves.

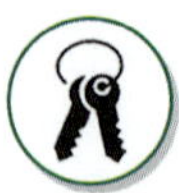

KEY POINTS

1. Chest compressions are indicated when heart rate (HR) remains <60 beats per minute (bpm) despite at least 30 seconds of effective positive pressure ventilation (PPV).

2. The steps to be taken before initiating chest compressions include, intubation, increasing FiO_2 to 100%, switching positions to create space for umbilical venous access and start preparing for umbilical venous access.

3. The recommended technique to provide chest compression is the 2-thumb technique with hands and fingers encircling the chest.

4. Chest compressions and PPV should be provided in ratio of 3:1 (90 chest compressions and 30 breaths in 1 minute).

5. Chest compressions can be discontinued once heart rate improves to ≥60 bpm, and PPV alone is continued.

6. If HR remains <60 bpm despite coordinated chest compressions and PPV for 60 seconds, one must establish a venous access to administer epinephrine.

■ REFERENCES

1. Wyckoff MH, Perlman JM, Laptook AR. Use of volume expansion during delivery room resuscitation in near-term and term infants. Pediatrics. 2005;115(4):950-5.

2. Soraisham AS, Lodha AK, Singhal N, Aziz K, Yang J, Lee SK, et al. Neonatal outcomes following extensive cardiopulmonary resuscitation in the delivery room for infants born at less than 33 weeks gestational age. Resuscitation. 2014;85(2):238-43.

3. Handley SC, Sun Y, Wyckoff MH, Lee HC. Outcomes of extremely preterm infants after delivery room cardiopulmonary resuscitation in a population-based cohort. J Perinatol. 2015;35(5):379-83.

4. Georgiou M, Papathanassoglou E, Xanthos T. Systematic review of the mechanisms driving effective blood flow during adult CPR. Resuscitation. 2014;85(11):1586-93.

5. Garcia-Hidalgo C, Schmölzer GM. Chest Compressions in the delivery room. Children (Basel). 2019;6(1):4.

6. Aziz K, Lee CHC, Escobedo MB, Hoover AV, Kamath-Rayne BD, Kapadia VS, et al. Part 5: Neonatal Resuscitation 2020 American Heart Association Guidelines for Cardiopulmonary Resuscitation and Emergency Cardiovascular Care. Pediatrics. 2021;147(Suppl 1):e2020038505E.

7. Wyckoff MH, Wyllie J, Aziz K, de Almeida MF, Fabres J, Fawke J, et al. Neonatal Life Support: 2020 International Consensus on Cardiopulmonary Resuscitation and Emergency Cardiovascular Care Science with Treatment Recommendations. Circulation. 2020

8. Douvanas A, Koulouglioti C, Kalafati M. A comparison between the two methods of chest compression in infant and neonatal resuscitation: a review according to 2010 CPR guidelines. J Matern Fetal Neonatal Med. 2018;31(6):805-16.

9. Yang D, Kim KH, Oh JH, Son S, Cho J, Seo KM. Development and evaluation of a new chest compression technique for cardiopulmonary resuscitation in infants. Pediatr Cardiol. 2019;40(6):1217-23.

10. Smereka J, Szarpak L, Smereka A, Leung S, Ruetzler K. Evaluation of new two-thumb chest compression technique for infant CPR performed by novice physicians: a randomized, crossover, Manikin trial. Am J Emerg Med. 2017;35(4):604-9.

11. Paek SH, Kim DK, Lee JH, Kwak YH. Comparison of standard and alternative methods for chest compressions in a single rescuer infant CPR: a prospective simulation study. PLoS One. 2019;14(12):e0226632.

12. Solevåg AL, Cheung PY, O'Reilly M, Schmölzer GM. A review of approaches to optimise chest compressions in the resuscitation of asphyxiated newborns. Arch Dis Child Fetal Neonatal Ed. 2016;101(3):F272-6.

13. Meaney PA, Bobrow BJ, Mancini ME, Christenson J, de Caen AR, Bhanji F, et al. Cardiopulmonary resuscitation quality: improving cardiac resuscitation outcomes both inside and outside the hospital—a consensus statement from the American Heart Association. Circulation. 2013;128(4):417-35.

14. Johnson PA, Cheung PY, Lee TF, O'Reilly M, Schmölzer GM. Novel technologies for heart rate assessment during neonatal resuscitation at birth: a systematic review. Resuscitation. 2019;143:196-207.

15. Voogdt KG, Morrison AC, Wood FE, van Elburg RM, Wyllie JP. A randomised, simulated study assessing auscultation of heart rate at birth. Resuscitation. 2010;81(8):1000-3.

16. Luong D, Cheung PY, Barrington KJ, Davis PG, Unrau J, Dakshinamurti S, et al. Cardiac arrest with pulseless electrical activity rhythm in newborn infants: a case series. Arch Dis Child Fetal Neonatal Ed. 2019;104(6):F572-4.

17. Patel S, Cheung PY, Solevåg AL, Barrington KJ, Kamlin COF, Davis PG, et al. Pulseless electrical activity: a misdiagnosed entity during asphyxia in newborn infants? Arch Dis Child Fetal Neonatal Ed. 2019;104(2):F215-7.

18. American Academy of Pediatrics, American Heart Association, Weiner GM, Zaichkin J (Eds). Textbook of Neonatal Resuscitation, 8th edition. Elk Grove Village, IL: American Academy of Pediatrics; 2022.

# Self Assessment

1. The indication to initiate chest compressions is when heart rate (HR) remains less than ____ beats per minute (bpm) despite effective positive-pressure ventilation (PPV).

2. If the first assessed HR (soon after the "initial steps") is <60 bpm, the next step is to:
   a. Initiate PPV alone
   b. Initiate chest compressions alone
   c. Perform coordinated chest compressions and PPV
   d. Continue "initial steps" for some more time

3. If HR is not improving and chest is not moving with PPV, the next step to be taken is:
   a. Take ventilation corrective steps
   b. Initiate chest compressions
   c. Continue PPV in the same way
   d. Initiate coordinated chest compressions and PPV

4. The recommended FiO_2 while administering chest compressions is _____.

5. The recommended technique to administer chest compressions is __________.

6. The ideal site to provide chest compressions is over the ____________.

7. Coordinated chest compressions and PPV are provided in ____ ratio for a duration of ___ seconds with a total of _____ events per minute.

8. Once the HR improves to >60 bpm.
   a. Coordinated chest compressions and PPV is continued.
   b. Chest compressions are stopped and only PPV is continued.

State TRUE or FALSE

9. In pulseless electrical activity, ECG may show a normal HR when the heart is in asystole.

10. As soon as the HR improves and pulse oximeter picks up a reliable signal, the FiO_2 must be reduced and titrated to achieve oxygen saturations within the target range.

Answers

For answers, go to the end of the Book, Page no. 322

Medications During Neonatal Resuscitation

Satvik C Bansal

Lessons to Learn

- Indications for use of medications during neonatal resuscitation
- Medications that are used during neonatal resuscitation
- Dose, route, and administration of medications
- Major knowledge gaps regarding use of medications
- Securing access for administering drugs

Majority of asphyxiated neonates would respond to positive pressure ventilation. Very few would require chest compression and use of medication such as epinephrine in the delivery room. It is estimated that <1 in 1,000 newborn would require epinephrine in the delivery room.[1] However in some facilities, the use of epinephrine may be higher when it is associated with ineffective ventilation of asphyxiated neonates.[2] The limited data that are available suggest that neonates requiring intensive resuscitation including use of multiple epinephrine doses have a higher risk of death and poor neurodevelopment outcome.[3,4]

The current evidence for use of epinephrine for neonatal resuscitation is largely based on animal models and limited human data.[5] This chapter reviews the available literature and summarizes the current recommendations. **Box 8.1** has an illustrative case of a neonate needing medication during resuscitation in the delivery room. You can follow it as you read through this chapter. *Figure* **8.1** highlights the section of the resuscitation algorithm when medication use has to be considered.

EPINEPHRINE (ADRENALINE)

Epinephrine is the only vasopressor drug currently recommended for use in neonatal resuscitation.[6] It is an endogenously produced catecholamine that stimulates all adrenergic receptors.

Mechanism of action in cardiopulmonary resuscitation (CPR): Epinephrine stimulates α_1, α_2, β_1, and β_2—adrenergic receptors.

BOX 8.1: ILLUSTRATIVE CASE

A 28-year second gravida is admitted at 38 weeks' gestation with seizures and high blood pressure. The woman is diagnosed to have eclampsia and the obstetric team records fetal bradycardia and decides to deliver her by emergency cesarean section. The neonatal team is informed. The team has a briefing session, and it (team) carries out a check of equipment and supplies.

The neonate at delivery is limp. The umbilical cord is clamped immediately, and the baby is shifted to a radiant warmer. The heart rate is noted to be 30 bpm. Initial steps of resuscitation are carried out by the neonatal team. The baby is still limp and has a heart rate of 30 bpm. Positive pressure ventilation (PPV) is initiated with room air. Pulse-oximeter sensor is applied on the right hand of baby and connected to a pulse oximeter. Even after 30 seconds of PPV with adequate chest rise, the baby has no breathing and heart rate is still at 30 bpm and pulse oximeter shows no reliable signal. The baby is intubated and coordinated chest compression and ventilation with 100% oxygen is carried out for 60 seconds.

After 60 seconds of coordinated chest compressions and PPV, baby's heart rate is noted to be 20 bpm. Another team member quickly inserts an umbilical venous catheter and injects epinephrine followed by a saline flush. ECG electrodes are placed on the baby. After 60 seconds of PPV and chest compression the heart rate is noted to be 50 bpm on the monitor. Chest compression and PPV is continued for another 1 minute. The heart rate is noted to be 80 bpm on the monitor. Chest compressions are discontinued and PPV alone is continued. After another 30 seconds of PPV, heart rate rises to 100 bpm and the oximeter has reliable signals. At 10 minutes, the baby is noted to have irregular breathing efforts and the heart rate is 130 bpm. FiO$_2$ is gradually reduced titrating with the target saturations. The family is counselled regarding the baby's status, and the baby is shifted to neonatal intensive care unit (NICU) for post-resuscitation care. Thereafter the team members have a debriefing session to review how they had planned and managed the baby.

The effects of alpha- and beta-receptors can be contrasting. The overall *in-vivo* effect of epinephrine is dependent upon factors such as density of different receptors on the target tissue and the binding affinity of these different receptors to epinephrine. **Table 8.1** summarizes the effects of epinephrine.

Initially, it was believed that effectiveness of epinephrine during resuscitation was primarily based on the myocardial stimulant effect of the drug through the β_1 adrenergic receptors. However, limited data from adult human and animal studies have now established that it is the coronary perfusion pressure (CPP) that determines the success of resuscitation.[7] CPP is the pressure gradient of blood flow (difference between diastolic aortic pressure and left ventricular diastolic pressure) to the coronary arteries during relaxation phase (diastole) of the cardiac cycle.

Inadequate blood flow and oxygen supply to the cardiac muscles results in energy depletion and decreased myocardial contractility and decreased pumping by the heart. In asphyxiated neonates who are acidotic, there is peripheral vasodilation, which leads to decreased peripheral vascular tone. During chest compression, blood preferentially flows to the low resistance peripheral circulation via the aorta rather than the high resistance coronary arteries. Use of epinephrine results in peripheral vasoconstriction; this results in increased aortic pressure and CPP which results in increased blood flow and oxygen supply to the myocardium. The re-establishment of

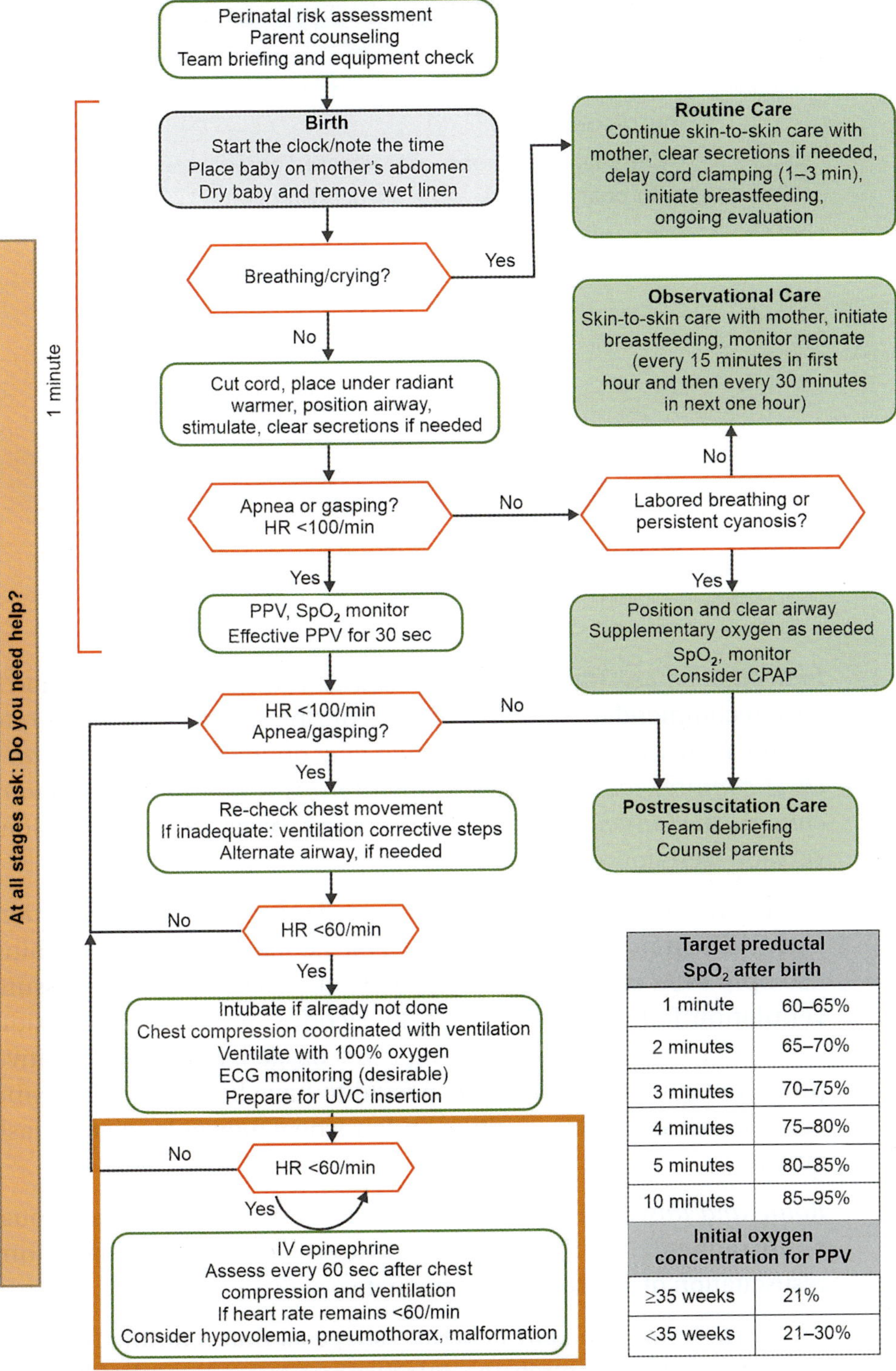

FIG. 8.1 Neonatal resuscitation algorithm *(boxed area indicates the steps related to providing medication).*

myocardial energy supply facilitates return of spontaneous circulation (ROSC). However, most of this information has come from studies on adult animal models or adult humans and not from asphyxiated neonatal models. The exact mechanism of epinephrine in asphyxiated newborn remains speculative.

TABLE 8.1: RECEPTORS OF EPINEPHRINE IN A NEWBORN

Receptor	Location	Action
alpha 1	Vascular smooth muscle cells	Vasoconstriction
alpha 2	• Presynaptic neurons • Coronary arteries	• Decreased norepinephrine release • Vasoconstriction
beta 1	Myocardium	• Chronotropy (increased heart rate) • Inotropy (increased contractility) • Dromotropy (increase conduction velocity) • Lusitropy (increased rate of myocardial relaxation)
beta 2	Vascular smooth muscle	Smooth muscle relaxation

Indication for use: International Liaison Committee on Resuscitation's 2020 recommendation for use of epinephrine states, "*If the heart rate has not increased to 60/min or greater after optimizing ventilation and chest compressions, we suggest the administration of intravascular epinephrine (adrenaline) (0.01–0.03 mg/kg)*" (weak recommendation, very low-certainty evidence).[8]

In terms of its use in practice in accordance with the resuscitation algorithm, epinephrine is indicated if the neonate's heart rate remains <60 bpm even after at least 30 seconds of effective positive pressure ventilation followed by another 60 seconds of chest compression coordinated with ventilation using 100% oxygen. Most often positive pressure ventilation (PPV) is expected to have been provided using either a well secured in-position endotracheal tube or laryngeal mask airway.

Route and dose: Epinephrine can be administered by intravenous, endotracheal, or intraosseous routes during delivery room resuscitation of an asphyxiated neonate.

   i. *Intravenous:* Current evidence suggests that administration of epinephrine through the intravenous route is probably more efficacious than the other routes. The recommended venous access for newborn at birth is the umbilical vein. This route would ensure that the medication reaches the central circulation rapidly.

   One must ***avoid*** attempting a peripheral venous access in states of circulatory collapse as the failure rates are likely to be high and it would delay administering medication in this life-threatening emergency condition.

Dose: The recommended intravenous dose is 0.02 mg/kg (equal to 0.2 mL/kg of prepared stock solution). The dose can vary from 0.01 to 0.03 mg/kg. The limited evidence shows no benefit of using higher doses, rather a greater incidence of adverse effects.

ii. *Endotracheal:* The current recommendations of the International Liaison Committee on Resuscitation (ILCOR) for use of endotracheal route for epinephrine states, *"If intravascular access is not yet available, we suggest administering endotracheal epinephrine (adrenaline) at a larger dose (0.05–0.1 mg/kg) than the dose used for IV administration"* (weak recommendation, very low certainty evidence).[8,9] It further goes on to state that the administration of endotracheal epinephrine should not delay attempts to establish vascular access (weak recommendation, very low-certainty evidence).[8] They have also recommended that if the *response to endotracheal epinephrine is inadequate, an intravascular dose be given as soon as vascular access is obtained, regardless of the interval after any initial endotracheal dose* (weak recommendation, very low-certainty evidence). The pharmacokinetic data available from animal studies coupled with the limited clinical improvement observed in a small number of newborn studies, conclude that there is a reduced bioavailability of the drug when given through endotracheal tube. The major limiting factors which could affect its bioavailability being: dilution of the drug itself by the fluid in the lungs, high pulmonary vascular resistance and thick epithelial lining of the respiratory tract, and pulmonary capillaries.

Dose: The suggested endotracheal dose is 0.1 mg/kg (equal to 1 mL/kg of prepared stock solution). The recommended dose range is from 0.05–0.1 mg/kg.

iii. *Intraosseous:* The primary vascular route recommended for drug and fluid administration during delivery room resuscitation of the newborn is by umbilical vein catheterization. However, if umbilical venous access is not feasible, intraosseous route could be considered as an alternative (weak recommendation, very low-certainty evidence).[8] The use of this route would depend on availability of equipment and expertise of the healthcare personnel.

Dose: The dose recommended is the same as for intravenous route, i.e., 0.02 mg/kg (equal to 0.2 mL/kg of prepared stock solution), with the dose varying from 0.01–0.03 mg/kg.

Available concentration and preparation: For neonatal resuscitation, the recommended concentration of epinephrine to be used is 1 mg/10 mL. However, in India, generally the available product has higher concentration of epinephrine, i.e., 1 mg/1 mL. It is desirable that two stock solutions of epinephrine are prepared prior to any resuscitation.

1. *For intravenous epinephrine:* It should be prepared in a 2-mL syringe. To prepare the stock solution for intravenous use, draw 0.2 mL of 1 mg/mL epinephrine solution into a 1 mL syringe and transfer into 2 mL syringe using a sterile connector or three-way connector/stopcock. Then draw normal saline to make up 2 mL of the diluted solution. It is important to remember to label the syringe indicating its concentration (0.1 mg/mL) and indicated use (intravenous).

2. *For endotracheal epinephrine:* It should be prepared in a 5-mL syringe. To prepare the stock solution for endotracheal use, draw 0.5 mL of 1 mg/mL epinephrine into a 1-mL syringe and transfer into a 5-mL syringe using a sterile connector or three-way connector/ stopcock. Then draw normal saline to make up 5 mL of the diluted solution. It is important to remember to label the syringe indicating its concentration (0.1 mg/mL) and indicated use (intratracheal).

Administration: The method of administering epinephrine through various routes is summarized here:

i. *Intravenous/intraosseous:* Epinephrine should be given rapidly. The dose should be followed by a quick flush of 3-mL normal saline to ensure that no part of the medication is left in the umbilical vein and reaches the heart quickly. **Box 8.2** summarizes the steps for securing an umbilical venous access (*Figs.* **8.2A to F**). **Box 8.3** summarizes the steps for inserting an intraosseous needle (*Fig.* **8.3**).

ii. *Endotracheal:* Epinephrine should be carefully administered directly into the tube. It is important to avoid leaving the drug in the tube connector. The drug dose should be followed by

---

BOX 8.2: STEPS FOR **U**MBILICAL **V**ENOUS **C**ATHETERIZATION (*Figs.* **8.2A to F**).

1. Follow appropriate aseptic precautions.
2. Use a 5- or 10-mL syringe. Fill it with normal saline. Attach a 3-way stopcock to this syringe. Now flush a 3.5 F or 5 F umbilical venous catheter with normal saline by connecting the catheter to the stopcock. Once the catheter is flushed, close the stopcock to the catheter to prevent fluid loss and air entry.
3. Next, clean the umbilical stump. A loose tie can be placed at the base of the stump above the skin margin. This tie can be tightened in case of bleeding.
4. Now the umbilical stump is cut using a scalpel. This is one of the most important steps which can ensure good visualization of umbilical vein and thereby quick catheterization. Remember to cut in a straight line around 1–2 cm above the skin margin.
5. Identify the umbilical vein on the cut section. It is a comparatively dilated, single, thin-walled structure usually located at 12 o'clock position.
6. The flushed catheter is inserted into the umbilical vein only up to 2–4 cm. Watch out for free back flow of blood in the catheter. At this point, the stop cock can be shifted to open and gentle aspiration of blood should be done. This confirms the position of catheter in the umbilical vein.
7. Administer the drug followed by saline flush. The catheter can be removed or temporarily secured to ensure availability of venous access till the baby is transported to the newborn care unit.

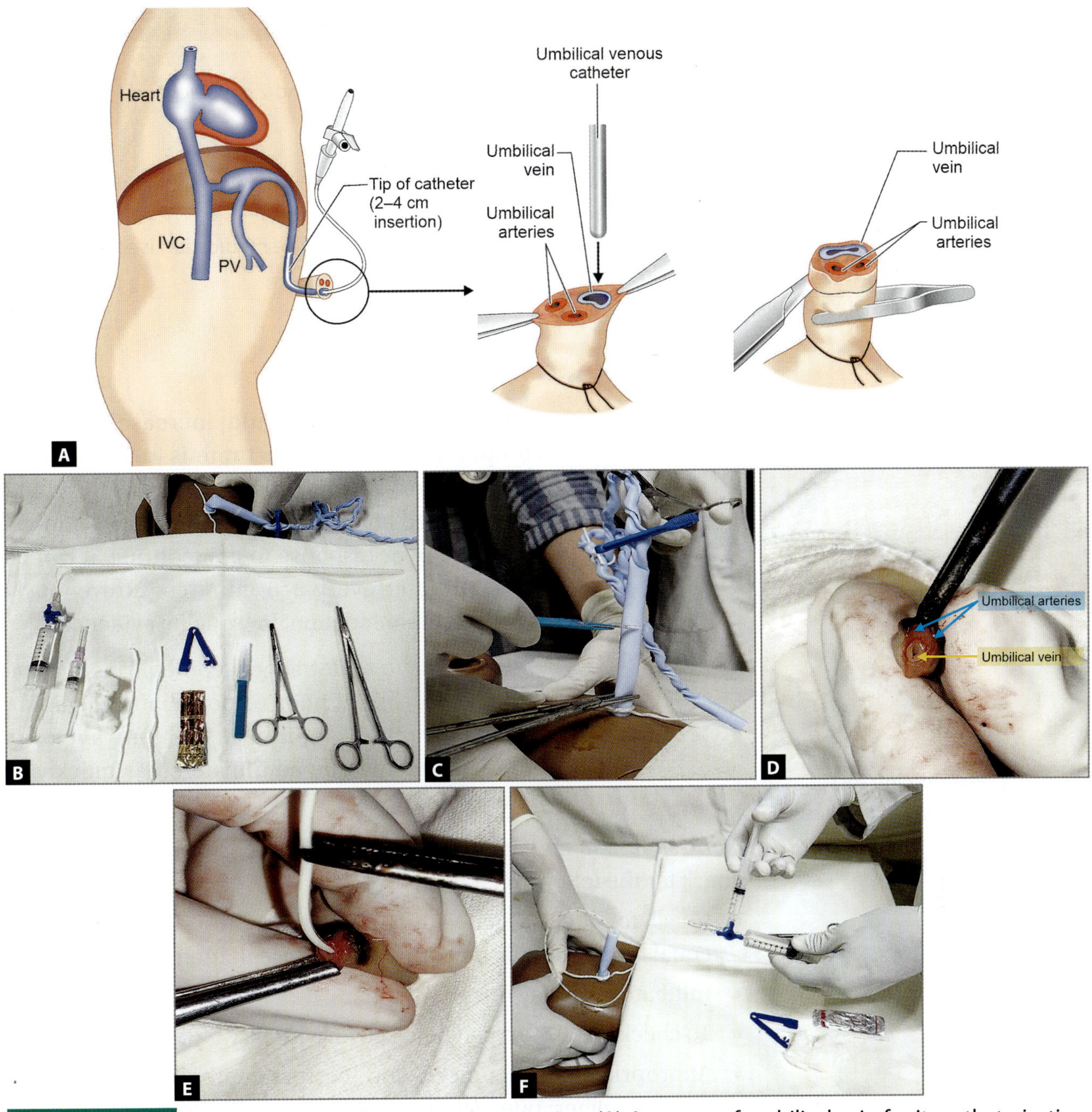

FIGS. 8.2A TO F Steps of umbilical venous catheterization. (A) Anatomy of umbilical vein for its catheterization; (B) Preparation of umbilical catheter for emergency cannulation; (C) Umbilical cord should be cut 1–2 cm above the skin margin; (D) The cut section of umbilical cord showing one umbilical vein (yellow arrow) and two umbilical arteries (blue arrow); (E) Insertion of saline-filled catheter inserted into the umbilical vein; (F) Catheter should be advanced until blood can be aspirated. Flush the catheter and administer the medication as indicated.

several positive-pressure breaths to ensure proper distribution. Administration of flush is not required.

Expected response to epinephrine: The baby should be assessed 1 minute after administering intravenous epinephrine while PPV with 100% oxygen and chest compression is continued. It is expected

> **BOX 8.3: STEPS FOR INSERTING INTRAOSSEOUS NEEDLE** (*Fig.* 8.3).
>
> 1. Follow appropriate aseptic precautions.
> 2. The site for the insertion of the intraosseous needle is the surface of the tibia lying 2 cm below and 1–2 cm medial to the tibial tuberosity.
> 3. Clean the insertion site.
> 4. The intraosseous needle is inserted perpendicular to the surface and advanced using twisting motion. As the needle enters the marrow space there is a sudden "give away" of resistance.
> 5. Infusion set along with a stopcock is then attached to the intraosseous needle. The medication is administered followed by a saline flush, as done during intravenous administration.
> 6. Monitor the site for any complications.

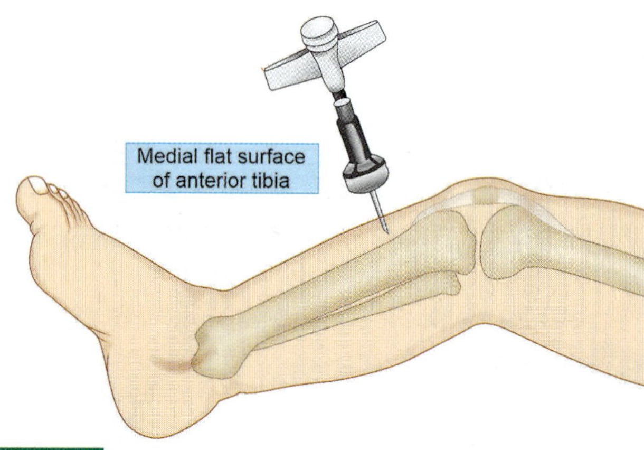

FIG. 8.3 Securing intraosseous access.

that the heart rate should increase to above 60 bpm. In case, the heart rate is <60 bpm, PPV with 100% oxygen and chest compression should be continued and reassessed after every 1 minute. In case of poor response to epinephrine, it can be repeated after every 3–5 minutes intravenously (weak recommendation, low quality evidence).[6]

Response to endotracheal epinephrine may be variable. In case of poor response after 1 minute of endotracheal epinephrine, intravenous epinephrine must be administered as quickly as possible.

Nonresponse to epinephrine should alert the healthcare providers to check for the following:

- Check for adequacy of ventilation (visible chest rise on PPV) and equal breath sounds on both sides on auscultation
- Intubate if already not done earlier
- To check if 100% oxygen being given with PPV
- Appropriate chest compression (correct depth—one-third of AP chest diameter; rate of 90/minute)
- To check for appropriate placement of umbilical venous catheter
- Also consider shock and/or pneumothorax

■ VOLUME REPLACEMENT

The need for volume replacement during neonatal resuscitation at birth is a rare event (reported as 0.04% of neonates in delivery room in a retrospective study).[10] The same study also reported that neonates who had received volume replacement in delivery room had lower blood pressure on arrival at the NICU; suggesting that factors other than hypovolemia are probably operative in neonatal shock at birth.

There is at present insufficient evidence for the routine use of volume expansion in neonates unresponsive to chest compression and epinephrine.

When to use volume replacement: Current recommendations state, *"It may be reasonable to administer a volume expander to newly born infants with suspected hypovolemia, based on history and physical examination, who remain bradycardic (heart rate <60/minute) despite ventilation, chest compressions, and epinephrine"* (weak recommendation, low quality evidence).[6]

Blood loss may occur due to antepartum hemorrhage, acute feto-maternal transfusion, fetal/neonatal trauma, and sudden umbilical cord rupture. The clinical features suggestive of shock in the baby include pallor, prolonged capillary filling time (CFT) and/or low volume pulses.

International guidelines have also suggested that a trial of volume replacement may be considered in neonates unresponsive to resuscitation even in the absence of history of blood loss as blood loss may be occult.[6,8,11] However, one must be cautious in use of volume replacement in the absence of blood loss, as volume load may be detrimental to an already depressed myocardium, especially in a preterm infant.

Type of fluid for volume replacement: There is insufficient evidence to recommend one type of fluid over another (blood, crystalloid, colloid). The current recommendation states, *"It may be reasonable to provide volume expansion with normal saline (0.9% sodium chloride) or blood at 10–20 mL/kg"* (weak recommendation, low quality evidence).[6]

The crystalloid solution recommended for use is normal saline (0.9% NaCl). However, one can also use Ringer's lactate. As it contains calcium it cannot be used through the same line through which blood is administered. In cases of blood loss or suspected fetal anemia, type O Rh-negative packed red cells can be used. Wherever possible the donor unit should be cross-matched to the mother (in cases of anemia diagnosed before birth). Otherwise, unmatched type O Rh-negative packed red blood cells can also be used for transfusion.

Dose: The initial dose of the volume expander should be 10 mL/kg which should be taken into a 20 mL or 50 mL syringe and infused through the umbilical venous catheter over 5–10 minutes. An additional dose of 10 mL/kg may be considered in case of large blood loss and if the neonate is not responsive to the initial dose. Volume bolus must be used with caution in preterm babies <32 weeks as large volume boluses have been associated with intraventricular and pulmonary hemorrhages.

■ SODIUM BICARBONATE

There is at present no substantive evidence for the use of sodium bicarbonate during neonatal resuscitation in the delivery room. ILCOR in its 2020 recommendations states, *"Sodium bicarbonate is discouraged during brief CPR but may be useful during prolonged arrests after adequate ventilation is established and there is no response to other therapies."*[8]

When to Stop Resuscitative Efforts

There is no definite single time point for discontinuation of resuscitative efforts in an asphyxiated newborn in the delivery room. Several factors would have to be considered prior to arriving at a decision to discontinue resuscitation efforts. These could include appropriateness of all steps as per the neonatal resuscitation algorithm, gestation of the baby, presence of major congenital anomalies, duration of asystole, facilities for post-resuscitation care and family's preferences.

The current recommendation states that *if there is no heart rate and all the steps of resuscitation have been performed, cessation of resuscitation efforts should be discussed with the team and the family.* A reasonable time frame for doing so would be around 20 minutes after birth (failure to establish spontaneous circulation by 10–20 minutes is associated with high risk of mortality and amongst survivors with high risk of significant neurodevelopment impairment).[6,8] However, the decision to continue or discontinue must be evaluated on a case-to-case basis and the family's decision.

■ KNOWLEDGE GAPS

- The current knowledge on use of medication is primarily extrapolated from small retrospective adult studies and clinical trials in animals. The major hurdles being—a very low incidence of use of medications during neonatal resuscitation and ethical concerns.

- Data about dose, route, timing, efficacy, and complications of drugs are majorly lacking especially in preterm neonates.

- The resuscitation guidelines for medications are not formulated based on gestational age, however drugs such as epinephrine are likely to have gestational age-dependent effects and pharmacokinetics.

- Alternative vasoconstrictor drugs with better safety profile that can be used during neonatal resuscitation.

- Pharmacokinetics and bioavailability of drugs administered through different routes.

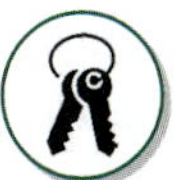 **KEY POINTS**

1. Epinephrine is indicated if the newborn's heart rate remains <60 bpm even after at least 30 seconds of effective positive pressure ventilation followed by another 60 seconds of chest compressions coordinated with ventilation using 100% oxygen.

2. Epinephrine should be used only after adequate ventilation is provided as evidenced by adequate chest rise.

3. The preferred route for administration of epinephrine is either intravenous or intraosseous.

4. Volume expansion should only be considered if the newborn is unresponsive to the steps of resuscitation and is in shock or has history of acute blood loss.

5. Cessation of resuscitative efforts should only be considered if there is documented absence of heartbeat after all resuscitative steps have been carried out appropriately for at least 20 minutes after discussing with the family.

■ REFERENCES

1. Kapadia VS, Wyckoff MH. Epinephrine use during newborn resuscitation. Front Pediatr. 2017;5:97. Erratum in: Front Pediatr. 2018;6:399.

2. Kapadia VS, Wyckoff MH. Drugs during delivery room resuscitation: what, when and why? Semin Fetal Neonatal Med. 2013;18(6):357-61.

3. Chawla S, Foglia EE, Kapadia V, Wyckoff MH. Perinatal management: what has been learned through the network? Semin Perinatol. 2016;40(6):391-7.

4. Foglia EE, Langeveld R, Heimall L, Deveney A, Ades A, Jensen EA, et al. Incidence, characteristics, and survival following cardiopulmonary resuscitation in the quaternary neonatal intensive care unit. Resuscitation. 2017;110:32-6.

5. Vali P, Sankaran D, Rawat M, Berkelhamer S, Lakshminrusimha S. Epinephrine in Neonatal Resuscitation. Children (Basel). 2019;6(4):51.

6. Aziz K, Lee CHC, Escobedo MB, Hoover AV, Kamath-Rayne BD, Kapadia VS, et al. Part 5: Neonatal Resuscitation 2020 American Heart Association Guidelines for Cardiopulmonary Resuscitation and Emergency Cardiovascular Care. Pediatrics. 2021;147(Suppl 1):e2020038505E.

7. Wyckoff MH. Neonatal cardiopulmonary resuscitation: critical hemodynamics. Neoreviews. 2010;11(3):e123-9.

8. Wyckoff MH, Wyllie J, Aziz K, de Almeida MF, Fabres JW, Fawke J, et al. Neonatal Life Support 2020 International Consensus on Cardiopulmonary Resuscitation and Emergency Cardiovascular Care Science with Treatment Recommendations. Resuscitation. 2020;156: A156-87.

9. Isayama T, Mildenhall L, Schmölzer GM, Kim HS, Rabi Y, Ziegler C, et al. The route, dose, and interval of epinephrine for neonatal resuscitation: a systematic review. Pediatrics. 2020;146(4):e20200586.

10. Wyckoff MH, Perlman JM, Laptook AR. Use of volume expansion during delivery room resuscitation in near-term and term infants. Pediatrics. 2005;115:950-55.

11. Madar J, Roehr CC, Ainsworth S, Ersdal H, Morley C, Rüdiger M, et al. European Resuscitation Council Guidelines 2021: Newborn Resuscitation and Support of Transition of Infants at Birth. Resuscitation. 2021;161:291-326.

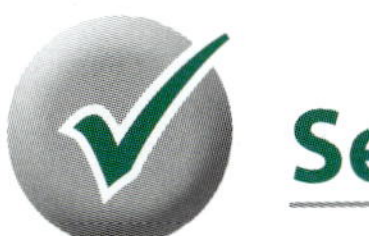 **Self Assessment**

1. The use of medications is recommended when heart rate remains <....... bpm despite effective ventilation with coordinated chest compressions.

2. The recommended dose of intravenous epinephrine (in mg/kg) administration during neonatal resuscitation is ....

3. The intravenous dose of epinephrine should be given rapidly followed by a bolus of ....mL of ....

4. The recommended dose of endotracheal epinephrine (in mg/kg) administration during neonatal resuscitation is ....

5. Volume expansion should be considered during neonatal resuscitation only if the following conditions are met [Choose correct option(s)]:
   a. Baby is in shock
   b. Heart rate <60 bpm
   c. Delivery by cesarean section
   d. Maternal antepartum hemorrhage
   e. All of the above

6. Volume expanders during neonatal resuscitation should be given over .... minutes.

7. Decision for discontinuation of resuscitation in a baby should be considered if there has been asystole for about ...... minutes.

Answers

For answers, go to the end of the Book, Page no. 322

SECTION

4

Special Scenarios in Resuscitation

Resuscitating the Preterm Baby

Reeta Bora

Lessons to Learn

- Reasons why a preterm neonate is at higher risk for needing resuscitation at birth
- The additional requirements that are needed for preterm care in the delivery room
- Measures to maintain temperature in preterm babies in the delivery room
- Managing umbilical cord in preterm babies at birth
- Considerations for use of oxygen during resuscitation
- Use of continuous positive airway pressure (CPAP) in preterm baby in delivery room
- Precautions to be taken to prevent brain injury to preterm babies

Preterm neonates (born before 37 completed weeks of gestation) are at higher risk of not effectively adapting to the transition at birth from fetal to neonatal state. Hence, they are more likely to require resuscitative assistance at birth as compared to babies born at term. They are also more likely to experience adverse events related to the resuscitation process. This chapter will deal with the additional efforts and resources needed to manage the preterm neonate at birth. **Box 9.1** provides an illustrative case of a preterm baby needing assistance for transition after birth. You could read it and relate it to the description provided in this chapter.

FACTORS PREDISPOSING PRETERM FOR RESUSCITATION NEED

There are several factors that make it difficult for the preterm neonates to establish effective ventilation after birth. These include a compliant rib cage with weak muscles of the chest wall, and immature lungs with decreased surfactant which makes it hard to expand the lungs both spontaneously and during positive pressure ventilation (PPV). The preterm infant is also susceptible to potential adverse outcomes

BOX 9.1: ILLUSTRATIVE CASE

A woman is admitted to the delivery room with rupture of membranes for 12 hours and a gestation of 30 weeks. The obstetric team assesses that the woman will progress to deliver and informs the neonatal team. The neonatal team asks for additional risk factors and then counsels the family of the possible outcomes for the baby. Other members of the team check the equipment and their functionality. They particularly check for the availability of a preterm face mask, laryngoscope blade size 0, plastic sheets, continuous positive airway pressure (CPAP) circuits, T-piece resuscitator, and they turn on the radiant warmer.

The baby is delivered vaginally. The obstetrician receives the baby in a warm linen, places the baby on the mother's abdomen, and notes that the baby is limp and not breathing. The baby is dried and wet linen is removed. The baby is provided gentle stimulation by rubbing the back. The baby is noted to have breathing efforts. The umbilical cord is cut after 1 minute of birth, and the baby is wrapped and handed over to the neonatal resuscitating team. The baby is placed under the radiant warmer. The linen in which the baby is wrapped is removed and the baby is wrapped in plastic sheets. The temperature sensor of the servo-controlled radiant warmer is placed on the baby's skin. Another team member places a pulse oximeter sensor on the baby's right hand. The baby is noted to have labored breathing (chest in-drawing), heart rate is 110 bpm and the oxygen saturation is below the target saturation. CPAP is initiated with 21% oxygen using a T-piece resuscitator and face mask. As the oxygen saturation remains below the target saturation, FiO_2 is gradually increased up to 0.35. The oxygen saturation starts to rise and remains in the target range. The baby is shifted to CPAP by nasal prongs and after about 20 minutes the oxygen requirements start to come down to FiO_2 of 0.25. The family is counseled about the baby's status and then the baby is shifted in a prewarmed incubator on nasal CPAP to the neonatal intensive care unit (NICU). The team thereafter holds a debriefing meeting to discuss the management of the preterm baby.

related to resuscitation procedures. These include risk of hypothermia due to excessive heat loss from the thin skin with small amounts of subcutaneous fat during the resuscitation process, risk of oxygen toxicity due to use of high oxygen concentrations, and increased risk of intraventricular hemorrhages due to capillary rupture on establishment of circulation after resuscitation. The lesser the gestational age, higher are the above referred to risks and adverse outcomes.

ADDITIONAL REQUIREMENTS FOR PRETERM RESUSCITATION

The following need to be taken care of while preparing for resuscitation in an anticipated preterm delivery.

- A servo-controlled radiant warmer
- Polythene bag/wrap (especially for babies <32 weeks)
- Preterm face mask
- Laryngoscope blades of size "0" and "00" of size
- Oxygen blender and pulse oximeter with appropriate size sensor
- A resuscitation device that provides both positive end-expiratory pressure (PEEP) and continuous positive airway pressure (CPAP) (such as a T-piece resuscitator)
- Surfactant in case a very preterm birth (<30 weeks) birth is anticipated

■ SPECIAL REQUIREMENTS

Thermal Control Measures

Low admission temperature to neonatal intensive care unit (NICU) has been shown to be a strong predictor of poor outcome.[1] Therefore, it is recommended that additional measures need to be undertaken to reduced thermal and metabolic stress and maintain the body temperature between 36.5 and 37.5°C. For preterm infants born ≤32 weeks additional interventions that are recommended for thermoregulation include *use of radiant warmers in the delivery, raising delivery room ambient temperature to 23–25°C, use of plastic wrappings without drying, warm blanket, thermal mattress* (weak recommendation, very low quality of evidence.[2]

The following measures should be undertaken prior to an anticipated birth of preterm baby:

- Preheat the radiant warmer
- Babies <32 weeks should be wrapped in plastic bags/wraps up to their neck without drying (*Fig.* **9.1**). The baby should be kept fully covered during resuscitation. If umbilical lines are to be inserted a small hole may be cut in the plastic sheet.
- Place the temperature sensor of the radiant warm on the baby to monitor the baby's temperature. Overheating is as much as a risk for adverse outcome as is hypothermia.

Umbilical Cord Management

For preterm neonates <34 weeks gestation, a recent meta-analyis by the International Liaison Committee on Resuscitation (ILCOR) which compared immediate cord clamping with a delay of at least 30 seconds concluded that delayed cord clamping may marginally improve survival, improved cardiovascular stability with decreased need for inotropic support, resulted in higher mean blood pressure in the first 12–24 hours, resulted in better hematological indices and the infants required fewer blood transfusions. There was no effect on severe intraventricular hemorrhage (IVH), necrotizing enterocolitis (NEC), or chronic lung disease.[3] Umbilical cord milking either on intact cord or cut cord has not been shown to have survival advantage in preterm newborn over early cord clamping or delayed cord clamping. Rather there is some evidence to suggest that intact cord milking increases the risk of severe IVH in very preterm neonates (<28 weeks).[4]

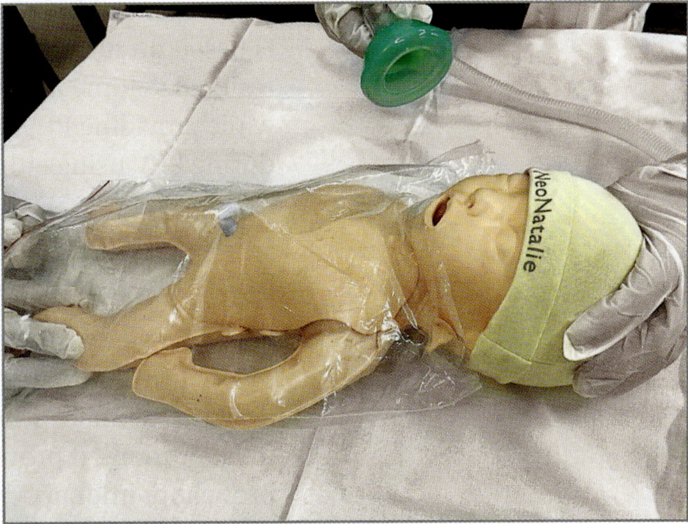

FIG. 9.1 Preterm baby wrapped in plastic wrap.
Courtesy: Dr Satvik C Bansal, Gwalior.

TABLE 9.1: TARGETED OXYGEN SATURATIONS	
	Target postductal SpO$_2$ after birth
1 minute	60–65%
2 minutes	65–70%
3 minutes	70–75%
4 minutes	75–80%
5 minutes	80–85%
10 minutes	85–95%

At present there is insufficient evidence to recommend delayed cord clamping in preterm infants needing resuscitation and cord milking is not recommended in preterm infants born at <28 weeks gestation.

Use of Oxygen during Resuscitation

For preterm neonates <35 weeks, resuscitation should be initiated with 21–30% oxygen. For newborn ≥35 weeks of gestation resuscitation should be commenced with 21% oxygen. A blender and a pulse oximeter in the labor room is a must. Additional oxygen supplementation should be based on minute specific preductal target oxygen saturation[5] **(Table 9.1)**.

▪ PROVIDING ASSISTED VENTILATION

Positive End-expiratory Pressure during Positive Pressure Ventilation

The current ILCOR recommendations suggest that PEEP be used for initial ventilation of preterm babies during resuscitation in the delivery room (weak recommendation, low quality evidence).[2] This is based on the observations that PEEP helps maintaining functional residual volume and hence would help inflating preterm lungs better while providing PPV. PEEP can be provided with a T-piece resuscitator during PPV using either a face mask or an endotracheal tube.

Continuous Positive Airway Pressure for a Spontaneously Breathing Preterm Baby

Several reviews have evaluated the use of CPAP in initial stabilization of preterm neonates in delivery room. These have shown that in preterm neonates who have labored breathing or persistent cyanosis in labor room, if provided with CPAP, have decreased rate of death or bronchopulmonary dysplasia (BPD) in contrast to those intubated.[6,7]

The current ILCOR recommendations state *"For spontaneously breathing preterm newborn infants with respiratory distress requiring respiratory support in the delivery room, we suggest initial use of CPAP rather than intubation and intermittent PPV"* (weak recommendation, moderate certainly of evidence).[2]

If a spontaneously breathing preterm baby with a heart rate of 100 bpm or more and has either difficult breathing or has an oxygen saturation below the target range, consider providing CPAP to the baby. CPAP can be provided initially using a T-piece resuscitator with face mask (*Fig. 9.2*). Provide a CPAP of at least 5 cmH$_2$O and titrate inspired oxygen concentration sufficient to keep the oxygen saturation in the target range **(Table 9.1)**. If the baby needs CPAP for a longer duration, it can be provided by nasal prongs.

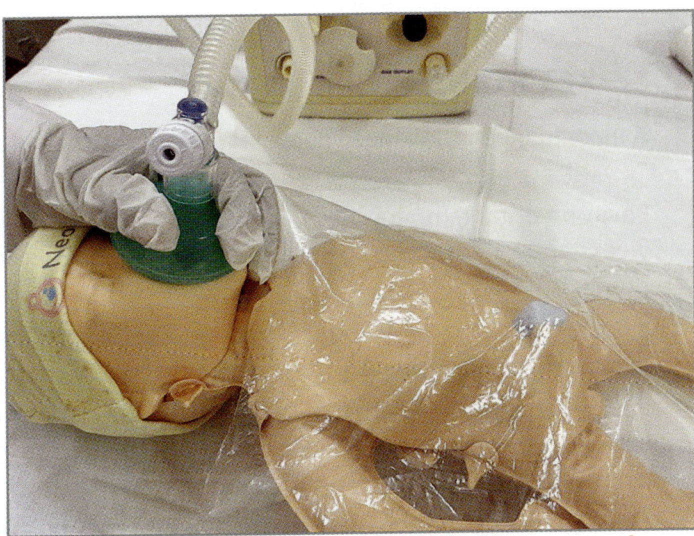

FIG. 9.2 Preterm baby being provided CPAP in delivery room with T-piece resuscitator and face mask. *Courtesy:* Dr Satvik C Bansal, Gwalior.

▉ PREVENTION OF BRAIN INJURY

As already mentioned, preterm neonates, especially those <32 weeks are at increased risk of neurologic injury consequent to the procedures we carry out during resuscitation. Some of the following precautions can help minimize this risk.

- The baby should be handled gently during resuscitation.

- One should avoid multiple painful stimuli such as repeated suction or repeated attempts to intubate the baby.

- One should avoid positioning the baby in head down position.

- During PPV the lowest pressure required for achieving a chest rise should be used.

- Avoid using excessive PEEP/CPAP.

- If supplemental oxygen is required, the lowest oxygen concentration required to maintain oxygen saturation in the target range should be used while monitoring with a pulse oximeter.

- If volume expansion is required for managing shock, rapid infusion of fluid should be avoided.

- After resuscitation the neonate should be monitored for his/her temperature, blood sugar (to prevent hypoglycemia), apnea associated with low heart rate and/or hypoxia, and perfusion. The infant should be provided appropriate fluid therapy to maintain fluid and electrolyte balance.

KEY POINTS

1. A team trained in advanced neonatal resuscitation should be available for all preterm deliveries.

2. To prevent thermal stress a servo-controlled warmer must be used to manage preterm babies at birth. Environmental temperatures in delivery room should be maintained between 23 and 25°C. In babies <32 weeks, the babies should be wrapped in plastic sheets without drying and placed under the radiant warmer during resuscitation.

3. If positive pressure ventilation (PPV) is required for preterm babies, it is recommended a T-piece with face mask and positive end-expiratory pressure (PEEP) is used.

4. Positive pressure ventilation should be initiated with 21% oxygen for newborn with gestational age ≥35 weeks and 21–30% oxygen for newborn with gestational age <35 weeks. Pulse oximetry should be used to titrate oxygen requirements.

5. Preterm babies with labored breathing and heart rate >100 bpm should be provided CPAP in the delivery room.

6. Precaution should be taken to prevent brain injury in newborns due to resuscitation procedures in the delivery room.

■ REFERENCES

1. Madar J, Roehr CC, Ainsworth S, Ersdal H, Morley C, Rüdiger M, et al. European Resuscitation Council Guidelines 2021: Newborn resuscitation and support of transition of infants at birth. Resuscitation. 2021;161:291-326.

2. Wyckoff MH, Wyllie J, Aziz K, de Almeida MF, Fabres JW, Fawke J, et al. Neonatal Life Support 2020 International Consensus on cardiopulmonary resuscitation and emergency cardiovascular care science with treatment recommendations. Resuscitation. 2020;156:A156-87.

3. Seidler T, Gyte GML, Rabe H, Díaz-Rossello JL, Duley L, Aziz K, et al. Umbilical cord management at preterm birth (<34 weeks): systematic review and meta-analysis. Pediatrics. 2021;147(3):e20200576.

4. Katheria A, Reister F, Essers J, Mendler M, Hummler H, Subramaniam A, et al. Association of umbilical cord milking vs delayed umbilical cord clamping with death or severe intraventricular hemorrhage among preterm infants. JAMA. 2019;322(19):1877-86.

5. Aziz K, Lee CHC, Escobedo MB, Hoover AV, Kamath-Rayne BD, Kapadia VS, et al. Part 5: Neonatal Resuscitation 2020 American Heart Association Guidelines for Cardiopulmonary Resuscitation and Emergency Cardiovascular Care. Pediatrics. 2021;147(Suppl 1):e2020038505E.

6. Subramaniam P, Ho JJ, Davis PG. Prophylactic nasal continuous positive airway pressure for preventing morbidity and mortality in very preterm infants. Cochrane Database Syst Rev. 2016;6:CD001243.

7. Schmolzer GM, Kumar M, Pichler G, Aziz K, O'Reilly M, Cheung PY. Non-invasive versus invasive respiratory support in preterm infants at birth: systematic review and meta-analysis. BMJ. 2013;347:f5980.

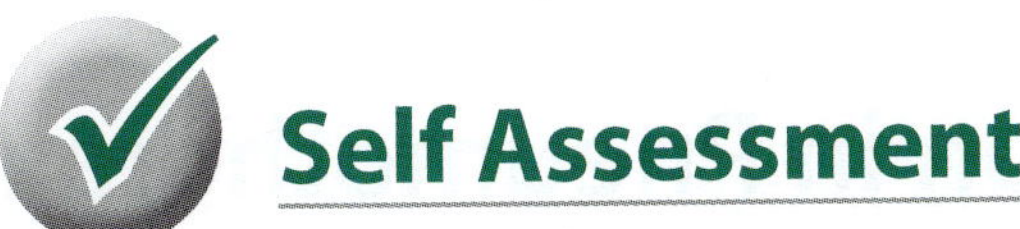

Self Assessment

Tick the Correct Statements (Multiple answers may be correct):

1. Which of the following factors make it difficult for the preterm newborn (born at <37 completed weeks of gestation age) to establish respiration at birth?
   a. Compliant rib cage with weak muscles of the chest wall
   b. Deficiency of surfactant
   c. Frequent hypothermia developed during resuscitation
   d. Associated meconium staining of liquor

2. Additional requirement during preterm resuscitation include:
   a. Polythene bag/wrap
   b. Preterm mask
   c. Laryngoscope blade 0 and 00 size
   d. T-piece resuscitator
   e. Oxygen blender
   f. None of the above

3. In preterm neonates at birth, cord clamping should be done:
   a. Immediately
   b. At 30 seconds to 1 minute
   c. Cord milking should be done rather than delayed cord clamping

4. Target saturation at 5 minutes after birth in preterm neonates is:
   a. 65%
   b. Same as for term neonates
   c. Should not be considered in case of preterm neonates

5. For preterm neonates less than 35 weeks, resuscitation should be started with:
   a. 21–30% oxygen
   b. 50% oxygen
   c. 100% oxygen

6. In a spontaneously breathing preterm neonate with a heart rate of ≥100/minute, if breathing is difficult or target saturation is not reached, provide:
   a. Free flow oxygen
   b. CPAP
   c. Bag and mask ventilation

Answers

For answers, go to the end of the Book, Page no. 322

Resuscitation in Pneumothorax and Pleural Effusion

VC Manoj

Lessons to Learn

- Causes of failure to establish ventilation after birth despite corrective measures of ventilation.
- Suspecting pneumothorax and pleural effusion.
- Confirm the presence of pneumothorax or pleural effusion.
- Managing pneumothorax or pleural effusion during neonatal resuscitation.

A newborn infant might fail to establish adequate ventilation despite all the corrective measures during positive pressure ventilation (PPV) (readjusting the face mask, repositioning, suction, opening the mouth, increasing ventilation pressure, and use of alternate airway) (*Fig.* **10.1**). This may be either due to a blocked airway or impaired lung function **(Table 10.1)**. One of the causes of impaired lung function may be the presence of air (pneumothorax) or fluid collection (pleural effusion) in the pleural cavity which is amenable to intervention in the delivery room. **Box 10.1** provides an illustrative case of a neonate with pneumothorax which you may follow as you read through this chapter.

▪ PNEUMOTHORAX

It is a condition where air escapes out of the ruptured alveoli into the pleural space (between the parietal and visceral pleura). Presence of air collection inside the pleural space if in large quantities, results in hypoxia, increased work of breathing and failure of improvement on PPV during resuscitation of infants. It may occur from 0.05 to 0.1% of all live births. Pneumothorax may occur spontaneously or on initiation of PPV. Other causes include respiratory distress syndrome, meconium aspiration syndrome, or malformations (e.g., pulmonary hypoplasia).[1]

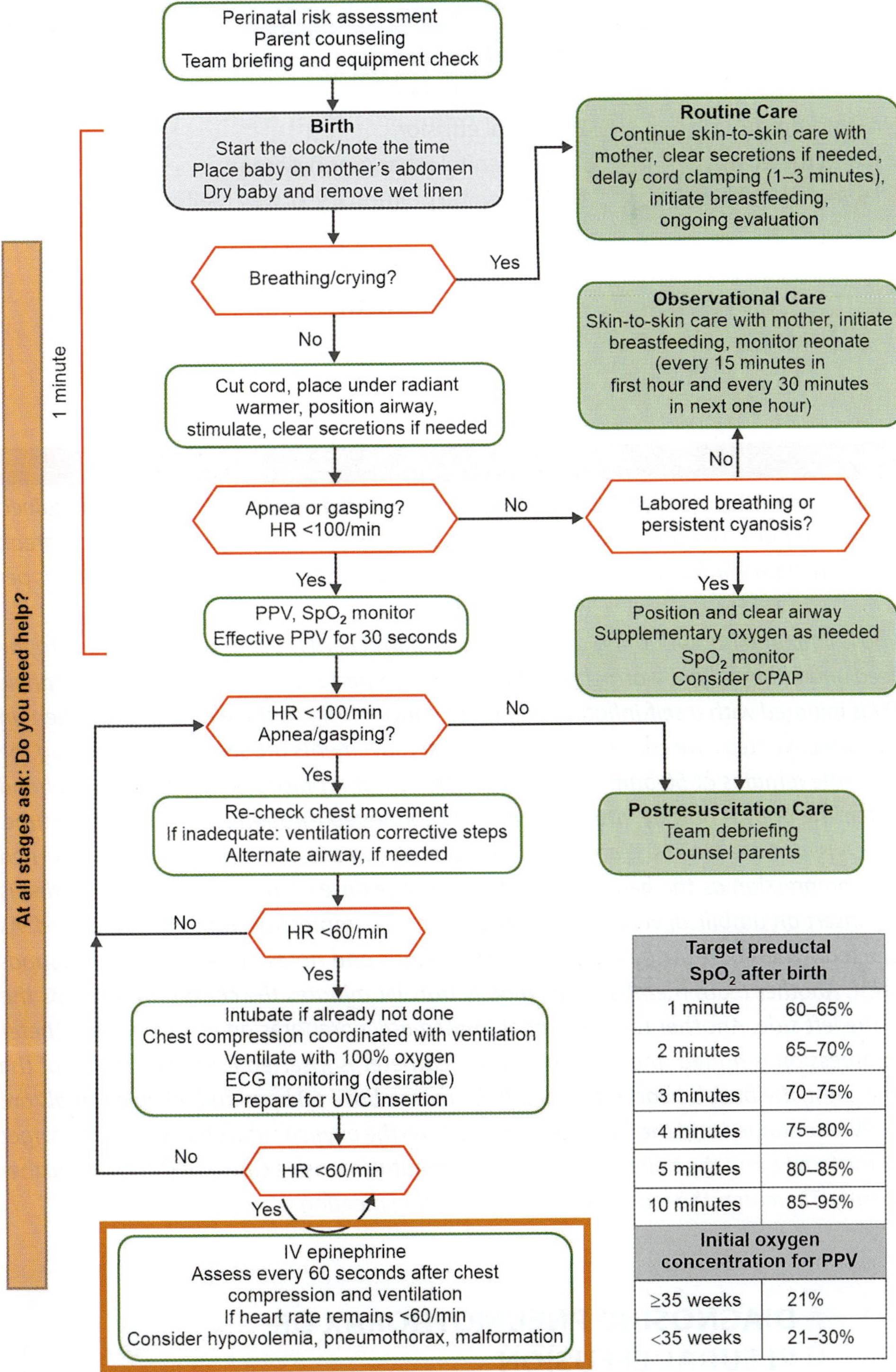

FIG. 10.1 Neonatal resuscitation algorithm *(boxed area indicates the steps related to pneumothorax).*

■ PLEURAL EFFUSION

The collection of fluid into the pleural space is termed as pleural effusion. It is rare in neonates and the most common causes at birth include hydrops fetalis and chylothorax.

TABLE 10.1: Causes of Failure to Establish Ventilation, after Ventilation Corrective Steps in Neonatal Resuscitation	
Blocked airway	**Impaired lung function**
1. Choanal atresia	1. Pneumothorax
2. Airway malformation (Robin syndrome)	2. Pleural effusion
3. Meconium or mucus obstructing the airway	3. Congenital lobar emphysema
4. Other rare conditions (e.g., laryngeal web)	4. Congenital pulmonary airway malformation
	5. Congenital diaphragmatic hernia
	6. Pulmonary hypoplasia
	7. Extreme prematurity
	8. Congenital pneumonia

BOX 10.1: Illustrative Case

A woman with 38 weeks pregnancy is admitted in labor. The membranes are ruptured and there is meconium-stained amniotic fluid, and the fetal heart is 90 bpm. The obstetric team decides to deliver the baby by emergency cesarean section and the neonatal resuscitation team is informed. The neonatal team checks the equipment and supplies as per the checklist.

A female baby is delivered who is limp and not breathing at birth. The umbilical cord is cut and baby handed to the neonatal team. The baby is placed under the radiant warmer and the initial steps performed. As the baby is still apneic with a heart rate of 60 bpm, PPV is initiated with a self-inflating bag using a face mask. As there is no improvement in the baby's condition, ventilatory corrective steps are carried out. Visible chest movements are seen after increasing the ventilation pressure, but the heart rate remains at 50 bpm. A pulse oximeter sensor is placed on the baby's right hand and connected to a pulse oximeter. The baby is quickly intubated and PPV continued through the endotracheal tube. As there is no improvement, the FiO_2 is increased to 100% and coordinated chest compression and ventilation is carried out. Even after 1 minute of chest compression as the heart rate is <60 bpm, one dose of intratracheal epinephrine is administered while preparing to insert an umbilical venous catheter and chest compression with PPV continued. As there is improvement, one of the team members auscultates for breath sounds and notes decreased breath sounds on the left side of the baby's chest. Another team member immediately transilluminates the chest and confirms the presence of pneumothorax on the left side. Another team member immediately prepares an intravenous catheter aspiration device. The chest compression is halted and the intravenous catheter is inserted into the left side of the chest. As air is aspirated from the chest, the baby's heart rate starts to increase above 60 bpm and reliable signals are detected on the pulse oximeter. PPV is continued and the FiO_2 is adjusted to keep the oxygen saturation within the target range. A team member counsels the family, and the baby is shifted to the neonatal intensive care unit (NICU) for further management including a chest X-ray. Thereafter the team conducts a debriefing meeting.

DIAGNOSING PNEUMOTHORAX OR PLEURAL EFFUSION

- Pneumothorax and pleural effusion should be suspected when despite adequate corrective measures for providing PPV, the neonate fails to improve, and a blocked airway is ruled out.
- Pleural effusion in the fetus may also have been diagnosed by an antenatal ultrasound.
- Decreased/absent breath sounds on the side of pneumothorax or pleural effusion should raise the suspicion.

However, one must also consider other causes of decreased breath sounds despite effective ventilation techniques—malpositioned endotracheal tube (insertion into right main bronchus can result in decreased breath sounds on the left side), congenital diaphragmatic hernia, and lung hypoplasia. Transillumination using a high intensity fiberoptic light source can aid in the diagnosis at the bedside.[2]

Transillumination Test

This is a bedside test used to identify pneumothorax. A high intensity fiberoptic light source is placed along the posterior axillary line on the side where the condition is suspected, after dimming the lights in the room. Pneumothorax is identified when the "the whole hemithorax lights up" (*Fig.* **10.2**) as compared to a negative test when only a ring of light is seen around the light source. The light is then moved up and down to assess the extent of the air leak. Transillumination test has a reported sensitivity of 87–100% and specificity of 95–100%.

The severity of the clinical signs of pneumothorax and pleural effusion depend on (1) volume of air/fluid collected in the pleural space, (2) site of the collection, and (3) rate of filling up of air/fluid in the space. The definitive diagnosis of pneumothorax/pleural effusion is by a chest X-ray (*Fig.* **10.3**).

■ MANAGEMENT IN THE DELIVERY ROOM

While a transillumination test or chest X-ray is desirable, these are not mandatory to initiate treatment in an emergency as severe collections of air or fluid could result in shock and death if not drained on time. Drainage of the air or fluid from the chest (*thoracentesis*) using an intravenous catheter generally results in prompt improvement in ventilation.[2,3]

Procedure for Drainage

The following are the steps for emergency thoracentesis:

- For emergency drainage of pneumothorax or pleural effusion, one would require an 18G or 20G intravenous catheter connected to a three-way stop-cock and a 10 mL syringe (*Fig.* **10.4**).

- The site for drainage of air is the 4th intercostal space in the anterior axillary line or the 2nd intercostal in the midaxillary line. For drainage of fluid, it is the 5th/6th intercostal space in the posterior axillary line.

- Disinfect the skin surface over the site located for thoracentesis.

- An 18 or 20G intravenous catheter is inserted perpendicular to the chest wall just above the rib.

- On entry into the pleural space, a 10 mL syringe with an attached three-way stopcock is used to aspirate the accumulated air from the pleural space by the intravenous catheter.

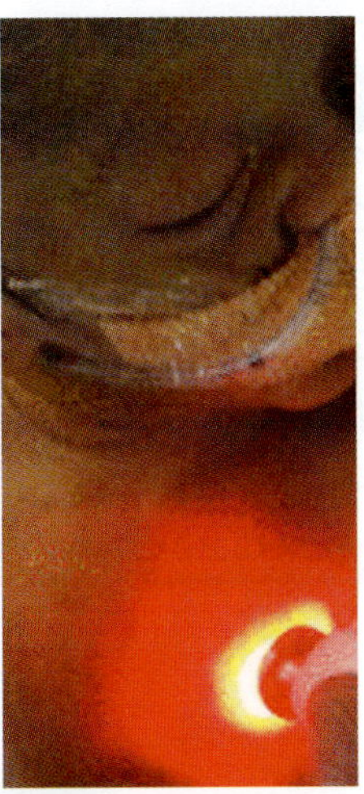

FIG. 10.2 Transillumination revealing a pneumothorax.

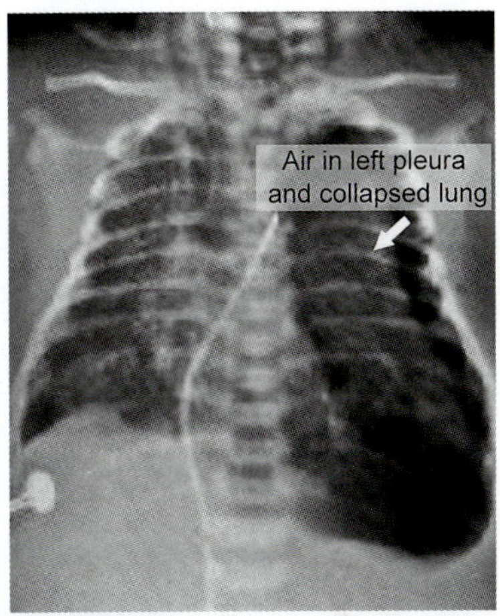

FIG. 10.3 X-ray chest revealing a pneumothorax on the left side with collapsed left lung
Courtesy: Dr Siddarth Ramji.

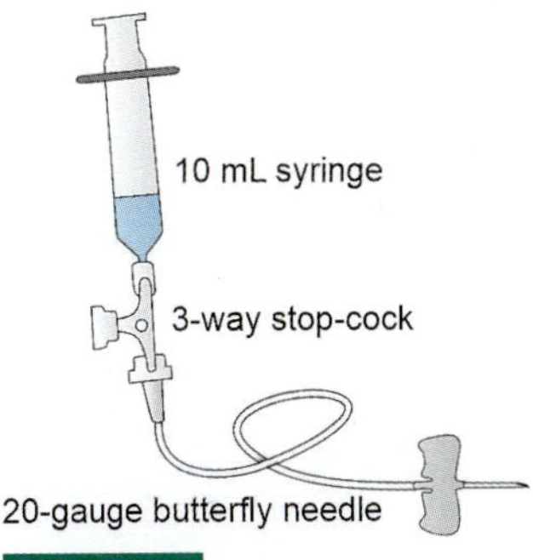

FIG. 10.4 Intravenous catheter with three-way stop-cock connected to a syringe for emergency thoracentesis.

KEY POINTS

1. Collection of air or fluid in the pleural space could result in the failure of establishment of adequate ventilation despite corrective measures during resuscitation of the newly born.

2. Breath sounds on auscultation are usually diminished of the side of pneumothorax/pleural effusion.

3. Transillumination using a high intensity fiberoptic light source aid in the diagnosis of pneumothorax at the bedside.

4. Immediate drainage of the air or fluid collection generally results in prompt improvement in ventilation.

■ REFERENCES

1. Duong HH, Mirea L, Shah PS, Yang J, Lee SK, Sankaran K. Pneumothorax in neonates: Trends, predictors and outcomes. J Neonatal Perinatal Med. 2014;7(1):29-38.

2. Parekh UR, Maguire AM, Emery J, Martin PH. Pneumothorax in neonates: Complication during endotracheal intubation, diagnosis, and management. J Anaesthesiol Clin Pharmacol. 2016;32(3):397-9.

3. Bruschettini M, Romantsik O, Ramenghi LA, Zappettini S, O'Donnell CP, Calevo MG. Needle aspiration versus intercostal tube drainage for pneumothorax in the newborn. Cochrane Database Syst Rev. 2019;2(2):CD011724.

Self Assessment

1. One should suspect ____________ when the baby cannot be ventilated adequately even after performing corrective steps of ventilation.

2. An important finding on auscultation in pneumothorax/or pleural effusion is _________ breath sounds on the side of the lesion.

3. The quickest way to confirm pneumothorax is by _______________.

4. Transillumination results in______________ in pneumothorax.

5. The site of insertion of intravenous catheter needle for drainage of pneumothorax is _______ intercostal space in the anterior axillary line.

Answers

For answers, go to the end of the Book, Page no. 322

Resuscitating a Newborn with Congenital Malformation

Prakash Amboiram

Lessons to Learn

- Congenital malformations causing delay in postnatal transition
- When to suspect congenital malformations during neonatal resuscitation
- Modification of the neonatal resuscitation in various malformations
- Preparation required for specific conditions

Congenital malformation can pose significant challenges during resuscitation. In many instances there may be a need to perform specific steps to improve resuscitation. The most common malformation that requires special resuscitation efforts include those of the airways and lungs (e.g., Pierre Robin sequence, congenital diaphragmatic hernia). There are others which may not need resuscitative assistance but need special care at birth for improving the disease outcome (e.g., omphalocele, neural tube defect). It is possible that information pertaining to presence and type of fetal malformation may be available prior to delivery from antenatal ultrasonography. This would help you being better prepared for handling such births.

SUSPECTING CONGENITAL MALFORMATIONS DURING RESUSCITATION

Even if one does not have an antenatal diagnosis of malformation in the fetus, one can suspect their existence, if one or more of the following problems are noted during resuscitation at birth:

- No chest movement is seen during positive pressure ventilation (PPV) through endotracheal tube.
- Difficulty in intubation or visualizing the larynx
- Respiratory distress or cyanosis in a baby with facial dysmorphism
- Heart rate remains low despite all efforts.
- Persistent cyanosis despite ventilation with 100% oxygen
- Baby remains apneic and floppy despite good response to PPV and no evidence of asphyxia.

Malformations of the Airways

Anomalies of the airways leading to obstruction are important causes contributing to difficulty in establishing ventilation in the delivery room. High index of suspicion helps in early airway stabilization. Congenital high airway obstruction syndrome (CHAOS) detected antenatally needs a multidisciplinary approach. Various anomalies of the airways which need special attention are described in **Table 11.1**.

TABLE 11.1: PRESENTATION AND DELIVERY ROOM MANAGEMENT OF MALFORMATIONS INVOLVING AIRWAYS		
Presentation	*Likely malformation*	*Delivery room management*
• Baby is normal when crying but becomes cyanosed or apneic if not crying.	Choanal atresia	• Place an oral airway[1] • Ryle's tube of size 5 Fr will not pass through nares of both sides.
• Babies with micrognathia or retrognathia and associated with respiratory distress or obstructive apnea and with difficulty in ventilation/intubation. • Presenting in the antenatal period with: – Polyhydramnios – Small stomach – Small jaw – Mass lesions in the oral cavity and neck	• Pierre Robin sequence (PRS)—retrognathia with posterior cleft palate [*Figs*. **11.1, 11.2 (A) and (B)**] • Tracheoesophageal fistula (TEF) with esophageal atresia • Cystic hygromas	Pierre Robin sequence with respiratory distress needs the following steps performed sequentially:[1] • Prone position • Insert the nasopharyngeal airway using a 2.5 mm size endotracheal tube to a length that would bypass the tongue (*Fig*. **11.2C**). To reduce the dead space the tube can be cut and flowered out (*Fig*. **11.3**) with the petals of the endotracheal tube (ETT) fixed over the lips and over the nose. • Laryngeal mask airway (LMA) can be used. In PRS, difficulty in establishing airway can be anticipated in the presence of Jaw Index[2] less than five (fetal MRI), polyhydramnios, and a small stomach bubble, then prepare a team who should be available for performing tracheostomy at birth. Mass in the neck with difficult intubation may also need an approach as mentioned for PRS for establishment of the airway. TEF requires early placement of Ryle tube for continuous drainage of the esophageal pouch in esophageal atresia. Infant can be positioned prone with head end elevation to avoid aspiration. Avoid positive pressure ventilation (PPV) using bag and mask

Contd...

Contd...

Presentation	Likely malformation	Delivery room management
• Antenatal diagnosis of congenital high airway obstruction syndromes (CHAOS) is made in presence of fetal hyperechoic enlarged lung and trachea with flattening or inversion of the diaphragm. There may be associated oligohydramnios or polyhydramnios • Difficult intubation (as alternate airway) due to non-visualization of vocal cords or unable to pass endotracheal tube through laryngeal inlet.	• Laryngeal or tracheal atresia • Tracheal stenosis • Obstructing laryngeal cysts • Obstructing tumors of the oropharynx and the cervical region (*Fig.* **11.4**)	• Multidisciplinary team with experts should be available for tracheostomy in case airways cannot be established. PPV with a mask may not be successful. • Intubation with a smaller tube may help negotiate a narrowed segment. If not, inserting a large bore needle/intravenous cannula in the larynx can help ventilation. Sometimes PPV can be successful with esophageal intubation due to fistula connecting the esophagus and trachea.[3]

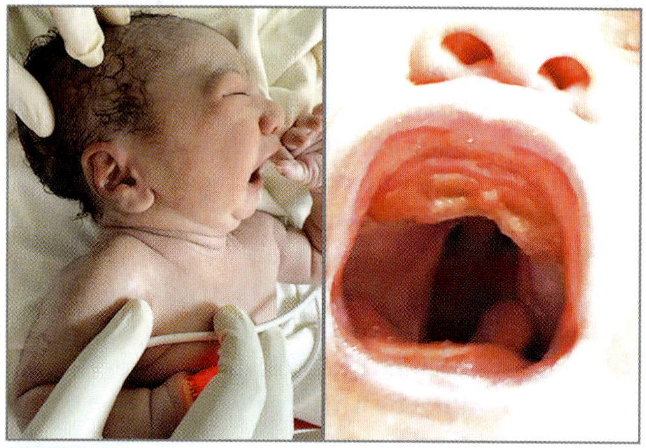

FIG. 11.1   Pierre Robin sequence showing retrognathia (left) and posterior cleft palate (right).

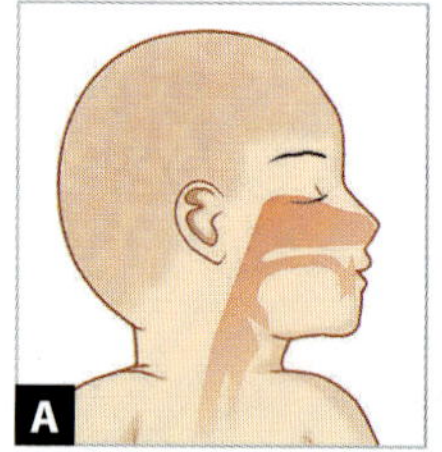
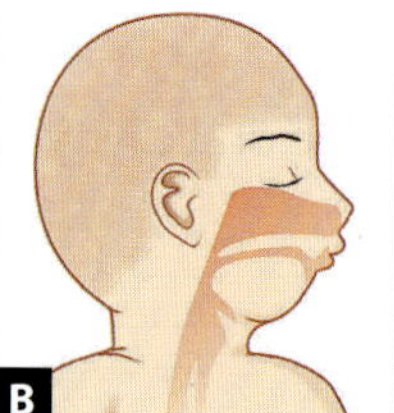
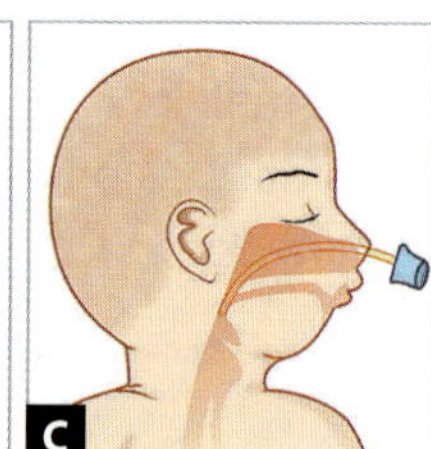

FIGS. 11.2A TO C   (A) Normal neonate; (B) Pierre Robin sequence: Retrognathia and tongue obstructing the airway; (C) Pierre Robin sequence with nasopharyneal airway using endotracheal tube.

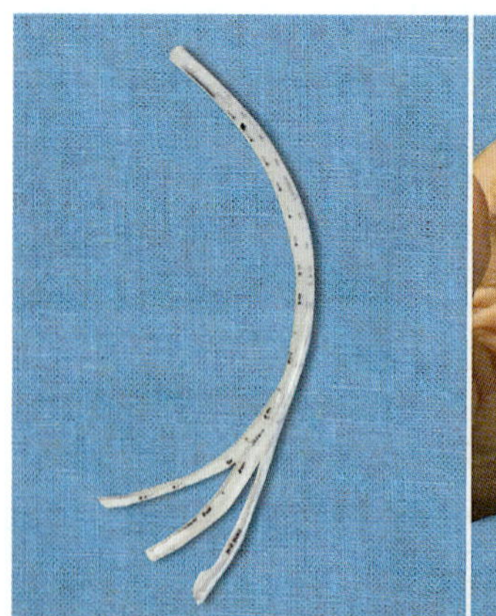
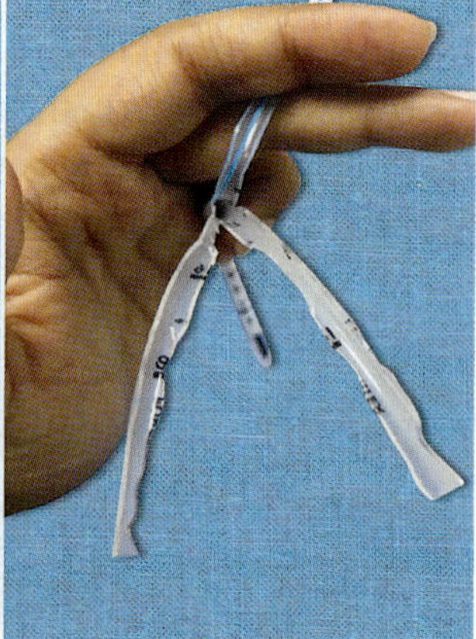

FIG. 11.3   Nasopharyngeal airway using endotracheal tube.

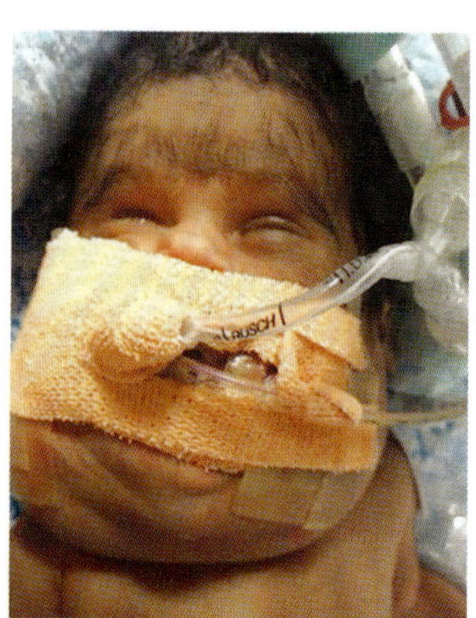

FIG. 11.4   Large cystic hygroma in the neck.

Malformations of the Lungs

Severe malformation of the lungs can be challenging for establishing ventilation and oxygenation in the delivery room. One of the most common conditions encountered is congenital diaphragmatic hernia (CDH). **Table 11.2** describes the presentation and delivery room management for lung malformations.

Malformations Needing Special Precautions at Birth

There are certain malformations that need special attention to the lesion to improve the outcome of the disease. The details of such malformations and the care to be taken at birth are provided in **Table 11.3**.

Malformation Associated with Failure to Initiate Breathing

At birth, neonates with neuromuscular disorders and severe brain malformation, may not breathe and remain floppy. These babies usually have good chest rise and heart rates >100 bpm in response to PPV but continue to have poor respiratory effort. Other clues to suspect or anticipate these conditions are presence of polyhydramnios, decreased fetal movement during pregnancy or presence of arthrogryposis and cannot be explained by other reasons such as maternal intake of opiates.[1]

TABLE 11.2: Presentation and Delivery Room Management for Lung Malformations[4]		
Presentation	**Likely malformation**	**Delivery room management**
• Respiratory distress, scaphoid abdomen, heart sound heard on the right side and decreased air entry on the left side • Generalized edema • Potter facies *Antenatal finding where resuscitation is anticipated:* • Lung malformation such as congenital diaphragmatic hernia (CDH), congenital pulmonary airway malformation (CPAM) • Pleural effusion due to hydrops fetalis • Severe oligohydramnios—lung hypoplasia	• Congenital diaphragmatic hernia (CDH) • Congenital pulmonary airway malformation (CPAM) • Hydrops • Lung hypoplasia	*CDH:* It is preferable to intubate as soon as the baby is born and insert an orogastric tube for continuous drainage of the gastric contents. Avoid PPV with bag and mask. Gentle ventilation to maintain oxygen saturation above 85% (after 5 minutes of life) with minimal ventilatory pressures. *Pleural effusion:* Chest drainage is indicated when positive pressure ventilation (PPV) through the endotracheal tube is not effective. Fluid in the chest can be drained using large bore cannula attached to 3-way stopcock and syringe. *CPAM:* Avoid PPV with intubation as CPAM can worsen. PPV after intubation, especially into the affected lung, can cause tension pnueumothorax. *Lung hypoplasia:* PPV with higher pressures may be required to move the chest. If required, the pop-off valve of the self-inflating bag can be occluded to move the chest with PPV. However, this can predispose to pneumothorax, and one must be prepared for managing it.

TABLE 11.3: MALFORMATIONS THAT NEED SPECIAL CARE AT BIRTH[1,5]

Malformation	Problem	Specific management at birth
Gastroschisis and omphalocele	Bowel when exposed can lead to excessive fluid loss and intestines are prone for injury and necrosis	• Delay the cord clamping and cut the umbilical cord further away as much as possible, from the baby. • Place the baby in plastic wrap covering the lower part of the body up to the chest. • Place the baby in the right lateral position. This aids in a better perfusion of the exposed bowel. • Insert Ryle's tube for continuous drainage of the stomach. • Avoid nasal continuous positive airway pressure (nCPAP). • If positive pressure ventilation (PPV) is required, then PPV is preferably given through endotracheal tube to prevent bowel distension and injury due to ischemia.
Neural tube defect (*Fig.* **11.5**)[3]	• When placed supine then the spinal myelomeningocele can be injured. • These babies, when compared to those without any congenital anomaly, are at higher risk of delivering preterm and with low 5 minute APGAR score. The APGAR score is based on appearance, pulse, grimace, activity and respiration.	• Place the baby in lateral or prone position. Use non-latex gloves. • Lesion is covered using saline-soaked gauze or cover with plastic sheet, to avoid drying • Avoid handling the myelomeningocele • If baby needs PPV in supine position, the meningomyelocele at the back is accommodated into a circular ring (like doughnut) made of cloth in order to avoid injury to the lesion.

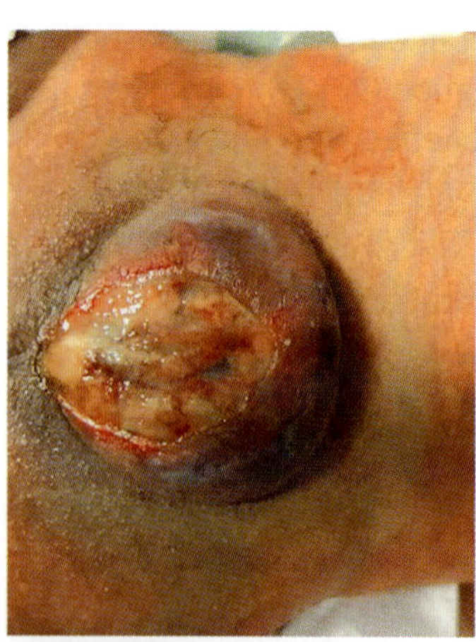

FIG. 11.5 Baby with meningomyelocele.

■ CONCLUSION

If the neonate does not improve with resuscitation, then congenital anomalies of the respiratory system should be suspected. In the present era with most of the major congenital malformations being detected antenatally, resuscitation team can be well prepared. As congenital malformations are uncommon, prior simulation exercises can improve the team performance during resuscitation in real time.

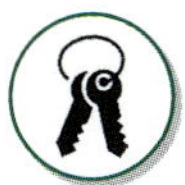

KEY POINTS

1. Antenatal diagnosis of congenital malformation in the fetus can help to anticipate the need for resuscitation at birth and plan accordingly.

2. One must consider presence of congenital malformation if the infant is not responding to resuscitation at birth, Airway can be established by simple measures like inserting an oral airway in babies with choanal atresia.

3. Pierre Robin sequence is one of the most common airway anomalies that need assistance for breathing. Such babies need to be placed prone and an nasopharyngeal airway needs to be inserted.

4. Congenital high airway obstruction syndromes (CHAOS) may require tracheostomy in the delivery room.

5. Specific care is required in malformations such as gastroschisis or omphalocele (placing the baby into plastic sheet covering abdomen) and meningomyelocele (covering with saline gauze and plastic sheet).

■ REFERENCES

1. American Academy of Pediatrics, American Heart Association. Textbook of Neonatal Resuscitation, 8th edition. In: Weiner GM, Zaichkin J, Kattwinkel J (Eds). Elk Grove Village, IL: American Academy of Pediatrics; 2021.

2. Tay SY, Krishnasarma R, Mehta D, Mehollin-Ray A, Chandy B. Predictive factors for perinatal outcomes of infants diagnosed with micrognathia antenatally. Ear Nose Throat J. 2021;100(1):NP16-20.

3. da Silva SA, de Almeida MF, Moron AF, Cavalheiro S, Dastoli PA, Guinsburg R. Resuscitation at birth in neonates with meningomyelocele. J Perinat Med. 2014;42(1):113-9.

4. Keller BA, Hirose S, Farmer DL. Surgical Disorders of the Chest and Airways. Gleason CA, Juul SE (Eds), Avery's Diseases of the Newborn, 10th edition. Elsevier. 2018;695-723.e9.

5. Kunisaki SM. Narrative review of congenital lung lesions. Transl Pediatr. 2021;10(5):1418-31.

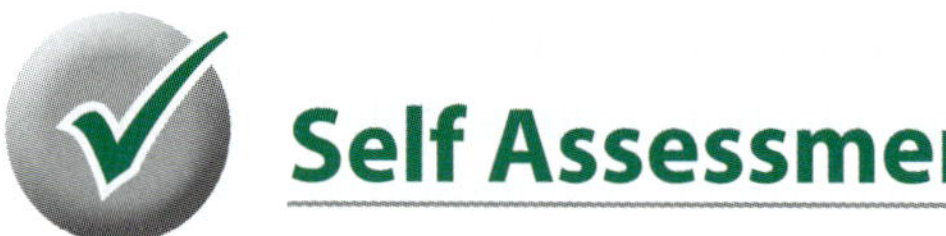

Self Assessment

1. In a baby who is cyanosed when not crying but whose color improves on crying most likely has______________________.

2. All of the following are true with respect to resuscitation of a baby with Pierre Robin sequence except:
   a. Place the baby supine
   b. Insert oral airway
   c. Laryngeal mask airways (LMA) is preferred over intubation for providing PPV
   d. Insert orogastric tube to prevent aspiration

3. All of the following are true regarding a neonate with lung hypoplasia except:
   a. High pressures may be needed while providing PPV.
   b. Pneumothorax may occur.
   c. May have antenatal oligohydramnios.
   d. LMA is preferred to endotracheal intubation.

4. All of the following are true regarding delivery room management of congenital diaphragmatic hernia (CDH) except:
   a. Electively intubate after birth
   b. Gentle ventilation should be used to stabilize the ventilation
   c. Insert orogastric tube for continuous drainage of the stomach
   d. Selective intubation of right bronchus

5. Following are true regarding the management of a neonate with meningomyelocele at birth except:
   a. Baby should to be kept in lateral or prone position after birth.
   b. Avoid drying of the meningomyelocele
   c. Latex gloves should not be used.
   d. Provide PPV in lateral or prone position

6. Following are true regarding management of baby with omphalocele/gastroschisis in the delivery room except:
   a. Nurse the baby in a supine position
   b. Umbilical cord to be clamped further away from the baby
   c. Cover the baby's abdomen and lower limbs with a plastic wrap
   d. Insert a Ryle's tube

Answers

For answers, go to the end of the Book, Page no. 322

Resuscitating Newborns of Multiple Pregnancy

Umamaheswari Balakrishnan

Lessons to Learn

- Preparing for birth of multiple babies
- Umbilical cord management in multiple births
- Resuscitation steps that may need modification during multiple birth
- Resuscitation in conjoined twins

The incidence of multiple pregnancy has been rising mainly due to assisted reproductive techniques. Twins and higher order pregnancies are at increased risk of morbidity and mortality compared to their singleton counterpart. Moreover, the chances of premature delivery and fetal growth restriction are higher in multiple pregnancy. Around 20% of births between 20 and 25 weeks of gestation are of multiple gestation. The rate of congenital malformations is higher in monozygotic twins compared to singleton.

There are a few circumstances which are unique to the twin pregnancies, especially among monochorionic twins—Twin-to-twin transfusion syndrome (TTTS), twin reversal arterial perfusion (TRAP) sequence, twin anemia polycythemia sequence (TAPS) as well as umbilical cord complications, which pose challenge during resuscitation. The second twin is at increased risk of perinatal asphyxia due to difficulty encountered in monitoring the second twin, premature separation of placenta, cord prolapse, and fetal distress. As the majority of the resuscitation related trials did not include twin gestation or multiple order gestation, evidence on certain steps of resuscitation is lacking. This chapter will discuss some of the relevant steps in the neonatal resuscitation algorithm important from the perspective of multiple births.

■ PREPARATION FOR BIRTH

Focus on Teamwork

One team leader should be identified for every baby and team briefing should be performed to ensure that everyone is prepared, and their

TABLE 12.1: Key Behavioral Skills[1]

Behavior	Situations applicable in resuscitation of multiple births
Know your environment	Know where the device such as intraosseous needle is available.
Use available information	Information regarding the presence of vascular malformation.
Anticipate and plan	• Working in a multidisciplinary team to practice a systematic approach. • Umbilical cord management planning with obstetrician.
Clearly identify team leader	Team briefing with individual team leaders.
Communicate effectively	Obstetric and neonatal team to share the assessment of neonate clearly. Response to treatment clearly verbalized.
Delegate the workload optimally	Multiple procedures may be needed simultaneously.
Allocate attention wisely	If team leader is involved in doing a skill, the next person should be prepared to take the role of team leader.
Use available resources	Ensuring the presence of adequate personnel based on risk factors.
Call for additional help when needed	When resuscitation gets complex, need additional help who can step in as needed.
Maintain professional behavior	Sharing the mental model and team debriefing after completion of resuscitation.

roles and responsibilities are defined. Resuscitation of multiple births requires the team to acquire and implement several important behavioral skills. Some examples as applicable in the context of multiple birth are highlighted in **Table 12.1**.

Equipment Check

The standardized equipment check list performed for any resuscitation should be carried out except that depending on the number of babies expected, the number of equipment and supplies should be separately prepared and checked for each baby. Additional thermoregulatory mechanism should be in place, in case premature babies are expected.

Preparation for birth is the first step to execute the key behavioral skill namely anticipation and planning. Any multiple gestation should per se be considered as a high-risk delivery. Even the known factors identified to be associated with delayed transition in the baby at birth, occur more commonly in a multiple pregnancy **(Table 12.2)**. Multiple gestation poses a higher need of resuscitation due to associated placental abnormality, cord blood flow compromise, and mechanical complication, especially during delivery of nonvertex second twin.[1] Preterm delivery is common in multiple gestation, whether it is spontaneous or induced.

When delivery of multiple fetuses is anticipated, at least two qualified care providers exclusively responsible for care of each baby should be

TABLE 12.2: FACTORS OCCURRING MORE FREQUENTLY IN MULTIPLE GESTATION[1]	
Antepartum factors	*Intrapartum factors*
1. Preterm	1. Delay in delivery of second twin
2. Maternal hypertension	2. Cord prolapse
3. Preeclampsia/eclampsia	
4. Maternal diabetes	
5. Fetal growth restriction	
6. Fetal anemia	
7. Fetal malformation	

available, e.g., in twin births at least four providers trained in neonatal resuscitation should be available at the time of birth. Additional resources should be identified prior to the delivery and prompt call for help initiated at appropriate time. In the presence of additional risk factors such as TTTS, a complete team of four would be desirable for each baby.

■ SPECIFIC MANAGEMENT

Umbilical Cord Management

Evidence for appropriate timing of cord clamping in multiple births is limited and hence the lack of standard guidelines for such births. Ruangkit et al.[2] reported the results of a randomized controlled trial (RCT) comparing delayed cord clamping (DCC) and immediate cord clamping (ICC) which enrolled 101 preterm infants (28–36 weeks) born of multiple pregnancy (twins and triplets) most of whom were delivered by cesarean section. While all infants outcome variables [hematocrit and superior vena cava (SVC) flow] were comparable, postpartum hemorrhage was significantly higher in DCC group (25%) as compared to the ICC group (4.3%). In a retrospective study, Jegatheesan et al.[3] observed that neonatal outcomes in preterm infants receiving DCC were comparable between *"singletons and multiples, first and second order multiples and monochorionic and dichorionic/ trichorionic multiples"*. Liu et al.[4] in a retrospective cohort study of 58 women delivering dichorionic diamniotic (DCDA) twins at gestations of 23–32 weeks observed similar neonatal outcomes (Apgar scores, temperatures, hematocrit, jaundice, etc.) in those who received DCC and ICC.

In view of the limited data, it may be prudent to consider several factors while planning for umbilical cord management which is summarized in **Table 12.3**. All the factors should be discussed and a plan about the execution of DCC should be made between obstetrician and pediatrician. If the twins are DCDA and appropriately grown, it is reasonable to delay the cord clamping for 60 seconds.

TABLE 12.3: UMBILICAL CORD MANAGEMENT IN MULTIPLE BIRTHS

Factor	Assessment	Situations for deferring delayed cord clamping (DCC)
Chorionicity and amnionicity	Dichorionic (DC) or monochorionic (MC); diamniotic (DA) or monoamniotic (MA)	MC twins are at higher risk for vascular malformations. MA twins are at increased risk of cord entanglement.
Growth	Fetal growth restriction (FGR) or appropriately grown. FGR could be because of selective growth restriction due to placental insufficiency or part of vascular malformations.	FGR fetus is at increased risk of polycythemia. Doppler changes of umbilical artery or ductus venosus can occur in FGR.
Growth discordancy	Growth discordancy calculated from the estimated fetal weight of the twins (MC or DC).	Growth discordancy of >20% is significant.
Doppler	Doppler of umbilical artery (UA), middle cerebral artery (MCA) and ductus venosus assessed	• Umbilical artery reversal or ductus venosus changes reflect the fetal hypoxia and acid-base status. • High MCA peak systolic velocity (PSV) in fetal MCA indicates fetal anemia.
Vascular malformations	Presence of twin-to-twin transfusion syndrome (TTTS), twin anemia polycythemia sequence (TAPS), or twin reversal arterial perfusion (TRAP) sequence	Presence of vascular malformation might reduce the benefit of DCC.
Survival	Single fetal demise	Surviving twin is at increased risk due to exposure to same factors responsible for single fetal demise.

Italian guidelines on transfusion recommend DCC for at least 30–60 seconds in vaginally or cesarean delivered term or preterm twin from dichorionic pregnancy.[5] In other circumstances, the decision should be individualized considering the risk versus benefit of DCC.

Resuscitation Steps

Initial steps, positive pressure ventilation, intubation, chest compression, and medication administration are similar as for singleton births. The steps that may need to be modified are listed in **Table 12.4**.

Positive Pressure Ventilation

In the presence of bilateral pleural effusion as may be seen in hydrops in TTTS, effective ventilation may not be achieved without draining the pleural fluid. Placement of intercostal drainage in 5th intercostal space helps in fluid drainage and lung expansion.[1] Ascitic tap may be needed. Donor twins can have hypoplastic lungs due to oligohydramnios which can result in difficulty in ventilating the lungs.

TABLE 12.4: NEONATAL RESUSCITATION STEPS IN CONTEXT TO MULTIPLE BIRTHS

Steps	Remarks
Preparation	Knowing additional risk factors including fetal growth restriction, Doppler abnormality, fetal anemia, vascular malformations including TTTS, TAPS, and TRAP help in planning the delivery; O negative blood to be arranged in case of fetal anemia.
Umbilical cord management planning	• Immediate cord clamping in monochorionic twins. • Delayed cord clamping in DCDA twins who do not require resuscitation at birth.
Team briefing	Individual team leader and assigning the roles and responsibilities of the team members
Equipment	Standard equipment list to be arranged for individual babies.
Initial steps	Same as for singleton
Positive pressure ventilation and intubation	Difficulty in achieving chest rise with PPV (effective PPV) in twins with hydrops or donor twin of TTTS with hypoplastic lungs; Hydropic neonate might need intercostal drainage to achieve effective PPV.
Chest compression	Same as for singleton
Medication	Volume expansion might be needed in donor twin of TTTS or TAPS.

(DCDA: dichorionic diamniotic; TAPS: twin anemia polycythemia sequence; TRAP: twin reversal arterial perfusion; TTTS: twin-to-twin transfusion syndrome)

Volume Expansion

The need for volume expansion is higher in donor twin in TTTS in view of blood loss.[1,6] However, volume expansion should not be given routinely. Careful assessment for volume status including paleness, pulse volume, and delayed capillary refill time should be carried out before giving normal saline bolus of 10 mL/kg over 5–10 minutes. Care should be taken in the presence of hydrops as cardiac decompensation can happen with volume overload. If fetal anemia is diagnosed in utero (high peak systolic volume in fetal middle cerebral artery), then O negative packed red blood cell crossmatched to mother should be made available during resuscitation.

Resuscitation in Conjoined Twins

Resuscitation of conjoined twins can be challenging.[7,8] Steps of resuscitation need to be modified in conjoined twins and are summarized in **Table 12.5**. Ergonomics of resuscitation of conjoined twins can improve safety and performance of the team and a suggested model is depicted in *Figure* **12.1**.

TABLE 12.5: Steps of Resuscitation in Conjoined Twins[7]

Steps	Remarks
Preparation assess perinatal risk factors	Preparation should start in the antenatal period itself. Antenatal diagnosis and 3D reconstruction would help the team to get prepared well. In-situ simulation (with modified manikin) can help the entire team to deliver efficient resuscitation. Babies can be identified by color code (orange/purple) rather than as twin 1 and 2.
Umbilical cord management planning	Immediate cord clamping
Team briefing	A team of at least 10 members are essential for effective resuscitation. Team leader can be one person coordinating events of both the babies. Team briefing, co-ordination between multiple teams, and attention to ergonomics are important.
Equipment checks	Standard equipment list to be arranged and color coded. Intraosseous needle to be kept ready.
Initial steps	Immediate cord clamping and initial steps in the warmer. Suctioning and positioning are difficult, especially in craniopagus twins.
Positive pressure ventilation and intubation	Pulse oximetry to be tied on the available hands, not necessarily on the right hand. Auscultation can be difficult in thoracopagus; pulse oximetry can be used to assess HR. Airway issues can be anticipated in craniopagus, thoracopagus, and omphalopagus twins. If PPV cannot be reliably administered, then early LMA insertion or endotracheal intubation can be performed. Ventilation can be difficult due to pendelluft effect in thoracopagus twins.
Chest compression	In case of spatial constrains, two-finger technique can be used. In thoracopagus twins, compression is done by placing one twin on top of the other with compressions on back of top twin.
Medication	Assessing umbilical vein can be difficult in omphalopagus. Intraosseous route can be used.

(LMA: laryngeal mask airway; PPV: positive pressure ventilation)

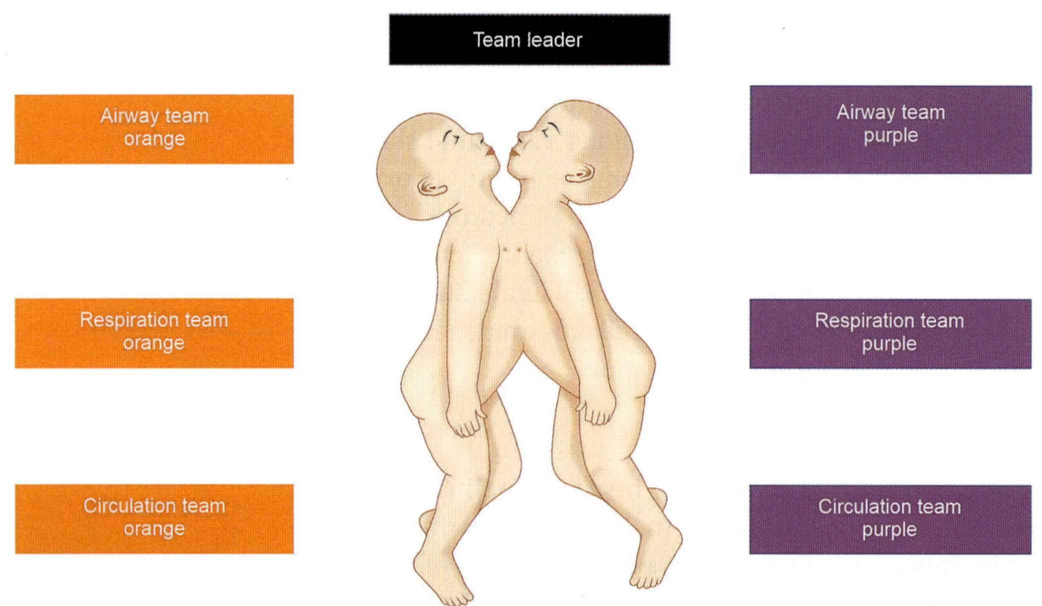

FIG. 12.1   Ergonomics of resuscitation for conjoined twins.

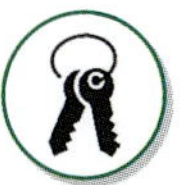

KEY POINTS

1. Twin gestation is common. Second twin is at increased risk of asphyxia.

2. Steps of resuscitation to be followed remain the same. However, any multiple gestation is considered as high risk.

3. For each baby, a team trained in neonatal resuscitation should be present at the time of delivery. Anticipation and planning are the important nontechnical steps in resuscitation, especially in the presence of vascular malformation such as twin-to-twin transfusion syndrome (TTTS).

4. Umbilical cord management should be individualized based on chorionicity, growth, Doppler changes, and presence of vascular malformations.

5. Ineffective positive pressure ventilation should raise the suspicion of lung hypoplasia or hydrops in the setting of TTTS.

6. Volume expansion can be considered with caution in case of anemic twin in TTTS.

■ REFERENCES

1. Weiner GM, Zaichkin J, Kattwinkel J. Textbook of Neonatal Resuscitation, 8th edition. Elk Grove Village, IL: American Academy of Pediatrics; 2021.

2. Ruangkit C, Bumrungphuet S, Panburana P, Khositseth A, Nuntnarumit P. A randomized controlled trial of immediate versus delayed umbilical cord clamping in multiple-birth infants born preterm. Neonatology. 2019;115(2):156-63.

3. Jegatheesan P, Belogolovsky E, Nudelman M, Song D, Govindaswami B. Neonatal outcomes in preterm multiples receiving delayed cord clamping. Arch Dis Child Fetal Neonatal Ed. 2019;104(6):F575-81.

4. Liu LY, Yee LM. Delayed cord clamping in preterm dichorionic twin gestations. J Matern Fetal Neonatal Med. 2019;26:1-5.

5. Ghirardello S, Di Tommaso M, Fiocchi S, Locatelli A, Perrone B, Pratesi S, et al. Italian Recommendations for Placental Transfusion Strategies. Front Pediatr. 2018;6:372.

6. Oygür N, Önal EE, Zenciroğlu A. National guidelines for delivery room management. Turk Pediatri Ars. 2018;53(Suppl 1):S3-17.

7. Sager EC, Thomas A, Sundgren NC. Conjoined twins: pre-birth management, changes to NRP, and transport. Semin Perinatol. 2018;42(6):321-8.

8. Yamada NK, Fuerch JH, Halamek LP. Modification of the neonatal resuscitation program algorithm for resuscitation of conjoined twins. Am J Perinatol. 2016;33(4):420-4.

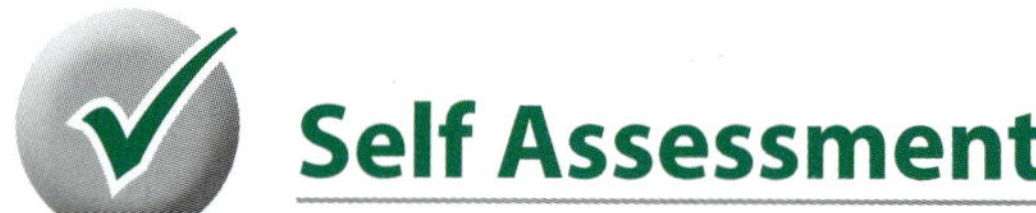

Self Assessment

1. Which one of the following is the best guideline for identifying the resuscitation team for a delivery when twins or triplets are anticipated?
    a. An individual should be able to multitask and care for all babies.
    b. Separate teams are essential for resuscitation of each baby.
    c. Additional risk factors need not be asked in multiple pregnancy.
    d. Additional resource personnel can be on-call at home.

2. Following are correctly matched except:
    a. Monochorionic twins—immediate cord clamping
    b. TTTS donor twin—volume expansion due to fetal anemia
    c. TTTS recipient twin—hypoplastic lungs due to oligohydramnios
    d. TTTS hydrops—intercostal drainage for pleural fluid drainage

3. Following are the modified steps in the resuscitation of conjoined twins except:
    a. Pulse oximetry for heart rate assessment
    b. Chest compression impossible in thoracopagus twins due to spatial constraints
    c. Two thumb technique acceptable for chest compression
    d. Intraosseous needle for medication administration in omphalopagus twins

Answers

For answers, go to the end of the Book, Page no. 323

Resuscitation of Neonate Born to a Mother with Human Immunodeficiency Virus Infection or SARS-CoV-2 Infection

Praveen Kumar

HUMAN IMMUNODEFICIENCY VIRUS-POSITIVE MOTHER

Lessons to Learn

- Prevention of mother-to-child transmission of human immunodeficiency virus (HIV).
- Protecting health workers from occupational exposure.

Mother-to-child transmission (MTCT), occurring during pregnancy, labor, or during breastfeeding accounts for over 90% of all HIV infections in children. The MTCT rate (including breastfeeding period) in 2020 was estimated at 27.4% (20.3–33.5%), down from 40.2% in 2010, but far above the target of 5%.

The major goals while attending the delivery of HIV positive pregnant women are to prevent MTCT and to prevent occupational exposure of healthcare workers, while providing respectful and nondiscriminatory care to the mother-infant dyad. The risk of MTCT of HIV is higher in the presence of recent HIV infection in the mother, high viral load, concurrent sexually transmitted infections, prolonged labor, prolonged rupture of membranes, multiple vaginal examinations, instrumental delivery, invasive fetal monitoring procedures, episiotomy, and prematurity.

This section will describe the activities that need to be undertaken to prevent MTCT of HIV.

ANTIRETROVIRAL THERAPY FOR THE PREGNANT WOMEN

Depending on the timing of the diagnosis and previous intake of antiretroviral therapy (ART), the obstetrician and delivery room nurse would need to ensure the intake of appropriate medicines and doses at admission, during labor and after delivery, without any interruption, as per the National acquired immunodeficiency syndrome (AIDS) control guidelines.[1]

■ CARE DURING DELIVERY

The risk of MTCT during delivery can be reduced by following standard (universal) precautions and avoiding nasogastric or orogastric suctioning, if not indicated. Baby's mouth and nostrils should be wiped as soon as the head is delivered. Infants should be handled with gloves until all blood and maternal secretions have been washed off. The cord should be clamped early, and not milked. The cord should be cut as soon as possible between clamps, while covering with gauze pieces to avoid splash of blood.

■ CARE AFTER BIRTH

All routine postpartum care services available for neonates born to HIV-negative mothers should also be provided to HIV exposed neonates. These include skin-to-skin contact soon after birth and early initiation of breastfeeding.

■ FEEDING

Breastfeeding with concurrent ART offers the greatest chance of HIV-free survival to HIV-exposed infants. Exclusive breastfeeding (EBF) initiated within 1 hour of birth and continued for at least 6 months is recommended. Even after starting complementary feeds at 6 months, breastfeeding should be continued for at least 12 months and preferably for up to 24 months or beyond (like the general population), while fully supporting mothers for ART adherence. Since breastfeeding does carry some risk of HIV transmission, individual pregnant women should also be informed about alternative infant-feeding options and their advantages and disadvantages as compared to breastfeeding. Exclusive replacement feeding may be considered only if the mother has died or has a terminal illness or decides not to breastfeed despite adequate counseling. The decision should be made using the affordable, feasible, acceptable, safe, and sustainable (AFASS) criteria.

Mixed Feeding

If mother is practicing mixed feeding, she should be counseled and motivated to exclusively breastfeed. When EBF is not possible for any reason (e.g., maternal sickness, twins), families can be reassured that maternal ART reduces the risk of postnatal HIV transmission in the context of mixed feeding as well and should be preferred over no breastfeeding at all. Breastfeeding should not be stopped in case of mixed feeding in the presence of antiretroviral (ARV) drugs.

TABLE 13.1: Risk Assessment of Infants Born to HIV-infected Mothers and Infant ARV Prophylaxis Options

Risk status	Option for ARV prophylaxis	Type of feeding opted	Duration of ARV
Low risk infants: Infants born to mothers with suppressed plasma viral loads (<1,000 copies/mL) assessed any time after 32 weeks of pregnancy up to delivery	*Single ARV* Nevirapine or zidovudine (where nevirapine will not be effective, i.e., mother with confirmed HIV-2 infection, mother who had received single dose of nevirapine during early pregnancy or delivery and infant born to a mother who is on protease inhibitor based ART due to treatment failure. If zidovudine is not available, nevirapine can be given for first 14 days after birth followed by lopinavir after 14 days of age.	Any (exclusive breastfeeding, mixed feeding or exclusive replacement feeding)	6 weeks
High risk infants: • Infants born to HIV-positive mother not on ART • Maternal viral load not done after 32 weeks of gestation • Maternal plasma viral load not suppressed after 32 weeks of pregnancy • Mother newly identified HIV-positive within 6 weeks of delivery	*Dual ARV* Nevirapine and zidovudine	Exclusive breastfeeding or mixed feeding	12 weeks
		Exclusive replacement feeding	6 weeks

(ART: antiretroviral therapy; ARV: antiretroviral; HIV: human immunodeficiency virus)

TABLE 13.2: Dosage of Antiretroviral (ARV) Prophylaxis for Infants

Birth weight	Nevirapine (NVP) (1 mL = 10 mg)		Zidovudine (AZT) (1 mL = 10 mg)	
	NVP daily dose (in mg)	NVP daily dose (in mL)	AZT daily dosage (in mg)	AZT daily dosage (in mL)
<2,000 g	2 mg/kg OD	0.2 mL/kg OD	5 mg/dose twice daily	0.5 mL twice daily
2,000–2,500 g	10 mg OD	1 mL OD	10 mg/dose twice daily	1 mL twice daily
>2,500 g	15 mg OD	1.5 mL OD	15 mg/dose twice daily	1.5 mL twice daily

ANTIRETROVIRAL PROPHYLAXIS FOR THE NEONATE (TABLES 13.1 AND 13.2)

This is must for all neonates born to HIV-positive mothers, irrespective of the breastfeeding status, to further decrease the risk of HIV infection after birth. The drug should be started within 1 hour of birth and continued for 6–12 weeks from the date of start as per **Table 13.1**. The family should be trained in hygienically administering the drugs in correct doses to the baby using a syringe or dropper. Family counseling for supporting and ensuring daily administration of the drugs for

6–12 weeks as per indication and EBF till a minimum of 6 months should be ensured.

Syphilis screening status of the mother should be checked and appropriate assessment, investigations and treatment undertaken as per the guidelines.

IMMUNIZATION

Birth doses of bacillus Calmette–Guérin (BCG), hepatitis B vaccine (HBV), and oral poliovirus vaccine (OPV) should be given as routine. Subsequently, live attenuated vaccines are contraindicated in severely immunocompromised infants and children with HIV infection (CD4 < 15% in <5 years; CD4 <200 cells/mm^3 in >5 years) because of the risk of disease caused by the vaccine strain. If BCG has not been given at birth, or for neonates with HIV infection confirmed by early virological testing, BCG vaccination should be delayed until ART has been started and the infant confirmed to be immunologically stable (CD4 >25%).

COTRIMOXAZOLE PROPHYLAXIS

All HIV-exposed infants should get cotrimoxazole prophylaxis from the age of 6 weeks in a dose of 5 mg/kg/day as a single daily dose.

HUMAN IMMUNODEFICIENCY VIRUS TESTING FOR THE NEWBORN

Human immunodeficiency virus deoxyribonucleic acid (DNA) polymerase chain reaction (PCR) should be done at 6 weeks of age by dried blood spot (DBS). If negative, it should be repeated at 6 months of age or earlier, if the infant becomes symptomatic. At 18 months, three rapid antibody tests should be performed.

OCCUPATIONAL SAFETY

The healthcare workers should practice universal precautions as for all deliveries. Universal precautions provide adequate protection against HIV as well as other blood borne diseases such as hepatitis B and C. Many women may be in the window period and a negative HIV test is no guarantee of noninfectivity. Hence, it is prudent to follow universal precautions for all deliveries. Universal precautions include personal protective equipment (PPE) **(Table 13.3)**, prevention of injuries due to sharps, hand hygiene, and safe decontamination of instruments.

In case of exposure, guidelines for management of occupational exposure should be followed. If blood or any other body fluid such as amniotic fluid splashes on unbroken skin, the area should be washed immediately with running water or soap and water. Do not use antiseptics. In case the contact is with eyes or mouth, they should be irrigated with water.

TABLE 13.3: PERSONAL PROTECTIVE EQUIPMENT FOR VARIOUS NEONATAL PROCEDURES

Procedure	Level of risk	Gloves	Apron	Goggles	Mask	Shoes
Injection	Low	Yes	No	No	No	No
Venipuncture, insertion of intravenous (IV) cannula	Medium—possibility of contact with blood or other body fluids, but without the risk of splash	Yes	May	No	No	No
Intubation	Medium plus—probable contact with a splash of blood or other body fluids	Yes	Yes	Yes	Yes	No

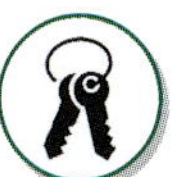 **KEY POINTS**

1. Prevention of mother-to-child transmission of HIV requires uninterrupted continuation of antiretroviral (ARV) treatment of the woman through labor and after delivery, as well as ARV prophylaxis for the neonate.
2. The exposed neonates should be provided all routine postnatal care as for neonates born to HIV-negative mothers. This includes early skin-to-skin contact and initiation of breastfeeding within 1 hour.
3. Exclusive breastfeeding (EBF) for 6 months is the recommended mode of feeding.
4. Universal precautions provide adequate protection to health workers against HIV as well as other blood borne diseases such as hepatitis B and C.

SARS-CoV-2 (COVID-19) INFECTION

Lessons to Learn

- Changes required in the resuscitation of neonates born to mothers with severe acute respiratory syndrome coronavirus-2 (SARS-CoV-2) [coronavirus disease-2019 (COVID-19)] infection.
- Precautions to protect the healthcare workers and the neonate from getting infected with SARS-CoV-2.

The novel COVID-19 caused by SARS-CoV-2 was first detected in late 2019 but spread rapidly to become a global pandemic. Though the virus and the disease have evolved, the pandemic threat continues. With the large experience gained from pregnant women infected with SARS-CoV-2, it is now known that neonates born to these women are more likely to be preterm and growth restricted, and hence may need resuscitation more frequently.

In general, the resuscitation of neonates born to women with suspected or confirmed COVID-19 should follow the standard neonatal resuscitation protocol. Special arrangements are required to protect the healthcare workers and the newborn infant from getting infected by the SARS-CoV-2 **(Box 13.1)**. A minimum number of personnel should attend resuscitation and wear a full set of PPE.

BOX 13.1: RECOMMENDATIONS RELATED TO RESUSCITATION OF NEONATES BORN TO MOTHERS WITH COVID-19

1. Minimum number of personnel should attend resuscitation (one person in low-risk cases and two in high-risk cases where extensive resuscitation may be anticipated) and wear a full set of personal protective equipment including N95 mask and face-shield or goggles.
2. Mother should perform hand hygiene and wear triple layer mask.
3. Neonatal resuscitation should follow standard guidelines. If positive pressure ventilation is needed, self-inflating bag and mask, or a T-piece resuscitator with disposable circuit may be used.
4. Indications for intubation shall not change because of maternal COVID-19 status.
5. Delayed cord clamping and early skin to skin contact should be practiced.
6. Perform oral or nasal suction only if indicated to clear the airway.
7. Endotracheal administration of medications should be avoided.
8. Bathing is not recommended in view of risk of hypothermia and hospital-acquired infections.

(COVID-19: coronavirus disease-2019)

There is no robust evidence indicating increased transmission of infection due to delayed cord clamping (DCC). On the other hand, the benefits of DCC are well established. Hence, DCC is recommended as per neonatal resuscitation guidelines even if mother is SARS-CoV-2 positive, and irrespective her being symptomatic or not. The practice of skin-to-skin care (SSC) immediately after birth should be continued as part of "routine care". During SSC, mother should follow the recommended infection prevention and control measures (hand hygiene, respiratory etiquette, and using a triple-layered mask).

This section will describe the management of neonates born to mothers testing positive for SARS-COV-2.[2]

■ INFECTION PREVENTION DURING RESUSCITATION

Personal Protective Equipment

The resuscitation team should wear an N95 mask, face shield or goggles, and full PPE for attending delivery of women with suspected or confirmed SARS-CoV-2 infection.

Equipment

A new set of disposables and disinfected reusables should be used for each delivery. Disposables such as endotracheal (ET) tubes, suction catheter, orogastric tube, tapes for fixing ET tube, umbilical catheter, and syringes placed near the resuscitation area should be discarded even if unused. Reusable equipment should be thoroughly disinfected as per hospital protocol. Protective clothing should be worn when dealing with contaminated equipment.

Airway

Oral or nasal suction should be performed only if indicated to clear the airway.

Respiratory Support

If positive pressure ventilation is needed, self-inflating bag and mask or a T-piece resuscitator with disposable tubing may be used. Indications for intubation are as per standard neonatal resuscitation protocol. The use of aerosol boxes during intubation and the use of filters attached to T-Piece/bag mask devices *are not recommended* during neonatal resuscitation.

The neonatal resuscitation team should doff the PPE after exiting the delivery area, discard the components in appropriate bins as per disposal policy and perform hand hygiene. Transfer of the neonate to the designated area can be performed by another healthcare worker wearing appropriate PPE. However, if there is a shortage of personnel, the resuscitation team member can doff partially and wear a fresh outer gown and gloves to transport the neonate. If the neonate is on respiratory support, transport personnel should wear an N95 mask.

◼ ROOMING-IN AND BREASTFEEDING

Table 13.4 shows that breastfeeding is protective for the neonate, possibly due to transfer of SARS-CoV-2 antibodies and other immunological factors.[3] Rooming-in is one of the most important interventions to promote the successful establishment of breastfeeding at birth and EBF till 6 months of age. Breastfeeding is the most effective intervention to reduce neonatal mortality. Hence, rooming-in and EBF must be promoted and supported **(Box 13.2)**. Though rooming-in marginally increases the incidence of neonatal COVID-19, the infection is mostly asymptomatic or mild with excellent outcomes. The risk of infection to the neonate can be decreased substantially by rigorous compliance to the conditions for safe breastfeeding.

Care Area for Symptomatic Unstable Neonates

Symptomatic neonates with suspected SARS-CoV-2 infection, who need special or intensive care, should be isolated from other healthy mothers and neonates and cared for according to recommended

TABLE 13.4: Risk of SARS-CoV-2 Infection Among Neonates based on the Mode of Feeding (NNF COVID-19 Registry)[3]

	Breastfed (n = 1,099)	Not breastfed (n = 182)	Relative risk (95% CI)
SARS-CoV-2 positive neonates	119 (10.8%)	20 (11.0%)	Unadjusted: 0.98 (0.63–1.54) Adjusted for rooming-in: 0.45 (0.23–0.87)

(CI: confidence interval; COVID-19: coronavirus disease-2019; SARS-CoV-2: severe acute respiratory syndrome coronavirus-2)

> **BOX 13.2: RECOMMENDATIONS REGARDING ROOMING-IN AND BREASTFEEDING OF NEONATES BORN TO MOTHERS WITH COVID-19**
>
> 1. *Stable neonates exposed to mothers or other persons with SARS-CoV-2 infection should be roomed-in with their mothers and be exclusively breastfed.*
>
>   For supporting lactation, nurses trained in essential neonatal care and lactation management should be provided. A healthy willing family member who is not positive for SARS-CoV-2, is not in direct contact with persons with suspected or confirmed infection and is asymptomatic may be allowed to stay with the mother-baby dyad to assist and provide support for breastfeeding.
>
> 2. *If rooming-in is not possible because of sickness in the neonate or the mother, the neonate should be fed expressed breastmilk (EBM) of the mother by a nurse or a trained healthy family member as described above.*
>
>   *Conditions to be met for safe breastfeeding:*
>
>   - Mothers should perform hand hygiene frequently, including before breastfeeding and touching the baby.
>   - Mothers should practice respiratory hygiene and wear a triple-layered mask while breastfeeding and providing care to the baby; they should routinely clean and disinfect the surfaces.
>   - Mothers can express milk after washing hands and wearing a mask. If possible, a dedicated breast pump should be provided. If not, it should be decontaminated as per protocol. This expressed milk can be fed to the baby without pasteurization. The collection and transport of EBM should be done very carefully to avoid contamination.
>
> (COVID-19: coronavirus disease-2019; SARS-CoV-2: severe acute respiratory syndrome coronavirus-2)

infection prevention and control practices. The care area for suspected cases should be separate from that of confirmed cases.

COVID TESTING IN NEONATES BORN TO COVID-19 MOTHERS

Perinatal transmission is suspected if COVID-19 was detected in the mother within 14 days before or within 2 days after delivery. Such neonates should undergo reverse transcription PCR (RT-PCR) test on swab samples taken from the nasopharynx between 24 and 48 hours of age. Rooming-in should not be postponed pending the testing. In case of earlier discharge, a predischarge sample should be taken. A repeat test is desirable at 5–7 days of age (or earlier if neonate becomes symptomatic). Repeat testing can help to prevent transmission from the neonate (who is likely to be asymptomatic even if infected) to other family members.

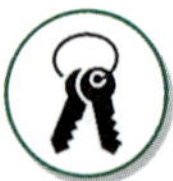

KEY POINTS

1. Resuscitation of neonates born to COVID-19 positive or suspect mothers should follow the standard Neonatal Resuscitation Protocol (NRP).
2. Stable neonates should be roomed-in and exclusively breastfed.
3. Health workers should use appropriate PPE.
4. Mothers should use triple layered surgical mask, follow hand hygiene and respiratory etiquettes.

■ REFERENCES

1. National AIDS Control Organization. National Guidelines for HIV Care and Treatment. Government of India: Ministry of Health; 2021.

2. National Neonatology Forum, Federation of Obstetric & Gynaecological Societies of India, Indian Academy of Pediatrics (2021). Perinatal-Neonatal Management of COVID-19. [online] Available from https://www.nnfi.org/cpg and https://www.fogsi.org/wp-content/uploads/gcpr/perinatal-neonatal-management-of-covid-19.pdf. [Last accessed January, 2023].

3. More K, Chawla D, Murki S, Tandur B, Deorari AK, Kumar P, et al. Outcomes of Neonates Born to Mothers with Coronavirus Disease 2019 (COVID-19)—National Neonatology Forum (NNF) India COVID-19 registry. Indian Pediatr. 2021;58(6):525-31.

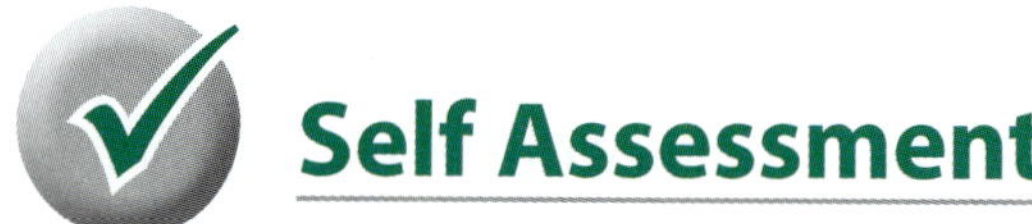

Self Assessment

State TRUE or FALSE

1. Breastmilk can transmit the HIV virus and hence neonates born to HIV positive mothers should be exclusively fed with formula milk.

2. The delivery of a HIV positive woman should be conducted in a separate labor room.

3. Antiretroviral prophylaxis should be initiated for all exposed neonates irrespective of mode of feeding.

4. Birth immunization should be deferred till the confirmation of HIV status of the neonate by HIV DNA PCR.

5. Pediatrician performing the resuscitation of a neonate born to HIV-positive woman is not at risk of occupational exposure.

6. Cord should be clamped within 10 seconds for a baby born to symptomatic mother with COVID-19.

7. Skin-to-skin contact should be done only after giving a bath to the baby born to COVID-positive mother.

8. COVID-positive women should wear a triple layered surgical mask during and after delivery.

9. The baby should be kept 2 meters away from the mother who is COVID positive.

10. All babies born to COVID-positive mothers should be isolated in COVID nursery for first 48 hours.

Answers

For answers, go to the end of the Book, Page no. 323

Postresuscitation Care

Postresuscitation Care: Management of Hypoxia and Other Issues

Sushma Nangia

Lessons to Learn

- Care to be offered to neonates after they have been resuscitated in the delivery room.
- Morbidities that are to be anticipated during postresuscitation phase.
- Supportive and organ-specific management following neonatal resuscitation.
- Role of therapeutic hypothermia in neonates during postresuscitation care, especially in low- and middle-income countries.
- Outcomes in asphyxiated neonates.

Approximately 10% of neonates require some assistance at birth but perinatal asphyxia accounts for nearly 20% of neonatal deaths.[1] Among the neonates that require support to initiate breathing, majority require basic steps of resuscitation whereas a minuscule group of neonates require advanced steps and aggressive resuscitation. All those requiring advanced resuscitation, get admitted to the neonatal intensive care unit (NICU) for further assessment and management, whereas most of the neonates requiring basic steps of resuscitation would be stable enough to be shifted with their mothers.

The current recommendations state *"Newly born infants who receive prolonged positive pressure ventilation (PPV) or advanced resuscitation (intubation, chest compressions, or epinephrine) should be maintained in or transferred to an environment where close monitoring can be provided"* (strong recommendation, low quality evidence).[2] However, some aspects are still not precisely defined such as the duration of PPV that qualifies as a significant criterion for admission to NICU and for how long should the monitoring continue. The evidence as to whether all neonates requiring resuscitation (basic or advanced steps) at birth need admission to NICU remains equivocal. If only some babies who needed resuscitation in the delivery room require NICU admission, we need to identify that subgroup. For those neonates, deemed to be stable enough by the treating physician to be shifted with their mothers, it is important to define what to monitor and at what frequency. The guidelines for postresuscitation care are not uniform and hence difficult to generalize. It may be pertinent to note that training healthcare professionals in neonatal resuscitation alone may not be sufficient to reduce neonatal mortality unless they are also equipped with the knowledge of postresuscitation care—this will have greater impact on intact survival rather than mere survival.

■ INTRODUCTION TO POSTRESUSCITATION CARE

Importance of Postresuscitation Care

The nature and duration of postresuscitation care required by a neonate may vary significantly depending on the degree of perinatal depression. Although some of these infants can be at high risk for further deterioration, others may be stable enough to require essential neonatal care.[3] Admission of all initially depressed low-risk infants for postresuscitation care may cause unnecessary separation of the mother-baby dyad leading to compromised bonding and breastfeeding and increasing parental anxiety. In addition, the higher number of resultant admissions can add a significant burden to hospital resources and the healthcare system along with the potential for added morbidity related to healthcare-associated infections. Moreover, most of the time, the nature, duration, and level of postresuscitation care provided are left to the clinician's discretion which largely depends on the experience of the care provider leading to marked variability in practice in part due to the availability of different guidelines. Hence, it is important to define the admission criteria for such neonates.

Defining Postresuscitation Care

Babies needing postresuscitation care generally would require supplemental oxygen, continuous positive airway pressure (CPAP) or positive pressure ventilation (PPV), after delivery. Such neonates will need closer assessment as they may develop problems associated with abnormal transition and should be evaluated frequently during the immediate newborn period. Many will require admission to an NICU where continuous cardiorespiratory monitoring is available and vital signs can be measured frequently.[4]

Postresuscitation care could be defined as the care required by neonates, who received PPV for 1 minute or longer after birth or required more extensive resuscitation, as these infants are at a high risk of further deterioration. It also includes neonates with respiratory distress after birth or preterm infants in whom CPAP is needed for initial stabilization.

Neonates who required only initial steps at birth or PPV for less than 1 minute can be shifted with their mothers and provided *observational care* that includes monitoring of temperature, breathing, heart rate, and activity apart from the establishment of breastfeeding. Such

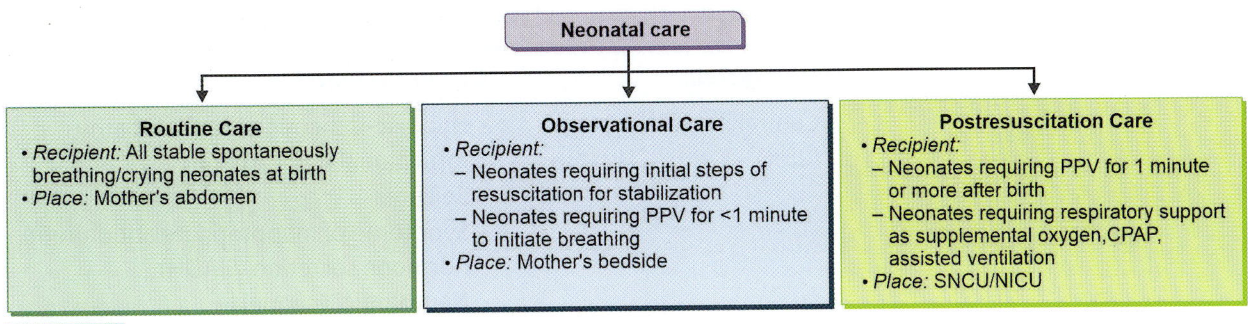

FIG. 14.1 Types of care after birth.
(CPAP: continuous positive airway pressure; NICU: neonatal intensive care unit; PPV: positive pressure ventilation; SNCU: special newborn care unit)

neonates can be monitored every 15–30 minutes during the first 2 hours of life. *Figure* **14.1** outlines the types of care that a neonate after delivery may be placed in.

Retrospective analysis has shown that neonates requiring PPV for even short duration (<1 minute) may require special newborn care unit (SNCU) admission if associated with high-risk factors such as placental abruption, assisted delivery, small-for-dates, gestational age <37 weeks, and low 5-minute APGAR score, etc. whereas, the neonates that require PPV for a longer duration (≥1 minute) are more likely to develop multiple morbidities and require specialized neonatal care.[5]

Setting for Providing Postresuscitation Care

The location for providing postresuscitation care is either SNCU or NICU. But more than the location, ensuring appropriate monitoring is the key to successful management. Prompt recognition of the signs that require immediate care is necessary for initiating treatment. To avoid missing out on such cases it is advisable to admit these neonates to the SNCU or NICU.

Consequences of Perinatal Asphyxia

Perinatal asphyxia is a multiorgan disorder affecting virtually every organ system of the body **(Table 14.1)**.[6] Knowledge and orientation towards determining the severity of organ dysfunction are essential for providing appropriate care as some of these complications are potentially fatal. The extent of multiorgan dysfunction determines the early outcome of an asphyxiated neonate. The most severely affected babies may manifest with stupor or coma, periodic breathing, or irregular respiration, hypotonia and loss of neonatal reflexes such as Moro reflex and sucking reflex. About 50% of the moderate-to-severely asphyxiated babies may have seizures. Severely affected babies may have progressive deterioration of their central nervous system function presenting as decreasing tone, increasing degree of sensorial alteration, and prolonged apnea over the next 48–72 hours.

TABLE 14.1: Organ Dysfunction in Perinatal Asphyxia	
Organ system	**Organ dysfunction**
1. Central nervous system (28%)[6]	• Hypoxic-ischemic encephalopathy • Intracranial hemorrhage • Seizures • Syndrome of inappropriate antidiuretic hormone secretion (SIADH) • Neurological sequelae
2. Cardiovascular (25%)[6]	• Poor myocardial and valvular function
3. Renal (50%)[6]	• Ischemic kidney injury • Acute tubular necrosis • Renal vein thrombosis
4. Gastrointestinal tract	• Ischemic bowel injury • Hepatic dysfunction
5. Pulmonary (25%)[6]	• Surfactant dysfunction • Delayed adaptation • Pulmonary hypertension • Meconium aspiration • Respiratory failure
6. Hematological	• Coagulation abnormality
7. Metabolic	• Hypocalcemia • Hypoglycemia • Hyponatremia • Acidosis

These neonates would eventually die or have permanent neurologic sequelae. Current evidence suggests that a cord "base deficit" of 12–16 mmol/L is associated with encephalopathy in 10% of neonates and with a base deficit of >16 mmol/L the risk of encephalopathy increases to 40%.[7]

■ MANAGEMENT DURING POSTRESUSCITATION CARE

Stepwise management of neonates requiring postresuscitation care consists of initial assessment and stabilization followed by prompt supportive care and organ-specific management.

Assessment

It includes monitoring vital parameters with special emphasis on temperature, oxygenation, perfusion, and neurological status of the neonate. This should be coupled with keeping a close watch for organ dysfunction. These infants should be monitored for:

- Temperature
- Airway, breathing, oxygenation (SpO_2, respiratory distress scoring)
- Circulation, perfusion

- Blood sugar
- For monitoring the neurological status, a staging system can be adopted as per the unit policy [Sarnat and Sarnat staging or Levene Staging **(Table 14.2)** or Thompson Score], which will guide in prompt recognition of the deteriorating neurological status of the neonate.

TABLE 14.2: CLASSIFICATION OF HYPOXIC ISCHEMIC ENCEPHALOPATHY (LEVENE STAGING)

Features	Mild	Moderate	Severe
Consciousness	Irritable	Lethargy	Comatose
Tone	Hypotonia	Marked hypotonia	Severe hypotonia (flaccid)
Seizures	No	Yes	Prolonged or uncontrolled
Sucking	Poor suck	Unable to suck	Absent suck
Respiration	Spontaneous	Periodic or irregular	Unable to sustain spontaneous respiration

Supportive Care

It aims to maintain temperature, perfusion, ventilation, and a normal metabolic state including glucose, calcium, and acid-base balance. Early detection by clinical and biochemical monitoring and prompt management of "deviations from normal range" of the above parameters must be done to prevent extension of cerebral injury. The primary insult may not be reversible but secondary extension of injury can be prevented by providing appropriate supportive care and organ-specific management. **Table 14.3** outlines the supportive care needed for such neonates.

TABLE 14.3: SUPPORTIVE CARE MANAGEMENT IN POSTRESUSCITATION CARE

Parameters	Management
Maintenance of temperature	• Temperature should be maintained in the normal range of 36.5–37.5°C. • Place the baby under a radiant warmer • Uncontrolled hypothermia and hyperthermia are both detrimental and worsen the outcome. • Passive cooling should be avoided as it may be harmful. • If facility for therapeutic hypothermia is available in a nearby tertiary care center, referral may be considered preferably within the first few hours (<6 hours).
Maintenance of airway and breathing	• Patent airway should be maintained by appropriate positioning and clearing any secretions if present. • Breathing should be monitored and supported as required. • Oxygenation should be kept in the normal range by monitoring oxygen saturation by pulse oximetry.

Contd...

Contd...

Parameters	Management
Maintenance of oxygenation and ventilation	• SpO$_2$ should be maintained between 91 and 95%. • Hypoxia should be treated with supplemental oxygen. • If hypoxia persists the neonate may need CPAP or mechanical ventilation in cases of inadequate spontaneous breathing efforts, apnea or in cases of hypercapnia. • Hypoxia and hypercarbia should be avoided as the resultant cerebral vasodilatation may lead to micro-hemorrhages increasing cerebral injury and worsen the outcome. • Hyperoxia and hypocarbia should also be avoided as the resultant cerebral vasoconstriction causes ischemic infarcts and worsens cerebral injury. • Maintain pCO$_2$ between 35 and 45 mm Hg and pO$_2$ between 60 and 90 mm Hg
• Maintenance of perfusion	• Ensure normal perfusion—maintain capillary refill time <3 seconds, absence of tachycardia, blood pressure within normal limits, and normal urine output • May require volume expanders and vasopressors to maintain the perfusion • *Blood pressure (BP):* In an asphyxiated neonate cerebral blood flow depends on systemic blood pressure. Hence, maintain systemic mean arterial BP at 40 mm Hg for term infants. The mean BP (in mm Hg) for preterm neonates should be maintained equal to gestational age in weeks. • If the neonate is in shock manage with fluid resuscitation followed by vasopressor support as required.
• Fluid therapy	• Start intravenous fluid (parenteral nutrition) depending on the clinical status of the neonate (in those with encephalopathy, severe respiratory distress, shock, and moderate-to-severe asphyxia) • Strictly monitor urine output • Do not restrict the fluid routinely except in cases of renal failure or SIADH.
• Enteral feeding	• *Not all babies require prolonged IV fluids and many can be fed enterally by gavage, spoon or at the breast.* • Assess for feeding every 4–6 hours. As soon as the baby is hemodynamically stable, there is no abdominal distension and the baby has passed meconium, start enteral feeds with expressed breast milk (EBM) @ 30 mL/kg/day and increase daily by 20–30 mL/kg/day or more as the baby tolerates
• Metabolic euglycemia	• Blood glucose should be monitored for at least first 48 hours. • If the baby is hypoglycemic, initiate treatment using glucose infusion @ 6 mg/kg/minute. • Avoid both hypo- and hyperglycemia
• Maintain normal calcium and hematocrit	• Administer calcium, only if there is documented hypocalcemia • In case of hypocalcemia, administer calcium as infusion in 1:1 dilution as a bolus, under cardiac monitoring • Maintain hematocrit in the range of 45–55% • Avoid both anemia and polycythemia
• Maintain acid-base balance	• Prevent metabolic acidosis by maintaining adequate perfusion • No evidence to support use of sodium bicarbonate to treat acidosis
• Additional supportive measures	• Ensure asepsis • Ensure gentle handling • Provide developmentally supportive care • Promote family participatory care

(CPAP: continuous positive airway pressure; SIADH: syndrome of inappropriate antidiuretic hormone secretion)

TABLE 14.4: ORGAN-SPECIFIC MANAGEMENT

Organ system	Clinical parameters	Investigational work-up	Management
Respiratory	Tachypnea, retractions, grunting, saturation lower than the target range	Consider sepsis screen, chest X-ray, and blood gas depending on the clinical status	• Maintain adequate oxygenation and ventilation • Consider surfactant therapy, if surfactant deficiency/dysfunction suspected (e.g., meconium aspiration syndrome) • Consider antibiotics if pneumonia suspected
	Oxygen lability: >5% difference in upper limb and lower limb saturation	2D echocardiography, if available, to rule out pulmonary hypertension and structural malformation of the heart	If pulmonary hypertension is present, after lung recruitment, treat with a pulmonary vasodilator (sildenafil/inhaled nitric oxide)
	Decreased air entry or chest rise	Transillumination test, chest X-ray, lung USG (if expertise is available)	Manage according to the diagnosis. May require immediate needle aspiration or intercostal tube drainage in case of significant pneumothorax
Cardiovascular	Signs suggestive of shock—tachycardia, low systemic perfusion, low blood pressure, metabolic acidosis, low urine output	• Invasive blood pressure monitoring if facility available • Blood gas analysis • Echocardiography, if available, helps in the assessment of cardiac function and in evaluating IVC collapsibility status • Echocardiography can also indicate cardiogenic shock—poor cardiac contractibility, ejection fraction and low cardiac output	• Consider use of volume expander and vasopressor as required • If cardiogenic shock, consider adding dobutamine or milrinone. Both these drugs are potent vasodilators, requires strict monitoring of blood pressure
Renal	Decreased urine output, peripheral edema	• Serum electrolytes, kidney function test, ultrasound KUB • Urine electrolytes, specific gravity	• Maintain urine output and electrolyte within normal range. • Monitor weight for volume overload. • Restrict fluid only if there is excess weight gain or signs suggestive of fluid overload or in cases of syndrome of inappropriate antidiuretic hormone (SIADH).

Contd...

Contd...

Organ system	Clinical parameters	Investigational work-up	Management
Gastrointestinal	Feed intolerance	• Sepsis screen • X-ray and ultrasound abdomen, as required	• Monitor closely for any signs of feed intolerance • Neonates with severe asphyxia may require gradual increase of feed volume along with parenteral nutrition for initial few days • Minimal enteral feeds can be initiated in neonates receiving therapeutic hypothermia
	Gastrointestinal bleeding	Liver function test, PT INR, APTT, d-dimer	• Continuous gastric aspirate • Injection vitamin K_1 • FFP, as required
Hematological	Bleeding, bruises, petechiae, pallor	• Complete blood counts (for anemia, thrombocytopenia) • PT INR, APTT, d-dimer • Liver function test	• Monitor closely for bleeding and any abnormality in the coagulation profile. • Injection vitamin K_1 • May require FFP and/or platelet transfusion
Neurological	• Encephalopathy, seizures, irritability, hyperalert state or hypotonia • Feeding coordination related difficulty	• Serum electrolytes, serum calcium and blood glucose • USG cranium, MRI brain, aEEG • Near Infrared spectroscopy (NIRS) for monitoring tissue oxygenation if facility available	• Seizures might be due to metabolic abnormalities such as hypoglycemia, hypocalcemia—correct accordingly • Seizures might require anticonvulsant therapy • Avoid hyperthermia • Consider therapeutic hypothermia, if the eligibility criteria is fulfilled and facility for the same is available. • Continue supportive care • Oro-motor stimulation exercises for better feeding coordination
Metabolic	Lethargy, poor feeding, seizures, jitteriness, stupor, shock	• Blood sugar • Serum calcium • Serum electrolyte • Blood gas analysis • ECG may be required	• If hypoglycemia, start glucose infusion @6 mg/kg/min to maintain euglycemia after initial bolus of glucose • If hypocalcemia, infuse calcium under cardiac monitoring • Manage sodium and potassium disturbances • Manage acid-base disturbances • Manage shock

Organ-specific Monitoring and Management

Table 14.4 outlines the organ-specific monitoring and management. Some specific management issues are detailed in this section.

Seizures

After initial stabilization of the neonate, identify the treatable causes as these should not be overlooked.

Hypoglycemia: If the blood sugar level is <45 mg/dL, give 2 mL/kg of 10% dextrose as a bolus and simultaneously start with continuous glucose infusion @6 mg/kg/min. Continue monitoring of blood sugar and increase glucose infusion rate as per the requirement, for maintenance of euglycemia.

Hypocalcemia: If the blood sugar is normal, send samples for serum calcium level estimation and simultaneously give 10% calcium gluconate as a bolus of 2 mL/kg IV over 10 minutes. This should be diluted in an equal volume of distilled water and is administered slowly using an infusion pump (withhold infusion if the heart rate is <100 beats/minute) along with cardiac monitoring.

Anticonvulsant medication:[8,9] These medications should be administered if no hypoglycemia or hypocalcemia is detected or if seizures persist even after correction of hypoglycemia and hypocalcemia:

- *1st line anticonvulsant:* Injection phenobarbitone 20 mg/kg IV should be given as an infusion over 20 minutes. If the baby has no further seizures, there is no need to start maintenance dose of the drug.

  If the seizures persist or recur after a loading dose of phenobarbitone, administer further boluses of 5 mg/kg as IV infusion, up to a total of 40 mg/kg. Start maintenance phenobarbitone at a dose of 3–4 mg/kg/day after 12 hours of the loading dose of phenobarbitone.

- *2nd line anticonvulsant:* The next choice of medication if seizures are persisting is injection phenytoin or fosphenytoin 20 mg/kg given as IV infusion over 20 minutes. Maintenance dose of phenytoin is initiated at a dose of 3–5 mg/kg/day after 12 hours of the bolus dose.

  Both phenobarbitone and phenytoin are administered at a maximum rate of 1 mg/kg/minute. Phenytoin should only be mixed with saline and not with dextrose as it precipitates in dextrose.

- *Levetiracetam* is popularly used in neonates as a second-line drug based on its safety profile in the pediatric population. There is need for further studies for providing more evidence for its use in the neonatal population.

- *Lidocaine* can also be used as a second-line agent but is less popularly utilized due to its limited availability and side effect profile.

- *Benzodiazepines* are used when the seizures cannot be controlled despite the use of a second-line agent. *Lorazepam and midazolam* are the most often used agents. Lorazepam is preferred due to its longer duration of action and lesser adverse events.

Table 14.5 provides a summary for the use of anticonvulsant drugs in neonates.

Discontinuation of the antiepileptic agent: It is preferable to stop anticonvulsants before the discharge of the neonate, but the overall duration depends on the neonatal neurological examination, cause of seizure/expected degree of control, and associated specialized investigations like electroencephalogram (EEG) **(Table 14.6)**.

Hypotension

There are multiple reasons accounting for low blood pressure in a neonate during the postresuscitation phase. These include: (i) hypoxia at the time of birth resulting in decreased cardiac function and tone of

TABLE 14.5: ANTICONVULSANT DRUGS IN NEONATES

Drug	Dosage	Remarks
1. Phenobarbitone	• 20 mg/kg IV as a loading dose followed by maintenance only in cases where there is a repeat episode of seizure requiring reloading of the drug • A maintenance dose is started after 12 hours of the first dose, 3–5 mg/kg IV	• Watch for sedation, hypotension, and respiratory failure • It can lead to electrochemical dissociation • Seems to increase neuronal apoptosis and may impair neurodevelopmental outcomes
2. Phenytoin or fosphenytoin	20 mg/kg followed by 3–5 mg/kg (maximum 8 mg/kg) IV	• 1.5 mg/kg of fosphenytoin is equivalent to 1 mg/kg of phenytoin • Fosphenytoin has less side effect as it causes less hypotension and cardiac abnormalities
Important points: • The rate of infusion for both phenobarbitone and phenytoin should not exceed 1 mg/kg/minute. • Cochrane review—comparable seizure control of phenobarbitone and phenytoin (with both controlling seizures in only half)[7] • WHO guidelines recommend phenobarbitone as the first-line agent for the management of neonatal seizures.[8]		
3. Midazolam	0.15 mg/kg bolus followed by infusion of 0.1–0.5 mg/kg/hour	• Known to have an impact on development • Faster acting, less respiratory depression, and sedation than lorazepam • Monitor for respiratory depression, apnea, and bradycardia
4. Lorazepam	0.05 mg/kg IV bolus every 8–12 hours	• Monitor for respiratory depression, hypotension, depressed consciousness
Do not use diazepam to control seizures in neonates		
5. Levetiracetam	40 mg/kg followed by 40 mg/kg every 8–12 hourly	Not approved by US Food and Drug Administration in neonates
6. Lidocaine	2 mg/kg IV bolus, then 6 mg/kg/hour drip, then titrate down by 2 mg/kg/hour every 12 hours until off	Commonly associated side effects such as arrhythmia, hypotension

TABLE 14.6: Duration of Anticonvulsant Therapy in Neonates	
Condition	**Plan of action**
Metabolic cause (hypocalcemia, hypoglycemia)	Treat the underlying cause. No need to continue antiepileptic agent
Seizures controlled with single-dose administration of phenobarbitone	No maintenance anticonvulsant is required Keep the baby under observation for further episode of seizures
Seizures controlled with multiple doses of phenobarbitone and are on maintenance dose of phenobarbitone	Stop phenobarbitone after 48 hours of seizure-free period
Multiple anticonvulsants required to control seizures	Start withdrawing anticonvulsants once the neonate is seizure free for 48 hours. This depends on the overall neurological state of the neonate
If neurological state is abnormal at discharge	May continue anticonvulsant in consultation with a pediatric neurologist
Assess neurological status at 1 month	If normal—stop phenobarbitone If abnormal—may continue anticonvulsant in consultation with a pediatric neurologist
If neurological status abnormal at 1 month or later	Consult pediatric neurologist or decide according to the neurological condition of neonates

the blood vessels; (ii) significant blood loss during delivery; and (iii) sepsis resulting in hypotension because of the dilation of blood vessels. Volume expansion may be required in cases of hypotension. Some babies may require medications such as dopamine, dobutamine, or epinephrine to maintain cardiac output and systemic blood flow.

▮ THERAPEUTIC HYPOTHERMIA

The current recommendations for therapeutic hypothermia (TH) state *"Newly born infants born at 36 weeks or more estimated gestational age with evolving moderate-to-severe hypoxic-ischemic encephalopathy (HIE) should be offered therapeutic hypothermia under clearly defined protocols"* (strong recommendation, high quality evidence)[2]. TH has demonstrated a significant reduction in death or disability at 18 months of age if initiated within 4–6 hours of birth and continued for 72 hours. Most of this data is from high-income countries (HIC) where health care is more organized than in low and middle-income-countries (LMIC). The International Liaison Committee on Resuscitation (ILCOR) in its 2020 guidelines had recommended as follows for the use of TH in settings with limited resources:

"We suggest that newborn infants at term or near-term with evolving moderate-to-severe hypoxic-ischemic encephalopathy in low-income countries and/or other settings with limited resources may be treated with therapeutic hypothermia (weak recommendation, low-quality evidence).

Cooling should only be considered, initiated, and conducted under clearly defined protocols with treatment in neonatal care facilities with the capabilities for multidisciplinary care and availability of adequate resources to offer intravenous therapy, respiratory support, pulse oximetry, antibiotics, anticonvulsants, and pathology testing. Treatment should be consistent with the protocols used in the randomized clinical trials in developed countries, i.e., cooling to commence within 6 hours, strict temperature control at 33–34°C for 72 hours and rewarming over at least 4 hours."[4]

However, the recent Hypothermia for Encephalopathy in Low and middle-income countries (HELIX) trial[10] which had enrolled 408 subjects reported that among neonates with HIE, TH has no effect on the primary outcome of death and/or moderate/severe disability at 18–24 months (RR: 1.06; 0.87–1.30); but it was observed that one of the many secondary outcomes—the risk of death before discharge was significantly increased in the hypothermia group (RR: 1.50; 95% CI: 1.10–2.04).

Therapeutic Hypothermia in India

In view of the inconclusive evidence with respect to use of TH in LMICs, particularly in the Indian context, the National Neonatology Forum released a position statement on the use of TH for HIE in India.[11] They concluded as follows:

- Therapeutic hypothermia is likely to decrease death or severe disability and cerebral palsy at 18–24 months even in LMICs as compared to HICs.

- There is significant heterogeneity in the studies from LMICs compared to HICs which reported mortality prior to discharge following TH in neonates with HIE. The pooled estimates for mortality prior to discharge showed a significant benefit in favor of TH (RR 0.77, 95%CI 0.62–0.94) in HICs. In the studies from LMICs there was uncertainty (RR: 0.74; 0.53–1.02); a possible reason could be the lack of certainty of the encephalopathy being due to an asphyxial insult.

- Mortality before discharge when analyzed for infants with moderate-severe HIE with cord pH <7.0 or did not report cord pH, there was considerable heterogeneity and no benefit in survival prior to discharge.

- In neonates with hypothermia at admission and unclear evidence of severe intrapartum asphyxia (cord pH ≥7.0 or cord pH not available—more often seen amongst outborn neonates in LMICs) there is uncertainty of the benefit from TH (ranging from benefit to harm).

- As the risk of death increases with severe encephalopathy, need for invasive ventilation, and inotropic support, availability of optimum neonatal intensive care facilities is essential if TH is to be offered at a health facility.

- Besides the factors alluded to earlier for the variations in outcomes between HIC and LMIC following TH in neonates with HIE, the possible effects of ethnicity, biologic factors, and differences in intrauterine exposures on outcomes of neonates with moderate-severe HIE would need further investigation.

Which Neonates should be Offered Therapeutic Hypothermia?

The National Neonatology Forum (NNF) position statement[11] has proposed the following criteria for identifying eligible neonates for TH:

Therapeutic hypothermia should be offered to neonates with a gestational age of ≥36 weeks within 6 hours of life with an admission temperature between 36 and 37.4°C, if they fulfill all of the following criteria:

1. pH <7 or BE >-16 on a cord or arterial blood gas done within 1 hour of life AND

    a. Apgar score <5 at 10 minutes or at least 10 minutes of PPV, AND

    b. History of acute perinatal event (such as but not limited to placental abruption, uterine rupture, and cord prolapse) along with

2. Evidence of moderate or severe encephalopathy.

■ PROGNOSIS

Addressing asphyxia timely is mandatory as it is associated with both short and long-term consequences. Some of them are listed in **Table 14.7**. The overall outcome of a neonate depends on the severity of the brain injury encountered at the time of birth, appropriate resuscitative measures offered, and optimum postresuscitation care provided. The overall mortality rate is about 20% and the frequency of neurodevelopmental sequelae amongst survivors is approximately 30%. More than 50% of infants with stage III HIE die; and those who survived have severe sequelae. Amongst those who experience HIE

TABLE 14.7: SHORT- AND LONG-TERM OUTCOME PARAMETERS OF THE NEONATE WITH ASPHYXIA	
Short term	Respiratory morbidity, cardiac dysfunction, electrolyte imbalance, HIE, seizures, death
Long term	*Motor:* Cerebral palsy, motor deficit
	Sensory: Hearing, speech, and visual impairment
	Cognitive: Delay and impairment
	Behavior: Short attention span, attention deficit hyperactivity disorder, autistic spectrum disorder, irritability, psychosocial issues, and lower academic performance.

(HIE: hypoxic ischemic encephalopathy).

II, up to 80% are reported to have normal outcome and the rest die or have abnormal neurodevelopmental outcomes. Prognosis can be refined using EEG and magnetic resonance imaging (MRI) studies to detect the severity of encephalopathy and seizures, and the severity and location of hypoxic-ischemic brain injury. This group may benefit the most from TH. Those neonates that have mild encephalopathy have a <1% mortality rate.

▇ QUALITY IMPROVEMENT INITIATIVE

For keeping track of how effectively recommendations have been incorporated into practice, standardized indicators must be used. Some suggested quality improvement indicators are provided here:

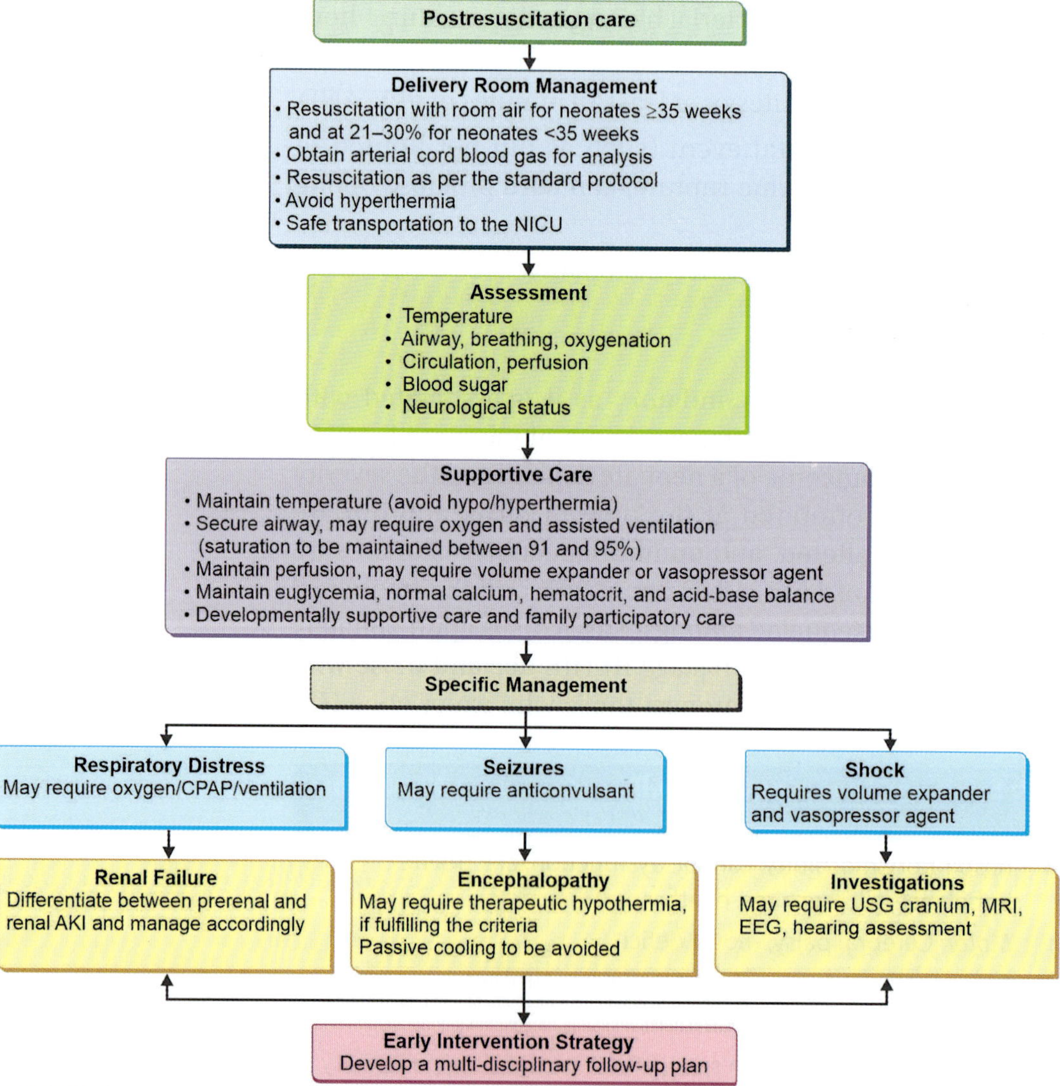

FIG. 14.2 Summary of postresuscitation care.
(AKI: acute kidney injury; CPAP: continuous positive airway pressure; EEG: electroencephalogram; NICU: neonatal intensive care unit; PPV: positive pressure ventilation).

- Proportion of neonates requiring postresuscitation care who are transported to NICU/SNCU.
- Proportion of neonates requiring postresuscitation care who are normothermic on admission to the NICU/SNCU.
- Proportion of neonates having complete documentation of their postresuscitation care.

When gaps are identified, every possible action must be considered to improve the quality of care.

CONCLUSION

The absence of definitive treatment for asphyxiated neonates despite extensive research once again poses the most fundamental question—what can be done better to prevent long-term sequelae or is there a neuroprotective strategy to reverse this process?

Neonatal resuscitation is the cardinal step in management of asphyxiated neonates but equally important is the timely and appropriate postresuscitation care of such neonates with constant vigil by healthcare providers so as to achieve intact survival. This requires not only good antenatal and intrapartum care but also quality care of the neonate during the postresuscitation phase and beyond. Allowing the parents to become part of the decision-making process is crucial. (*Fig.* **14.2**).

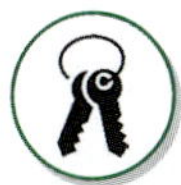 **KEY POINTS**

1. Neonates requiring positive pressure ventilation (PPV) for more than 1 minute and those requiring respiratory support as supplemental oxygen, continuous positive airway pressure (CPAP), and assisted ventilation, require admission to neonatal intensive care unit (NICU)/special newborn care unit (SNCU) for postresuscitation care. This care includes close monitoring of respiratory efforts, oxygenation, blood glucose, hemodynamic stability, neurological status, and temperature.
2. Multiorgan dysfunction is encountered frequently in neonates requiring extensive resuscitation. Close monitoring and assessment along with supportive care and organ-specific management are required for a good outcome.
3. Therapeutic hypothermia in low- and middle-income countries (LMICs) must be offered with caution. It must be offered only to those neonates fulfilling eligibility criteria, in units with capabilities for multidisciplinary care and availability of adequate resources to offer quality tertiary level neonatal care.
4. All asphyxiated neonates at discharge must have a multidisciplinary follow-up plan to ensure better long-term neurological outcome.

REFERENCES

1. American Academy of Pediatrics and American Heart Association. In: Weiner GM, Zaichkin J (Eds). Textbook of Neonatal Resuscitation, 8th edition. Illinois, USA: American Academy of Paediatrics; 2021.

2. Aziz K, Lee CHC, Escobedo MB, Hoover AV, Kamath-Rayne BD, Kapadia VS, et al. Part 5: Neonatal Resuscitation 2020 American Heart Association Guidelines for Cardiopulmonary Resuscitation and Emergency Cardiovascular Care. Pediatrics. 2021;147(Suppl 1):e2020038505E.

3. Ringer SA, Aziz K. Neonatal stabilization and post-resuscitation care. Clin Perinatol. 2012;39(4):901-18.

4. Wyckoff MH, Wyllie J, Aziz K, de Almeida MF, Fabres J, Fawke J, et al. Neonatal life support: 2020 international consensus on cardiopulmonary resuscitation and emergency cardiovascular care science with treatment recommendations. Circulation. 2020;142(16_suppl_1):S185-221.

5. Akinloye O, O'Connell C, Allen AC, El-Naggar W. Post-resuscitation care for neonates receiving positive pressure ventilation at birth. Pediatrics. 2014;134(4):e1057-62.

6. Perlman JM, Tack ED, Martin T, Shackelford G, Amon E. Acute systemic organ injury in term infants after asphyxia. Am J Dis Child. 1989;143(5):617-20.

7. Volpe JJ. Intrauterine, Intrapartum assessment in the term infant. In: Neurology of the Newborn. Philadelphia: WB Saunders; 2018. pp. 458-83.

8. Booth D, Evans DJ. Anticonvulsants for neonates with seizures. Cochrane Database Syst Rev. 2004;(4):CD004218.

9. WHO. Guidelines on neonatal seizures. Geneva: World Health Organization; 2011.

10. Thayyil S, Pant S, Montaldo P, Shukla D, Oliveira V, Ivain P, et al. Hypothermia for moderate or severe neonatal encephalopathy in low-income and middle-income countries (HELIX): a randomised controlled trial in India, Sri Lanka, and Bangladesh. Lancet Glob Health. 2021;9(9):e1273-85.

11. National Neonatology Forum, India. (2021). Position Statement and Guidelines for the Use of Therapeutic Hypothermia (TH) to Treat Neonatal Hypoxic Ischemic Encephalopathy (HIE) in India. [online] Available from http://nnfi.org/assests/pdf/ NNF_Position_statement_ and_Guidelines_for_TH%20_Final_(10112021)-converted. Pdf [Last accessed January, 2023].

Self Assessment

1. A male baby is delivered at 35 weeks of gestation. The baby did not cry immediately after birth and required initial steps of resuscitation followed by positive pressure ventilation (PPV) for 30 seconds to initiate breathing. Now the baby is breathing spontaneously and has a heart rate >100 bpm. What are your next steps for this baby?

2. A term baby did not cry immediately after birth and received positive pressure ventilation for 90 seconds. Where do you think this baby should be managed?

3. What parameters do you think need to be assessed in these neonates requiring prolonged PPV or advanced resuscitation?

4. What specific treatment would you offer for a neonate born by emergency cesarean section due to cord prolapse requiring PPV for 10 minutes after birth with cord arterial gas having a pH of –6.9 and BE –18 and has features of moderate encephalopathy?

5. What advice should be given to the parents of neonates with moderate-to-severe encephalopathy at the time of discharge?

Answers

For answers, go to the end of the Book, Page no. 323

Evidence-base for Neonatal Resuscitation Practices

Evidence-base for Neonatal Resuscitation Practices: Initial Steps

Shashi Kant Dhir, Dheeraj Shah, Piyush Gupta

Lesson to Learn

- To summarize the findings from published research papers that have guided the current neonatal resuscitation practices related to the initial steps of neonatal resuscitation—effect of initial briefing and debriefing, warming, routine suction, tracheal intubation and suction in non-vigorous infants with meconium-stained amniotic fluid, timing of cord clamping and heart rate monitoring

- To provide evidence-based conclusions on various components of initial steps of neonatal resuscitation

Evidence-based medicine (EBM) involves the "conscientious, explicit, and judicious use of current best evidence in making decisions about the care of individual patients." Making available evidence-based guidelines and policies through a process of systematic retrieval of the best evidence available and its critical appraisal is an important step for promotion of practice of EBM. Neonatal resuscitation is one area where the most recent and best available evidence has always fed and guided the guideline development process, and organizations have not shied away from bringing out drastic changes based on the evidence, often replacing the practices based on traditional beliefs.

Neonatal resuscitation has witnessed a large growing body of evidence in the last few years. In this and the next chapter, the current evidence for the neonatal resuscitation practices will be presented. Current Neonatal Resuscitation Program (NRP) guidelines use the American Heart Association nomenclature for the class of recommendation (COR) and the level of evidence (LOE).[1] The COR and LOE indicate the strength of recommendation by the writing group and quality of available evidence, respectively. These have been described in **Box 15.1**.

BOX 15.1: DESCRIPTION OF CLASS OF RECOMMENDATION AND LEVEL OF EVIDENCE

Class	Recommendation	Benefit vs. Risk
Class 1	Strong	Potential benefit greatly outweighs the risk
Class 2a	Moderate	Benefit most likely outweighs the risk
Class 2b	Weak	Unknown whether benefit will outweigh the risk
Class 3	No benefit (moderate)	Equal likelihood of benefit and risk
	Harm (Strong)	Risk outweighs the potential benefit

Level	Studies Included
Level A	• High-quality evidence from >1 randomized controlled trial (RCT) • Meta-analyses of high-quality RCTs • One or more RCTs corroborated by high-quality registry studies
Level B-R (randomized)	• Moderate—quality evidence from 1 or more RCTs • Meta-analyses of moderate-quality RCTs
Level B-NR (non-randomized)	• Moderate—quality evidence from 1 or more well-designed, well-executed nonrandomized studies, observational studies, or registry studies • Meta-analyses of such studies
Level C-LD (Limited data)	• Randomized or nonrandomized observational or registry studies with limitations of design or execution • Meta-analyses of such studies • Physiological or mechanistic studies in human subjects
Level C-EO (Expert opinion)	• Consensus of expert opinion based on clinical experience

(RCT: randomized controlled trial)

◾ 1. BRIEFING-DEBRIEFING

The Concept

Attending the delivery and performing the neonatal resuscitation as per protocol has many steps which need to be followed with absolute diligence to achieve the desired outcome. There are high chances of committing medical errors during neonatal resuscitation as the processes and communications have to be followed in a particular manner during the whole event. Deviations from the protocol may have direct implications on neonatal mortality and morbidity. Therefore, using a systematic structured approach to apprise the entire team of their roles and responsibilities, and later analyzing the behavior of the team during the event is of utmost importance for the NRP.

Briefing is defined as an act of giving precise instructions or essential information to the team members so that they can perform in a well-coordinated manner.[2] In NRP, the "briefing" comprises of discussing the available antenatal information, including the risk factors, to anticipate the likely complications arising during the NRP, planning a team response for these, identifying a team leader by mutual consensus, delegating specific tasks to individual team members (receiving baby, initial assessment, positive pressure ventilation (PPV), intubation, chest compression, vascular access, reporting events, etc.), discussing the necessary disposables and equipment during the event, and identifying the need of—and planning for—additional help if needed.[3]

Debriefing is defined as "a constructive review of actions and thought processes after an event to promote reflective learning and improve clinical performance".[3] The usual sequence is what went well, what did not go well and what could be improved. An early quick debriefing may be followed by detailed debriefing later to identify the potential areas of improvement in the team. Corrective actions can then be taken to address the issues deliberated during the debriefing sessions.[4]

The Evidence Base for NRP Guidelines

Savoldelli, et al. randomized 42 anesthesia residents to "no debriefing", oral feedback and oral plus video feedback, and it was reported that there was improvement in the technical skills after debriefing.[5] This randomized controlled trial (RCT) (LOE 1) and 17 observational studies (LOE 3–4) showed briefing-debriefing to have better acquisition of cognitive and psychomotor domains of learning, and better efficiency, coordination of care, and infant outcomes. On the basis of these studies, briefing-debriefing was mentioned as an optional need for the first time in the NRP 2010 guidelines.[6] It was recommended to use the briefing-debriefing sessions as one of the educational and training techniques for teaching, assessment, and maintenance of NRP protocol knowledge and skill during the simulated patients and clinical activities.[6] The topic was not included in NRP 2015 guidelines for review. Based upon data showing improved efficiency, better teamwork, communication among members and favorable clinical outcomes; *the current NRP 2020 guidelines strongly recommend (COR 1, LOE C-LD) the inclusion of briefing-debriefing, especially in a high-risk delivery.*[7] These studies are described in **Table 15.1**.

Other Evidence

Recently, Fawke, et al.[13] published a scoping review on briefing and debriefing in neonatal resuscitation using International Liaison Committee on Resuscitation (ILCOR) methodology and results from four eligible studies and reported that as of now there is insufficient new evidence for justifying the conduction of fresh systematic reviews or reviewing of current NRP recommendations of 2020 on this topic.[13] They also reported on basis of these studies that there were improved processes of care, short-term clinical outcomes and decreased communication issues while using briefing-debriefing using videos, checklists, and rapid cycle deliberate practice.

TABLE 15.1: SUMMARY OF INTERVENTIONAL STUDIES FOR BRIEFING-DEBRIEFING DURING NEONATAL RESUSCITATION

Author, Year	Number of participants	Participants	Intervention	Results
Bennet et al., 2016[8]	10,839 deliveries in 24 NICUs	Neonates admitted in the NICUs in the California Perinatal Quality Care Collaborative (CPQCC)	Addition of the sections of briefing-debriefing in the checklists in the readiness bundle (RB) during the high-risk deliveries over 18 months	9/17 (53%) NICUs rated briefing-debriefing as most effective component of the readiness bundle. The compliance to the readiness bundle increased from baseline 0% to median 71% during initial 6 months of implementation and further to 80% after 6 months of completion of the collaborative. Pooled and Sustenance Median (interquartile range) was 73.3 (42.9, 85.7) and 79.5 (61.7, 91.7) respectively. 14/17 (82%) NICUs recommended the use of the RB in other NICUs.
Balakrishnan et al., 2017[9]	1,113 infants from nine NICUs	Inborn high-risk neonates admitted to nine Florida Hospitals included in delivery room management plan	Implementation of adapted checklist[7] and implementation of briefing (having a system which enabled the team members to know their roles pre-hand) and debriefing	Briefing before delivery was significantly associated ($p <0.001$) with a more complete equipment checks, clearer role assignment, and optimal usage of radiant warmers. Debriefing helped in getting feedback as well as in analyzing the communication gaps between the obstetrical and the resuscitation personnel.
Talati et al., 2019[10]	3771 resuscitations from nine NICUs	Neonates admitted to nine NICUs from Tennessee Perinatal Quality Collaborative	Introduction of the briefing-debriefing in the toolkit of potentially better practices and role assignment to each member of the team	Special Cause Improvements for role assignment were achieved and sustained for the team briefings (80–92%) and post-resuscitation debriefings (68–81%). There was improvement in the clinical outcomes following the toolkit of potentially better practices.
Litke-Wager et al., 2021[11]	108 simulations by 65 participants	62 residents and three nurses	*Intervention Group:* Task-oriented role assignment (TORA) training and standard NRP training *Control Group:* Standard NRP training alone	The initial TORA training resulted in improved behavior skill scores in 8/10 NRP key behavioral skills and higher overall behavioral skill scores (30.1 [±7.2] vs. 34.9 [±4.8]; $p <0.001$).

Contd...

Contd...

Author, Year	Number of participants	Participants	Intervention	Results
Katheria et al., 2013[12]	445 checklists over 3 years	NICU Team, including nurses, pediatrics residents, respiratory therapists	Checklist containing the briefing and debriefing was completed after high-risk delivery and later discussed in video-based resuscitation quality assurance meetings among the team members.	As compared to the initial 2 years of introducing the checklist, communication issues during debriefing in the 3rd year decreased from 22–4% (p <0.001).

One of the studies included in this scoping review[12] has already been included in evidence cited by NRP guidelines, and another study[14] which reported the use of a pre-brief and debriefing component into the checklist, was a primary intervention of the comprehensive quality improvement initiative to improve delivery room management of high-risk deliveries (CPQCC),[7] also described in NRP guidelines as part of a larger collaborative. In a prospective pre-post intervention study involving midwives and doctors attending compromised neonates of a Norway teaching hospital, Skåre, et al.[15] reported that usage of video recording-based debriefing of the real-time scenario had led to the improvement in the Neonatal Resuscitation Performance Evaluation score (77% vs. 89%, p <0.001). Significant improvement was also seen in group function/communication (88% vs. 100%, p = 0.001), preparation and initial steps (75% vs. 90%, p <0.001), and PPV (70% vs. 100%, p <0.005).[15]

Magee, et al.[16] conducted a randomized controlled trial in 38 interns posted in labor room comparing the effect of rapid cycle deliberate practice (RCDP), a type of debriefing in which facilitator provides continuous debriefing throughout the process, to standard simulation debriefing during NRP teaching session. The authors reported that participants using RCDP had better immediate score on the Megacode Assessment Form (89% vs. 84%, p = 0.026), could initiate PPV within 1 minute (100% vs. 71%, p = 0.045), and could administer adrenaline early (152 s vs. 180 s, p = 0.039).[16]

The isolated effect of briefing or debriefing separately from other interventions and long-term clinical outcomes still needs to be seen.

Conclusion

Briefing-debriefing is helpful, especially in a high-risk delivery to improve team coordination and efficiency in dealing with potential complications during resuscitation (COR 1, LOE C-LD).

▌2. ROUTINE SUCTIONING AT BIRTH

The Concept

The recommendations for clearing of the oral, nasal, pharyngeal, and tracheal airway during neonatal resuscitation have substantially changed over time. Oral and nasopharyngeal suction on the one hand can assist in the initiation of breathing by physical clearing of the secretions, but at the same time, is shown to be associated with complications such as hypoxemia, bradycardia, apnea, and deranged cerebral hemodynamics. The suction guidelines also varied depending upon whether or not the neonate was born through meconium-stained liquor and was vigorous at birth or not [vigorous defined as having heart rate (HR) >100 and normal tone and having good respiratory effort].[17]

The Evidence Support for Neonatal Resuscitation Program Guidelines

The very early guidelines (NRP 2005 and earlier) had recommended routine suctioning of any fluid (meconium as well as clear fluid) from the oral and nasal airway in all neonates, irrespective of the respiratory status.[18] Gungor, et al.[19,20] conducted two RCTs (n = 140) to evaluate the impact of "suctioning" versus "no suctioning" in healthy term infants born through clear amniotic fluid, and reported that routine oro-nasopharyngeal suctioning (ONPS) did not provide any extra benefit and was associated with lower oxygen saturation values. Velaphi and Vidyasagar reviewed the available literature from 1971–2006 and concluded that routine ONPS has more harms than benefits and was associated with bradycardia, apnea, and disturbances in the achieved oxygen saturation.[21] Taking cognition of these reported adverse effects associated with routine ONPS, a practice review was undertaken.[17] Based upon this review, NRP 2010 guidelines, mentioned that routine suctioning was not recommended in vigorous neonates born through clear or meconium-stained liquor. ONPS was recommended only if there was obstructed airway by secretions in an apneic, gasping or hypotonic neonate; and if there was need for positive pressure ventilation.[6]

A Cochrane review involving eight RCTs [five with clear amniotic fluid, two meconium-stained amniotic fluid (MSAF), and one clear or MSAF] having 4,011 neonates reported inconclusive results neither supporting nor refuting the benefits or harms of routine oro/nasopharyngeal suction over no suctioning for the following outcomes—mortality (RR 2.29, 95% CI 0.94–5.53, n = 3023; two trials), need for resuscitation (RR 0.85, 95% CI 0.69–1.06, n = 3791; five trials), admission to neonatal intensive care unit (NICU) (RR 0.82, 95% CI 0.62–1.08, n = 997; two trials), and APGAR scores at 5 minutes (MD = –0.03, 95% CI 0.08–0.02, n = 330; three trials).[17]

The recent NRP 2020 guidelines have continued with their earlier recommendation that routine oral, nasal, oropharyngeal, or endotracheal suctioning of neonates is of no benefit (COR-3, LOE C-LD), and hence not recommended.[7]

Conclusion

Routine oro/nasopharyngeal suctioning at birth in a neonate is not beneficial and should not be done (COR-3, LOE C-LD).

3. TRACHEAL SUCTIONING IN NEONATES BORN THROUGH MECONIUM-STAINED AMNIOTIC FLUID

The Concept

Meconium, a sterile, complex substance consisting of water, fetal desquamated cells, enzymes, mucin, lanugo, antigens, free fatty acids and bile, is usually passed after birth. However, it could be passed antenatally into the amniotic fluid if the fetus experiences hypoxia, acidosis, or utero-placental insufficiency, and has the potential to be aspirated during deep gasping respiration by the compromised fetus.

Meconium aspiration syndrome (MAS) is an important cause of neonatal mortality and morbidity, and symptoms range from isolated short duration tachypnea to life-threatening respiratory failure requiring prolonged ventilation. Therefore, formulating strategies to prevent this complication has always remained a priority. Suctioning of the airway to prevent MAS at the time of delivery is one of the most studied interventions during neonatal resuscitation.

The Evidence Support for Neonatal Resuscitation Program Guidelines

Management of neonate born through MSAF by intrapartum suctioning of the oro/nasopharyngeal cavity at the delivery of head, but before the delivery of shoulder, followed by direct laryngoscopy, intubation and tracheal suctioning remained in practice for many decades.[22] However, based upon the results of a large multicentric randomized control trial by Vain, et al.[23] which included 2,514 term neonates born with MSAF in USA and Argentina, reporting no benefit of routine intrapartum suctioning in preventing MAS and other related clinical outcomes, this practice was not recommended in NRP 2005 guidelines (LOE-Class 1).[18,23]

Wiswell, et al.[24] in a large multi-centric RCT, randomized 2094 term vigorous neonates born through MSAF into groups of routine tracheal suctioning or no suctioning, and reported no significant difference in incidence of MAS (2.7% vs. 3.2%) in the two groups.[24] In a subsequent Cochrane systematic review on the effect of tracheal intubation and suction in vigorous neonates, comparable incidence of MAS was reported in the two groups [RR 1.29, 95% CI 0.80, 2.08; n = 2,884].[25] Based upon these data, the ILCOR and NRP Guidelines 2010 recommended that routine tracheal suctioning of neonates born through MSAF was not required in vigorous neonates. They also recommended that the available evidence was not sufficient to either support or refute the routine ET suctioning in non-vigorous/depressed neonates born through MSAF.[6]

In the 2015 NRP guidelines, there was a major departure from earlier recommendations and, based upon the preference for "Avoidance of Harm" (avoiding of potential delay in initiating positive pressure ventilation due to inadequate skills in caregivers, or likely injury from the intubation procedure itself) to unknown benefits of the endotracheal intubation and suctioning, it was recommended that routine endotracheal intubation and tracheal suctioning should not be done in non-vigorous neonates born through MSAF as there was insufficient evidence to support this practice. The guidelines also emphasized that all efforts should be made to initiate ventilation during the "first golden minute" in all neonates who have apnea or ineffective respiration.[26] These recommendations were based upon the results from one RCT,[27] and nine other very low quality evidence studies.[28-36] Some of these studies had used tracheal suctioning in non-vigorous or depressed neonates and reported the occurrence of MAS even after tracheal suctioning, and hence questioned the utility of this practice. The details of these individual studies are presented in **Table 15.2**.

Subsequent to the 2015 guidelines, three RCTs from India and two cohort studies (from USA and UK) have reported that "endotracheal suctioning" in the non-vigorous neonates born through MSAF does not provide any additional benefit in the clinical outcomes as compared to "No endotracheal suctioning".[37-41] The details of these studies are presented in **Table 15.3**. Based upon the results of systematic reviews of these studies, the American Heart Association (AHA) 2020 guidelines have recommended that routine endotracheal suctioning of non-vigorous neonates born through the MSAF is no longer recommended (COR-3-No benefit, LOE-C-LD), and it should be reserved only for those neonates who have evidence of airway obstruction (COR-2a, LOE C-EO).[7]

TABLE 15.2: SUMMARY OF STUDIES OF TRACHEAL SUCTIONING IN INFANTS BORN THROUGH MSAF

S. No.	Author Year	Number of participants/ Study type	Participants	Intervention	Outcomes	Results
1.	Chettri, et al., 2015[27]	122 RCT	Term, non-vigorous neonates born through MSAF	Endotracheal suction and no-suction groups	Risk of MAS, complications of MAS, mortality, duration of neonatal intensive care unit (NICU) stay, and neurodevelopmental outcome at 9 months	The incidence of MAS (33% vs. 31%), perinatal asphyxia (31% vs. 28%), or mortality (11% vs. 13%) was not significantly different in the two groups.
2.	Peng, et al., 1996[28]	638 Prospective observational study	Neonates born through MSAF	Intrapartum suction in all neonates followed by tracheal suction in the depressed neonates	Occurrence of MAS, Apgar scores at 1 and 5 minutes, cord pH and NICU admissions	The incidence of MAS (0 vs. 2.84%), umbilical artery pH (7.28 vs. 7.27), and NICU admissions (2.5% vs. 11.7%) was not significantly different in neonates not suctioned at birth and routinely suctioned at birth.
3.	Hageman, 1988[29]	464 Prospective	Neonates born through MSAF	Intrapartum suction in all neonates using bulb syringe, suction catheter or both followed by tracheal suction	APGAR scores, respiratory rates, presence, or absence of meconium on or below the vocal cords, and development of MAS	142/464 neonates had meconium below the vocal cords, 10% developed MAS, and all survived. No differences were seen in Apgar scores, respiratory rates, presence or absence of meconium on or below the vocal cords, or development of MAS in the three groups.
4.	Davis, 1985[30]	1420 Retrospective review	Neonates born through MSAF	Intrapartum suction of all followed by tracheal suction in non-vigorous babies	Incidence of MAS, Death, Autopsy of the infants suspected to have clinical diagnosis of MAS	30/1420 (2.1%) of the neonates developed MAS, 12/30 (40%) of these died. At autopsy, meconium aspiration was histologically proven to be present in only 50% of the deaths, 25% had only suspicion and 25% did not have evidence of aspiration.

Contd...

Contd...

S. No.	Author Year	Number of participants/ Study type	Participants	Intervention	Outcomes	Results
5.	Manganaro 2001[31]	361 Prospective	Term meconium-stained neonates	Endotracheal intubation done for non-vigorous neonates	MAS, 1- and 5-minute Apgar scores, metabolic acidemia or the percentage of depressed/asphyxiated infants	The authors reported a 9.6 % incidence of MSAF, and 0.28 % incidence of MAS in neonates having MSAF. There were no significant differences in low 1 and 5 minute Apgar scores, metabolic acidemia or the percentage of depressed/asphyxiated infants.
6.	Dooley et al., 1985[32]	272 Observational study	Babies born through MSAF divided into two groups presence or absence of meconium below the vocal cord	Intrapartum suction of all followed by tracheal suction in non-vigorous babies	Fetal heart rate abnormalities, cord blood gas analysis	58/272 neonates were found to have meconium below the vocal cords. No significant difference was noted in difference in mean pH (t = 1.53), PCO_2 (t = 1.64) or base deficit (t = 1.05), cumulative duration of variable deacceleration ($\chi2 >0.05$).
7.	Takroni et al., 1998[33]	11,344 510 intubated, 10,834 non-intubated vigorous retrospective review of 6 years record	Neonates born through MSAF	Intrapartum suction of all followed by tracheal suction in non-vigorous babies and no suction in vigorous babies	Incidence of MAS, ventilation requirement, NICU stay, mortality	The neonates in the tracheal suction group had more incidence of MAS (46% vs. 0.26%), deaths (7.2% vs. 0%), required ventilation (23.5% vs. 0.27%.).

Contd...

Contd...

S. No.	Author Year	Number of participants/ Study type	Participants	Intervention	Outcomes	Results
8.	Suresh et al., 1994[34]	294 Prospective observational study	Neonates born through MSAF	Intrapartum suction of all followed by tracheal suction in the depressed neonates	Occurrence of MAS	Despite of intrapartum suction, 43.8% of neonates had meconium in the trachea, and 18% of the neonates developed MAS.
9.	Yoder 1994[35]	799 prospective control study	Three-arm study; a control group of neonates with clear amniotic fluid matched for gestational age and year of birth, suctioned group and non-suctioned group	Neonates with light meconium and vigorous infants with moderate-to-thick meconium were selectively not suctioned.	Incidence of MAS, need for ventilator or oxygen support	The neonates undergoing tracheal suction as compared to non-tracheal suctioned had significantly greater rates of abnormal fetal heart rate patterns, fetal acidosis, low APGAR scores at 5 minutes, need for resuscitation, need of ventilation and neonatal intensive care unit admission ($p <0.05$). Incidence of MAS was more in suctioned infants as compared to those selectively not suctioned, those with light meconium, and those with clear fluid (11 vs. 3 vs. 0 vs. 0%; $p < 0.01$).
10.	Rossi et al., 1989[36]	238 Prospective observational study	Neonates born through MSAF divided	Intrapartum suction of all followed by tracheal suction in the depressed neonates	Occurrence of MAS, presence of meconium in trachea	Despite suctioning with a DeLee apparatus and endotracheal suctioning, meconium was present in the trachea in 87/238 (37%) and meconium aspiration syndrome developed in 22 (9.2%).

(MAS: meconium aspiration syndrome; MSAF: meconium-stained amniotic fluid).

TABLE 15.3: SUMMARY OF RECENT STUDIES OF TRACHEAL SUCTIONING IN INFANTS BORN THROUGH MSAF

S. No.	Author, Year	Number of participants/ Study type	Participants	Intervention Group	Control Group	Major Outcomes	Results
1.	Singh et al., 2018[37]	152 Open-label RCT	Full-term non-vigorous neonates born through MSAF	Endotracheal suctioning of meconium was done using a meconium aspirator device under direct laryngoscopy followed by oropharyngeal suctioning	Only oropharyngeal suction was done using a 12–14 Fr catheter followed by initial steps and PPV if required	Incidence of MAS, mortality, hospital stay	Lower hospital stay (9.91 ± 3.22 vs. 11.17 ± 3.73 days; MD −1.26 (−3.36 to −0.17); $p = 0.024$), and trend of lower incidence of MAS in ET suction group vs. no suction (41% vs. 57%, OR 0.53, 95% CI, 0.28, 1.01; $p = .05$), Similar mortality (5% vs. 9%,) was reported in ET suction vs. No suction. Lower hospital stay was reported.
2.	Oommen et al., 2020[38]	838 Observational	Non-vigorous neonates delivered through MSAF	*Prospective Group:* No routine ET suctioning done in the non-vigorous neonates born with MSAF	*Retrospective Group:* Chart review of routine ET suctioning was done in non-vigorous neonates born with MSAF from August 2015 to September 2016	MAS, oxygen therapy, NICU admission, need of mechanical ventilation	No significant difference in the incidence of MAS 95.6% vs. 4.3%, OR 1.30; 95% CI 0.70–2.20) and less NICU admissions were noted (19.1% vs. 55.6%, $p < 0.05$) in the prospective as compared to the retrospective group.
3.	Kumar et al., 2019[39]	132 Open-label RCT	Non-vigorous singleton neonates of gestational age >34 weeks delivered through MSAF	*Endotracheal Suction Group:* Endotracheal suctioning of meconium was done under direct laryngoscopy followed by oropharyngeal suctioning	*Control Group:* After oropharyngeal suctioning of meconium, the remaining initial steps of resuscitation were completed	Incidence of MAS, resuscitation in labor room, mortality, complications, need for mechanical ventilation, HIE	Incidence of MAS was comparable in both the groups 31.8% vs. 22.7% in ETS and no-ETS groups [RR 1.40, 95% CI, 0.79–2.47].

Contd...

Contd...

S. No.	Author, Year	Number of participants/ Study type	Participants	Intervention Group	Control Group	Major Outcomes	Results
4.	Nangia, et al., 2015[40]	175 Open-label RCT	Full-term non-vigorous neonates born through MSAF	Oropharyngeal suction was done using a 12–14 Fr catheter followed by ET suction.	Only oropharyngeal suction was done using a 12–14 Fr catheter followed by initial steps and PPV if required.	Incidence of MAS, mortality, complications, need for mechanical ventilation, HIE	No significant differences in incidence of MAS (ET suction vs. no suction, 32% vs. 26%, [OR 0.4 (0.12–1.4); $p = 0.14$)] or mortality (10% vs. 5% OR 0.75 (0.62–1.2), $p = 0.38$), and other outcomes.
5.	Chiruvolu, et al., 2018[41]	231 Observational	Non-vigorous neonates delivered through MSAF	*Prospective Group:* No routine ET suctioning done in the non-vigorous neonates born with MSAF	*Retrospective Group:* Chart review of routine ET suctioning was done in non-vigorous neonates born with MSAF from October 2015–September 2016	MAS, oxygen therapy, NICU admission, need of mechanical ventilation	Significantly more neonates admitted to the NICU for respiratory issues in the prospective group (no tracheal suctioning) compared to the retrospective (routine tracheal suctioning) group (40% vs. 22%; OR, 2.2; 95% CI, 1.2–3.9), required oxygen therapy more often (37% vs. 19%; OR, 2.5; 95% CI, 1.2–4.5); mechanical ventilation (19% vs. 9%; OR, 2.6; 95% CI, 1.1–5.8). Trend toward more infants developing MAS in the non-ET suctioned group (5% vs. 11%; OR 2.3; 95% CI, 0.83–6.2; $p = 0.14$).

(HIE: hypoxic ischemic encephalopathy; MAS: meconium aspiration syndrome; MSAF: meconium-stained amniotic fluid; NICU: neonatal intensive care unit).

Other Evidence

A Cochrane systematic review (including 581 non-vigorous neonates from four RCTs done in India) analyzing the effect of tracheal suctioning in the non-vigorous neonates born through MSAF reported no significant difference in the incidence of MAS [RR 1.00, 95% CI, 0.80–1.25], all-cause mortality [RR 1.24, 95% CI 0.76–2.02], any severity HIE [RR 1.05, 95% CI 0.68–1.63], need for mechanical ventilation [RR 0.99, 95% CI 0.68–1.44], pulmonary air leaks [RR 1.22, 95% CI 0.38–3.93], pulmonary hypertension [RR 1.29, 95% CI 0.60–2.77] and culture-positive sepsis [RR 1.32, 95% CI 0.48–3.57] in the endotracheal suctioning versus no endotracheal suctioning groups.[42] A more recent systematic review which incorporated two additional observational studies (USA, UK) to the Cochrane review involving 1,026 neonates, also did not find significant difference in neonatal mortality [RR 1.22, 95% CI 0.73–2.04], or occurrence of MAS [RR 1.08, 95% CI 0.76–1.53] in the routine tracheal suctioning versus no suctioning group.[43]

These systematic reviews conclude that there is uncertainty about the routine use of tracheal suctioning in the non-vigorous neonates born through MSAF. The Neonatal Life Support Task Force as well as systematic reviews have also underlined the need for a large well-powered randomized control trial to conclusively answer this question.[7,42,43]

Conclusion

Routine tracheal suction in the non-vigorous neonates born through MSAF has not been found useful and should not be performed (COR-3-No benefit, LOE-C-LD). Tracheal suctioning may be useful in neonates having evidence of airway obstruction during PPV (COR-2a, LOE C-EO). This approach would also help practice in low- and middle-income countries where the incidence of non-vigorous neonates born to MSAF is higher than in high-income countries. Emphasizing the initiation of PPV in low-resource settings during the first golden minute would be more pragmatic as skill and logistics required for intubating and endotracheal suctioning are relatively lower in these settings.

4. HEART RATE ASSESSMENT DURING RESUSCITATION

The Concept

Rapid and accurate assessment of heart rate (HR) during neonatal resuscitation is of critical importance as judgement of effectiveness of spontaneous respiration, decision to initiate PPV, and chest compressions, as well as response to the resuscitative measures are assessed using the HR. NRP guidelines recommend the initiation of PPV if the HR is <100 after initial steps and chest compressions if the HR is <60 after 30 seconds of effective PPV.[7] Increment in HR is considered to be the most sensitive indicator of a successful intervention during neonatal resuscitation.

The Evidence Support for Neonatal Resuscitation Program Guidelines

Traditionally, the clinical estimation of HR is done for 6 seconds and it is multiplied by 10 to estimate the total heart rate. The auscultation of the precordium using a stethoscope is recommended as the preferred method for the initial assessment of HR.[7] However, when continuous HR monitoring is required, both palpation of umbilical cord and auscultation of the precordium were found to be less reliable and associated with more likelihood of underestimation of the HR.[44] In addition, noise, HR variability, and human factors can also affect the clinical judgement. This led to the recommendations of use of adjuncts such as pulse oximeter with sensor placed on the right wrist to document preductal saturation (2010 NRP guidelines) and three lead electrocardiography (2015 NRP Guidelines) for more accurate, non-invasive, and reliable HR assessment when continuous monitoring of the HR was required.[6,26]

The pulse-oximeter readings usually tend to display slower heart rate in first 2 minutes of life as the systemic perfusion and reliable signal acquisition takes some time and therefore resuscitation team may resort to potentially unnecessary interventions such as chest compressions. Results from two RCTs and nine non-randomized studies, showed ECG to be faster and more accurate in detecting the HR in the initial minutes of life, when compared to pulse oximetry and clinical auscultation as a method of HR assessment. Although the evidence was of very low quality (COR 2b, LOE C-LD), use of ECG for the assessment of the neonatal HR in both term as well as preterm neonates was recommended in NRP 2020 guidelines.[7] The details of the studies have been described in **Table 15.4**.[44-54] The administration of ECG leads was also found to be feasible during the neonatal resuscitation. However, it should be noted that the ECG does not replace the use of pulse oximeter during resuscitation for determining the need of supplemental oxygen based upon saturation targets.

Conclusion

The use of electrocardiography might be considered while resuscitating the preterm as well as term neonates for rapid and accurate assessment of the neonate's heart rate (COR 2b, LOE C-LD).

TABLE 15.4: Summary of Studies of Heart Rate Assessment During Neonatal Resuscitation

S. No.	Author, Year	Number of participants, type of study	Participants and intervention	Outcomes	Results
1.	Kamlin, et al., 2006[44]	23 Observational	Independent assessment of the HR by auscultation, and umbilical cord palpation of stable neonates by health-care workers (doctors, nurses, residents). Findings were then compared with the ECG tracing.	Heart rate	Both auscultation and umbilical cord palpitation compared to ECG, underestimated the heart rate with a mean difference of 14 and 21 bpm, respectively.
2.	Kamlin, et al., 2008[45]	55 Observational	Video-based review done for the HR assessment by pulse oximeter (PO) and ECG	Difference in the HR	The HR by PO as compared to the ECG was −2 (± 26) bpm slower overall and −0.5 (± 16) bpm slower in those infants who received PPV ± chest compressions. The detection of bradycardia (HR <100) by PO as compared to by ECG had sensitivity of 89% and specificity of 99%, respectively.
3.	Katheria, et al., 2012[46]	46 Observational	Video-based review done for the HR assessment by PO and ECG	Time of placement of sensor or electrodes, Time to achieve Recordable signals from the devices	The median (IQR) times to acquire a signal from the ECG and PO were 4 seconds (1–6) and 32 s (15–40, $p = .001$), respectively. During the first minutes of resuscitation, 93% of infants had an ECG heart rate compared with only 56% for PO.
4.	Katheria, et al., 2017[47]	40 RCT	Intervention group had ECG HR displayed Control Group HR assessment by auscultation ± PO. Camera based review was later done of both the groups	Time taken for HR Assessment	PO HR assessment took longer time than ECG (114 vs. 66 s) ($p < 0.0001$).

Contd...

Contd...

S. No.	Author, Year	Number of participants, type of study	Participants and intervention	Outcomes	Results
5.	Shah, et al., 2019[48]	632 Before and after study	Clinical outcomes of neonates were compared between 1-year epochs of pre-HR assessment by ECG guidelines (retrospective cohort) and post HR assessment by ECG guidelines (prospective cohort)	Intubation rate, chest compressions, mortality	In the epoch, when HR assessment was done using ECG, the endotracheal intubations decreased significantly (36% vs. 48%, $p < .005$), 5-min Apgar scores were higher [7 (5–8) vs. 6 (5–8), $p < .05$], mortality was similar (8% vs. 9%), and had increased chances of receiving chest compressions [OR 3.6 (95% CI 1.4–9.5)].
6.	Mizumoto, et al., 2012[49]	20 Observational	Video-based review done for the HR assessment by PO and ECG	Time taken to display the values	The PO showed HR longer than the ECG (122 s vs. 38 s after delivery).
7.	Narayen, et al., 2015[50]	12,970 Readings from PO observational cohort	Detailed data collected from logs of readings of the Masimo PO from the normal neonates. The readings showing system messages was compared with the readings not showing them.	The readings of low heartrate with and without system messages were analyzed.	The means and SDs of heart rate with system messages were significantly lower than the heart rates obtained without system messages ($p < 0.001$). The HR was under estimated when there were system messages.
8.	van Vonderen, et al., 2015[51]	53 Observational	Review of digital recordings of the logs of PO and ECG was done.	Time taken to acquire stable data	Mean difference between ECG and PO HR was 56 bpm at 60 s ($p < 0.05$), 67 bpm at 90 s ($p < 0.01$), and 75 bpm at 120 s ($p < 0.001$) time for initial HR assessment: 99 s for PO and 82 s for ECG ($p = 0.001$).

Contd...

Contd...

S. No.	Author, Year	Number of participants, type of study	Participants and intervention	Outcomes	Results
9.	Dawson, et al., 2013[52]	8,000 pairs of observations from 40 infants Observational	Video-based review done for the HR assessment by Nellcor and Masimo PO and ECG	Difference in the HR	Although, the overall HR assessment was similar between the ECG and both types of PO, yet the PO did show a lower value during the bradycardia. HR was 7.8 (11.6) bpm and 1.6 (10.7) bpm lower in Nellcor and Masimo respectively as compared to the ECG.
10.	Iglesias, et al., 2017[53]	29 Observational	Video-based review done for the HR assessment by PO and ECG in the preterm neonates	Time for initial HR assessment, Latency during resuscitation, efficacy	PO accuracy decreased with progressing bradycardia, compared to ECG. PO HR assessment took longer than ECG (60 vs. 18 s) ($p < 0.0001$). PO was later than ECG a median time of 5 s for bradycardia start and end. PO did not detect bradycardia start 69% of times.
11.	Murphy, et al., 2019[54]	100 RCT	Video-based review done for the HR assessment by PO and ECG	Time for initial HR assessment, efficacy	PO took longer than ECG to first display HR (48 vs. 24 s) ($p < 0.001$) PO displayed an initial bradycardia compared to ECG. Auscultation underestimated ECG HR mean difference by 9 bpm and PO HR by 5 bpm (not statistically different, $p > 0.05$).

5. WARMING OF THE NEONATES DURING RESUSCITATION

The Concept

Neonates are at higher risk of becoming hypothermic (defined as core temperature <36.5 °C) at birth due to sudden exposure to cold delivery room temperature after birth, large surface area, and immature compensatory responses to hypothermia.

The Evidence Support for Neonatal Resuscitation Program Guidelines

On the basis of 36 observational studies, NRP task force observed increased association between death and on-admission hypothermia in neonates born without asphyxia across all gestations (Class I, LOE B-NR).[26] Hypothermia has been found to be associated with many severe adverse neonatal morbidities, more so in preterm neonates. In a study done on 5,277 low birth weight (LBW) neonates, it was shown that there was increase of 28% "mortality during hospital stay" and 11% late onset sepsis with each 1°C decrease in the on-admission temperature.[55]

The temperature of the neonates born without asphyxia should always be maintained between 36.5–37.5°C at admission as well as throughout the stabilization phase (Class I, LOE C-LD). While providing early skin-to-skin contact (SSC) by keeping the neonate on the mother's abdomen or chest, drying by warm towels, and starting early breastfeeding is usually adequate for term and some vigorous preterm neonates, additional sources for maintaining the temperature are warranted for the neonates born more preterm.[7]

The ILCOR guidelines recommend that the healthy neonates who do not require resuscitation should be provided skin-to-skin care after delivery (COR 2a, LOE BR).[7] These recommendations were in tandem with a Cochrane systematic review done on 38 RCTs from 21 countries to analyze the effect of the early skin-to-skin contact on maternal and infant outcomes. The authors reported that infants who had received SSC were more likely to be breastfed at 1–4 months postnatal age (RR 1.24, 95% CI 1.07–1.43, n = 887; 14 studies), had longer duration of breastfeeding (MD 64 days, 95% CI 38–90 days, n = 264; six studies), higher blood-glucose values (MD: 10.49, 95% CI 8.4–12.6, n = 144; three studies), and higher (but clinically insignificant) temperature (MD 0.30°C, 95% CI 0.13–0.47°C, n = 558; six studies).[56]

For the neonates born preterm or LBW, the ILCOR guidelines recommend that the usage of warming adjuncts such as prewarmed radiant heat warmers, polyethylene plastic wrap or bag, increased ambient delivery room temperature to >23°C, hats, warm humidified blended oxygen, prewarmed transport incubator (COR 2a, LOE BR), and usage of thermal mattress (COR 2b, LOE BR) is beneficial either individually or in combination "bundles" (COR 2b, LOE NR) to prevent the occurrence of hypothermia.[7] A Cochrane systematic review (n = 2433 from 25 trials) analyzed the effect of various warming techniques to prevent the occurrence of hypothermia in premature and/or LBW neonates. The authors reported that the use of plastic wrap led to increased core temperature (MD 0.58°C, 95% CI 0.5–0.66, n = 1633; 13 studies), and decreased incidence of hypothermia (RR 0.67, 95% CI 0.62–0.72, n = 1417; 10 studies) at admission to NICU or during first 120 minutes of life. The meta-analysis, however, did not show any difference in neonatal morbidity or mortality. Exothermic mattress was shown to result in higher temperature on-admission to NICU (MD 0.65°C, 95% CI 0.36–0.94°C n = 126 from two trials) in neonates <1,500 g.[57] One recent systematic review, involving 10 studies using the combination of the warming techniques, analyzed the effect of implementation of the QI bundles and reported a significant improvement (all p <0.01) after the interventions.[58]

In the resource-limited settings, the neonates may be put up to the neck into clean food grade plastic wrap or re-closable bags with cut-open bottom to prevent them from becoming hypothermic. The full resuscitation process can continue with the preterm neonate wrapped in the bag. Umbilical catheterization, if needed should be done by cutting a hole in the plastic sheet. It is very important to continuously monitor the temperature as the combination methods used for warming may overheat the neonate.[3]

Conclusion

Healthy neonates who do not require resuscitation should be provided skin-to-skin care after delivery (COR 2a, LOE BR). The use of warming adjuncts described above either alone (COR 2a, LOE BR), or in combination bundles (COR 2b, LOE NR) may be effective in preventing occurrence of hypothermia in neonates born preterm or with low birth weight.

▉ 6. TIMING OF THE CORD CLAMPING

The Concept

After delivery, blood flows from the placenta to the neonate via the umbilical cord till it stops pulsating or it is clamped by artificial means. This blood flow affects the absolute blood volume as well as the physiological transition in term and preterm neonates. The practice of clamping the umbilical cord as soon as the baby is born (called early or immediate cord clamping) has been the standard practice for many decades.

The Evidence Support for Neonatal Resuscitation Program Guidelines

The ILCOR guidelines till 2005, recommended only early cord clamping to be followed in each birth.[18] Subsequent studies documented that delaying the clamping of the umbilical cord improved short- and long-term outcomes for neonates of all gestational ages. Based upon the data from the preliminary studies, the ILCOR 2010 guidelines recommended delayed cord clamping (DCC) for at least 1 minute in neonates not requiring resuscitation and delaying by at least 30 seconds in the preterm neonates. In term neonates, it was shown to improve hematocrit, hemoglobin, and iron stores in late infancy; whereas preterm neonates were noted to require less inotropes as well as blood transfusion and had lower incidence of any grade intraventricular hemorrhage and necrotizing enterocolitis.[6] A comprehensive systematic review was undertaken by ILCOR in 2015 and based upon those findings it was recommended that DCC for >30 seconds is reasonable for both term and preterm infants who do not require resuscitation at birth (Class IIa, LOE C-LD).[26]

Based upon rigorous scientific review undertaken in view of emerging evidence on cord care management strategies by the ILCOR committee in 2020, it was recommended that it would be reasonable to practice DCC in preterm neonates not requiring resuscitation at birth for longer than 30 seconds (COR 2a, LOE BR). For term/late preterm neonates not requiring resuscitation, it may be reasonable to practice DCC for >30 seconds and cord may be clamped after assessing the neonate for respiratory efforts and activity while placed on the mother (COR2b, LOE C-LD). There is insufficient evidence to recommend either ECC or DCC in neonates requiring resuscitation (COR 2b, LOE C-EO).[7,59]

The summary of various systematic reviews published on the clamping of the umbilical cord is presented in **Table 15.5**.[59-62]

Conclusion

Delayed cord clamping for >30 seconds should be practiced in preterm neonates who do not require resuscitation at birth (COR 2a, LOE BR). In term/late preterm neonates who do not need resuscitation, it may be reasonable to practice DCC for >30 seconds and cord may be clamped after assessing the neonate for respiratory efforts and activity while on mother (COR2b, LOE C-LD). DCC may or may not be of benefit as compared to early clamping in neonates requiring resuscitation (COR 2b, LOE C-EO).

TABLE 15.5: SUMMARY OF INTERVENTIONAL STUDIES ADDRESSING DELAYED CORD CLAMPING IN NEONATES

S. No.	Author, Year	Number of participants, studies included	Participants	Major outcomes	Results
1.	Jasani, et al., 2021[60]	6,852 from 56 studies	Preterm	Mortality, intraventricular hemorrhage (IVH), need for pRBC transfusion	DCC had lower mortality (OR 0.64, 5% vs. 7.6%, n = 3,083 from 22 studies, 95% CI 0.39–0.99) lower intraventricular hemorrhage (OR 0.73, 17.8% vs. 15.4%; 95% CI 0.54–0.97, n = 3,316 from 25 studies), decreased need for pRBC transfusion (OR- 0.48, 38.3% vs. 46.9%, 95% CI 0.32–0.66, n = 2904 from 18 studies).
2.	Rabe, et al., 2019[61]	5,721 from 48 studies	Preterm <34 weeks	Mortality, IVH, chronic lung disease (CLD)	DCC led to lower mortality (aRR 0.73, 95% CI, 0.54–0.98, n = 2,680 from 20 trials, similar grade 3/4 IVH (aRR 0.94, 95% CI, 0.63–1.39, n = 2058 from 10 trials), mild decrease in any grade IVH (aRR 0.83, 95% CI, 0.7–0.99, n = 2,333 from 15 trials). There was similar incidence of CLD (aRR 1.04, 95% CI, 0.94–1.14, n = 1,644 from 16 trials).
3.	Wyckoff, et al., 2022[59]	2,988 from 18 studies	Preterm	Mortality	DCC led to 18/1,000 more survival in neonates (0–36 more/1,000), RR-1.02, 95% CI 1.00–1.02.
		2,972 from 14 studies	Preterm	Severe IVH	DCC led to 1/1,000 lesser incidence of severe IVH (10 fewer—10 more/1,000) 0.98 (0.67–1.42).
		196 from four studies	Preterm	Hb within 24 h	DCC had 1.24 g/dL more Hb as compared to ECC (0.01–2.47).
		1,022 from 14 studies	Preterm	HCT within 24 h	DCC had 2.6% more HCT as compared to ECC (1.85–3.42).
		351 from six studies	Preterm	Inotropic support for hypotension	In the DCC group, 91/1,000 neonates required lesser inotropes during first day of life.
		374 from seven studies	Preterm	Lowest mean airway pressure (MAP)	DCC had 1.79 mm Hg higher MAP as compared to ECC (0.53–23.05).
		2,910 from 12 studies	Preterm	Receiving BT	DCC led to 71/1,000 lesser transfusions (40–111 lesser/1,000), RR 0.83, 95% CI 0.77–0.90.
4.	McDonald, et al., 2013[62]	3,951 15 studies	Term and near term	Neonatal Mortality, Hb, likelihood of being iron deficient at 3–6 months	DCC group had higher Hb in neonates at 24–48 h (MD 1.49 g/dL, 95% CI, 1.21–1.78, n = 884), early cord clamping (ECC) were twice as likely to be iron deficient at 3–6 m (RR 2.65 95% CI, 1.04–6.73, n = 1,152 from five studies). Both groups had similar neonatal mortality (RR 0.37, 95% CI 0.04–3.41, n = 381 from two studies).

Contd...

Contd...

S. No.	Author, Year	Number of participants, studies included	Participants	Major outcomes	Results
5.	Wyckoff, et al., 2022[59]	537 from four studies	Term and late preterm	Mortality	DCC led to 8/1,000 more deaths in neonates (10 fewer–30 more/1000), RR 2.54, 95% CI 0.50–12.74.
		1,352 from nine studies	Term and late preterm	Hb within 24 h	DCC had 1.17 g/dL more Hb as compared to ECC (0.48–1.86).
		2,183 from 12 studies	Term and late preterm	HCT within 24 h	DCC had 3.38% more HCT as compared to ECC (2.08–4.67)
		1,335 from 13 studies	Term and late preterm	Polycythemia	DCC led to 50/1,000 more polycythemia in neonates (30–80 more/1,000), RR-2.26, 95% CI 1.56–3.28.
		695 from three studies	Term and late preterm	Hb within 7 days	DCC had 1.11 g/dL more Hb as compared to ECC (0.4–1.82).
		2,910 from 12 studies	Term and late preterm	HCT within 7 days	DCC had 5.84% more HCT as compared to ECC (2.74–8.95).
		2,972 from 14 studies	Term and late preterm	Anemia at 4–6 months	DCC and ECC had similar incidence of anemia at 4–6 months of age RR 0.75 95% CI (0.42–1.35).

(CLD: chronic lung disease; DCC: delayed cord clamping; ECC: early cord clamping; Hb: hemoglobin; HCT: hematocrit; IVH: intraventricular hemorrhage; MAP: mean airway pressure)

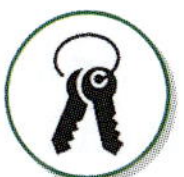

KEY POINTS

1. Briefing-debriefing is helpful, especially in a high-risk delivery to improve team coordination and efficiency in dealing with potential complications during resuscitation.

2. Routine oro/nasopharyngeal suctioning at birth in a neonate is not beneficial and should not be done.

3. Routine tracheal suction in the non-vigorous neonates born through meconium-stained amniotic fluid has not been found useful and should not be performed; however, tracheal suctioning may be useful in neonates having evidence of airway obstruction during positive pressure ventilation (PPV).

4. Electrocardiography might be used while resuscitating the preterm as well as term neonates for rapid and accurate assessment of the neonate's heart rate.

5. Healthy neonates not requiring resuscitation should be provided skin-to-skin care after delivery. Warming adjuncts (e.g., prewarmed radiant heat warmers, polyethylene plastic wrap or bag, increased ambient delivery room temperature, hats, warm humidified blended oxygen, prewarmed transport incubator, thermal mattress), either individually or in combination "bundles", may be effective in preventing hypothermia in preterm or low birth weight neonates.

6. Delayed (>30 s) cord clamping should be practiced in neonates who do not require resuscitation at birth, whereas it may or may not be of benefit as compared to early clamping in neonates requiring resuscitation.

■ REFERENCES

1. Magid DJ, Aziz K, Cheng A, Hoover AV, Mahgoub M, Panchal AR, et al. Part 2: Evidence Evaluation and Guidelines Development: 2020 American Heart Association Guidelines for Cardiopulmonary Resuscitation and Emergency Cardiovascular Care. Circulation. 2020;142:S358-65.

2. Merriam-Webster. Briefing Definition and Meaning. [online] Available form from: https://www.merriam-webster.com/dictionary/briefing [Last accessed January, 2023].

3. American Academy of Pediatrics and American Heart Association. In: Weiner GM, Zaichkin J (Eds). Textbook of Neonatal Resuscitation, 8th edition. Healdsburg, CA, USA: American Academy of Pediatrics; 2020.

4. Sawyer T, Loren D, Halamek LP. Post-event debriefings during neonatal care: why are we not doing them, and how can we start?. J Perinatol. 2016;36:415-9.

5. Savoldelli GL, Naik VN, Park J, Joo HS, Chow R, Hamstra SJ. Value of debriefing during simulated crisis management: oral versus video-assisted oral feedback. Anesthesiology. 2006;105:279-85.

6. Perlman JM, Wyllie J, Kattwinkel J, Atkins DL, Chameides L, Goldsmith JP, et al. Part 11: Neonatal resuscitation: 2010 International Consensus on Cardiopulmonary Resuscitation and Emergency Cardiovascular Care Science with Treatment Recommendations. Circulation. 2010;122:S516-38.

7. Aziz K, Lee HC, Escobedo MB, Hoover AV, Kamath-Rayne BD, Kapadia VS, et al. Part 5: Neonatal Resuscitation: 2020 American Heart Association Guidelines for Cardiopulmonary Resuscitation and Emergency Cardiovascular Care. Circulation. 2020;142:S524-50.

8. Bennett SC, Finer N, Halamek LP, Mickas N, Bennett MV, Nisbet CC, et al. Implementing delivery room checklists and communication standards in a multi-neonatal ICU Quality Improvement Collaborative. Jt Comm J Qual Patient Saf. 2016;42:369-76.

9. Balakrishnan M, Falk-Smith N, Detman LA, Miladinovic B, Sappenfield WM, Curran JS, et al. Promoting teamwork may improve infant care processes during delivery room management: Florida perinatal quality collaborative's approach. J Perinatol. 2017;37:886-92.

10. Talati AJ, Scott TA, Barker B, Grubb PH, Tennessee Initiative for Perinatal Quality Care Golden Hour Project Team. Improving neonatal resuscitation in Tennessee: a large-scale, quality improvement project. J Perinatol. 2019;39:1676-83.

11. Litke-Wager C, Delaney H, Mu T, Sawyer T. Impact of task-oriented role assignment on neonatal resuscitation performance: a simulation-based randomized controlled trial. Am J Perinatol. 2021;38:914-21.

12. Katheria A, Rich W, Finer N. Development of a strategic process using checklists to facilitate team preparation and improve communication during neonatal resuscitation. Resuscitation. 2013;84:1552-7.

13. Fawke J, Stave C, Yamada N. Use of briefing and debriefing in neonatal resuscitation, a scoping review. Resusc Plus. 2021;5:100059.

14. Sauer CW, Boutin MA, Fatayerji AN, Proudfoot JA, Fatayerji NI, Golembeski DJ. Delivery room quality improvement project improved compliance with best practices for a community NICU. Sci Rep. 2016;6:37397.

15. Skåre C, Calisch TE, Saeter E, Rajka T, Boldingh AM, Nakstad B, et al. Implementation and effectiveness of a video-based debriefing programme for neonatal resuscitation. Acta Anaesthesiol Scand. 2018;62:394-403.

16. Magee SR, Battle C, Morton J, Nothnagle M. Promotion of family-centered birth with gentle cesarean delivery. J Am Board Fam Med. 2014;27:690-3.

17. Foster JP, Dawson JA, Davis PG, Dahlen HG. Routine oro/nasopharyngeal suction versus no suction at birth. Cochrane Database Syst Rev. 2017;4:CD010332.

18. International Liaison Committee on Resuscitation. 2005 International Consensus on Cardiopulmonary Resuscitation and Emergency Cardiovascular Care Science with Treatment Recommendations. Part 7: Neonatal resuscitation. Resuscitation. 2005;67:293-303.

19. Gungor S, Teksoz E, Ceyhan T, Kurt E, Goktolga U, Baser I. Oronasopharyngeal suction versus no suction in normal, term and vaginally born infants: a prospective randomised controlled trial. Aust NZJ Obstet Gynaecol. 2005;45(5):453-6.

20. Gungor S, Kurt E, Teksoz E, Goktolga U, Ceyhan T, Baser I. Oronasopharyngeal suction versus no suction in normal and term infants delivered by elective cesarean section: a prospective randomized controlled trial. Gynecol Obstet Invest. 2006;61(1):9-14. doi:10.1159/000087604.

21. Velaphi S, Vidyasagar D. The pros and cons of suctioning at the perineum (intrapartum) and post-delivery with and without meconium. Semin Fetal Neonatal Med. 2008;13:375-82.

22. Chiruvolu A, Wiswell TE. Appropriate management of the nonvigorous meconium-stained newborn. NeoReviews. 2022;23(4):e250-61.

23. Vain NE, Szyld EG, Prudent LM, Wiswell TE, Aguilar AM, Vivas NI. Oropharyngeal and nasopharyngeal suctioning of meconium-stained neonates before delivery of their shoulders: multicentre, randomised controlled trial. Lancet. 2004;364:597-602.

24. Wiswell TE, Gannon CM, Jacob J, Goldsmith L, Szyld E, Weiss K, et al. Delivery room management of the apparently vigorous meconium-stained neonate: results of the multicenter, international collaborative trial. Pediatrics. 2000;105:1-7.

25. Halliday HL, Sweet DG. Endotracheal intubation at birth for preventing morbidity and mortality in vigorous, meconium-stained infants born at term. Cochrane Database Syst Rev. 2001;2001(1):CD000500.

26. Wyckoff MH, Aziz K, Escobedo MB, Kapadia VS, Kattwinkel J, Perlman JM, et al. Part 13: Neonatal Resuscitation: 2015 American Heart Association Guidelines Update for Cardiopulmonary Resuscitation and Emergency Cardiovascular Care. Circulation. 2015;132:S543-60.

27. Chettri S, Adhisivam B, Bhat BV. Endotracheal suction for nonvigorous neonates born through meconium stained amniotic fluid: a randomized controlled trial. J Pediatr. 2015;166:1208-1213.e1.

28. Peng TCC, Gutcher GR, Van Dorsten JP. A selective aggressive approach to the neonate exposed to meconium-stained amniotic fluid. Am J Obstet Gynecol. 1996;175:296-303.

29. Hageman JR, Conley M, Francis K, Stenske J, Wolf I, Santi V, et al. Delivery room management of meconium staining of the amniotic fluid and the development of meconium aspiration syndrome. J Perinatol. 1988;8:127-31.

30. Davis RO, Philips JB, Harris BA, Wilson ER, Huddleston JF. Fatal meconium aspiration syndrome occurring despite airway management considered appropriate. Am J Obstet Gynecol. 1985;151:731-6.

31. Manganaro R, Mamì C, Palmara A, Paolata A, Gemelli M. Incidence of meconium aspiration syndrome in term meconium-stained babies managed at birth with selective tracheal intubation. J Perinat Med. 2001;29(6):465-8.

32. Dooley SL, Pesavento DJ, Depp R, Socol ML, Tamura RK, Wiringa KS. Meconium below the vocal cords at delivery: correlation with intrapartum events. Am J Obstet Gynecol. 1985;153:767-70.

33. Al Takroni AMB, Parvathi CK, Mendis KBL, Hassan S, Reddy I, Kudair HA. Selective tracheal suctioning to prevent meconium aspiration syndrome. Int J Gynecol Obstet. 1998;63:259-63.

34. Suresh GK, Sarkar S. Delivery room management of infants born through thin meconium stained liquor. Indian Pediatr. 1994;3:1177-81.

35. Yoder BA. Meconium-stained amniotic fluid and respiratory complications: impact of selective tracheal suction. Obstet Gynecol. 1994;83:77-84.

36. Rossi EM, Philipson EH, Williams TG, Kalhan SC. Meconium aspiration syndrome: intrapartum and neonatal attributes. Am J Obstet Gynecol. 1989;161:1106-10.

37. Singh SN, Saxena S, Bhriguvanshi A, Kumar M, Chandrakanta, Sujata. Effect of endotracheal suctioning just after birth in non-vigorous infants born through meconium stained amniotic fluid: a randomized controlled trial. Clin Epidemiol Glob Health. 2019;7:165-70.

38. Oommen VI, Ramaswamy VV, Szyld E, Roehr CC. Resuscitation of non-vigorous neonates born through meconium-stained amniotic fluid: post policy change impact analysis. Arch Dis Child Fetal Neonatal Ed. 2021;106:324-6.

39. Kumar A, Kumar P, Basu S. Endotracheal suctioning for prevention of meconium aspiration syndrome: a randomized controlled trial. Eur J Pediatr. 2019;178:1825-32.

40. Nangia S, Sunder S, Biswas R, Saili A. Endotracheal suction in term non vigorous meconium stained neonates: a pilot study. Resuscitation. 2016;105:79-84.

41. Chiruvolu A, Miklis KK, Chen E, Petrey B, Desai S. Delivery room management of meconium-stained newborns and respiratory support. Pediatrics. 2018;142:e20181485.

42. Nangia S, Thukral A, Chawla D. Tracheal suction at birth in non-vigorous neonates born through meconium-stained amniotic fluid. Cochrane Database Syst Rev. 2021;6:CD012671.

43. Dikou M, Xanthos T, Dimitropoulos I, Iliodromiti Z, Sokou R, Kafalidis G, et al. Routine tracheal intubation and meconium suctioning in non-vigorous neonates with meconium-stained amniotic fluid: a systematic review and meta-analysis. Diagn Basel Switz. 2022;12:881.

44. Kamlin COF, O'Donnell CPF, Everest NJ, Davis PG, Morley CJ. Accuracy of clinical assessment of infant heart rate in the delivery room. Resuscitation. 2006;71:319-21.

45. Kamlin COF, Dawson JA, O'Donnell CPF, Morley CJ, Donath SM, Sekhon J, et al. Accuracy of pulse oximetry measurement of heart rate of newborn infants in the delivery room. J Pediatr. 2008;152:756-60.

46. Katheria A, Rich W, Finer N. Electrocardiogram provides a continuous heart rate faster than oximetry during neonatal resuscitation. Pediatrics. 2012;130(5):e1177-81.

47. Katheria A, Arnell K, Brown M, Hassen K, Maldonado M, Rich W, et al. A pilot randomized controlled trial of EKG for neonatal resuscitation. PloS One. 2017;12:e0187730.

48. Shah BA, Wlodaver AG, Escobedo MB, Ahmed ST, Blunt MH, Anderson MP, et al. Impact of electronic cardiac (ECG) monitoring on delivery room resuscitation and neonatal outcomes. Resuscitation. 2019;143:10-6.

49. Mizumoto H, Tomotaki S, Shibata H, Ueda K, Akashi R, Uchio H, et al. Electrocardiogram shows reliable heart rates much earlier than pulse oximetry during neonatal resuscitation. Pediatr Int. 2012;54:205-7.

50. Narayen IC, Smit M, van Zwet EW, Dawson JA, Blom NA, te Pas AB. Low signal quality pulse oximetry measurements in newborn infants are reliable for oxygen saturation but underestimate heart rate. Acta Paediatr 1992. 2015;104:e158-63.

51. van Vonderen JJ, Hooper SB, Kroese JK, Roest AA, Narayen IC, van Zwet EW, et al. Pulse oximetry measures a lower heart rate at birth compared with electrocardiography. J Pediatr. 2015;166:49-53.

52. Dawson JA, Saraswat A, Simionato L, Thio M, Kamlin CO, Owen LS, et al. Comparison of heart rate and oxygen saturation measurements from

Masimo and Nellcor pulse oximeters in newly born term infants. Acta Paediatr. 2013;102:955-60.

53. Iglesias B, Rodrí Guez MAJ, Aleo E, Criado E, Martí Nez-Orgado J, Arruza L. 3-lead electrocardiogram is more reliable than pulse oximetry to detect bradycardia during stabilisation at birth of very preterm infants. Arch Dis Child Fetal Neonatal Ed. 2018;103:F233-7.

54. Murphy MC, De Angelis L, McCarthy LK, O'Donnell CPF. Randomised study comparing heart rate measurement in newly born infants using a monitor incorporating electrocardiogram and pulse oximeter versus pulse oximeter alone. Arch Dis Child Fetal Neonatal Ed. 2019;104:F547-50.

55. Laptook AR, Bell EF, Shankaran S, Boghossian NS, Wyckoff MH, Kandefer S, et al. Admission temperature and associated mortality and morbidity among moderately and extremely preterm infants. J Pediatr. 2018;192:53-9.e2.

56. Moore ER, Bergman N, Anderson GC, Medley N. Early skin-to-skin contact for mothers and their healthy newborn infants. Cochrane Database Syst Rev. 2016;11:CD003519.

57. McCall EM, Alderdice F, Halliday HL, Vohra S, Johnston L. Interventions to prevent hypothermia at birth in preterm and/or low birth weight infants. Cochrane Database Syst Rev. 2018;2:CD004210.

58. Donnellan D, Moore Z, Patton D, O'Connor T, Nugent L. The effect of thermoregulation quality improvement initiatives on the admission temperature of premature/very low birth-weight infants in neonatal intensive care units: a systematic review. J Spec Pediatr Nurs. 2020;25(2):e12286.

59. Wyckoff MH, Singletary EM, Soar J, Olasveengen TM, Greif R, Liley HG, et al. 2021 International Consensus on Cardiopulmonary Resuscitation and Emergency Cardiovascular Care Science with Treatment Recommendations: Summary from the Basic Life Support; Advanced Life Support; Neonatal Life Support; Education, Implementation, and Teams; First Aid Task Forces; and the COVID-19 Working Group. Resuscitation. 2021;169:229-311.

60. Jasani B, Torgalkar R, Ye XY, Syed S, Shah PS. Association of umbilical cord management strategies with outcomes of preterm infants: a systematic review and network meta-analysis. JAMA Pediatr. 2021;175(4):e210102.

61. Rabe H, Gyte GM, Díaz-Rossello JL, Duley L. Effect of timing of umbilical cord clamping and other strategies to influence placental transfusion at preterm birth on maternal and infant outcomes. Cochrane Database Syst Rev. 2019;9:CD003248.

62. McDonald SJ, Middleton P, Dowswell T, Morris PS. Effect of timing of umbilical cord clamping of term infants on maternal and neonatal outcomes. Cochrane Database Syst Rev. 2013;7:CD004074.

 # Self Assessment

1. "A constructive review of actions and thought processes after an event to promote reflective learning and improve clinical performance" is called as:
   a. Briefing
   b. Debriefing
   c. Feedback
   d. Two-way communication

2. Routine tracheal suction in the non-vigorous neonates born through MSAF:
   a. Should be performed routinely as mortality and risk of MAS was less in the routine tracheal suctioning group.
   b. Should be performed routinely as similar mortality and MAS incidence was seen in the two groups.
   c. Should not be performed as similar mortality and MAS incidence was seen in the two groups.
   d. Should not be performed routinely as mortality and risk of MAS was higher in the routine tracheal suctioning group.

3. Which method is considered most accurate for continuous monitoring of the heart rate during initial minutes of resuscitation, as it has least chances of under estimation of heart rate?
   a. Umbilical cord palpation
   b. Stethoscope
   c. Pulse oximetry
   d. Electrocardiography

4. What is the recommended time for clamping of umbilical cord in term and preterm infants who do not require resuscitation at birth?
   a. Cord should be clamped immediately after birth
   b. Before 30 seconds of birth
   c. After 30 seconds of birth
   d. After the cord stops pulsating

5. What are the adjuncts which are helpful in preventing hypothermia in premature born neonates?

Answers

For answers, go to the end of the Book, Page no. 323

Evidence-base for Neonatal Resuscitation Practices: Beyond Initial Steps

Deepak Chawla, Siddarth Ramji

Lessons to Learn

○ Assessment and interventions during neonatal resuscitation have evolved over time with emergence of new evidence. Practices such as special airway clearance maneuvers in neonates born with meconium-stained amniotic fluid and use of 100% oxygen have gradually abated with accumulation of evidence of harm or of no benefit.

○ Addition of interventions or techniques such as use of pulse oximetry or electrocardiography to assess heart rate and oxygen saturation and the use of air-oxygen blenders and T-piece resuscitators to provide positive pressure ventilation have made the assessment more objective and the interventions safer and reliable.[1]

○ This chapter presents the evidence on interventions that are emerging or are well established but are perceived to need improvement—positive end-expiratory pressure (PEEP) versus no PEEP, T-piece versus self-inflating bag, monitoring oxygen therapy in term and preterm neonates, laryngeal mask airway (LMA) versus intubation, cardiopulmonary resuscitation (CPR) ratios and technique, epinephrine dose and route, intraosseous versus umbilical vein for emergency infusion, sodium bicarbonate for resuscitation.

▉ EVIDENCE GENERATION

The evidence for each intervention that is being discussed in this chapter is presented as a "Practice Question" in patient/population, intervention, comparison and outcomes (PICO) format. Subgroups of interest and outcomes that are likely to be impacted were identified *a-priori*. Outcomes were divided into two categories—resuscitation outcomes and postresuscitation outcomes. Literature search was then conducted to identify the evidence. If a systematic review that is published or updated during the last 2 years was found, it was used to present the evidence summary. If a recent systematic review was not available, randomized controlled trials (RCTs) were used to build the evidence summary. If RCTs were not available, observational studies followed by animal experiments were used to build the evidence summary. The level of evidence was classified using the grading of recommendations, assessment, development and evaluations (GRADE) method[2,3] if the included systematic review provided an evidence summary, or by Oxford Centre for Evidence-based Medicine (CEBM) level of evidence.[4]

1. POSITIVE END-EXPIRATORY PRESSURE VERSUS NO PEEP

Practice Question

Does addition of positive end-expiratory pressure (PEEP) in comparison to no PEEP improve the resuscitation and respiratory outcomes in neonates needing positive pressure ventilation (PPV) at birth?

This question does not include the following: Use of sustained inflation, and use of continuous positive airway pressure (CPAP) to stabilize respiration in a neonate not needing PPV.

The *subgroups of interest* were (i) Full term and late preterm neonates and (ii) Extremely preterm neonates.
The *outcomes* of interest were:

1. *Resuscitation outcomes:*
   a. Duration of PPV
   b. Need of intubation
   c. Need of advanced steps of resuscitation
2. *Postresuscitation outcomes:*
   a. Need and duration of any respiratory support (including non-invasive and invasive ventilation)
   b. Need and duration of invasive ventilation
   c. Need of surfactant
   d. Incidence of bronchopulmonary dysplasia
   e. Incidence of pulmonary air leaks
   f. Incidence of severe intraventricular hemorrhage

Evidence Summary

Application of PEEP during resuscitation can help in clearance of lung fluid and in the establishment of functional residual capacity (FRC). In turn, establishment of FRC, can affect the development of respiratory distress, need for surfactant, and need for or extent of respiratory support in preterm neonates. PEEP can be provided during resuscitation by using a self-inflating bag (SIB) with a PEEP valve, or a T-piece resuscitator (TPR). In compiling the evidence for this practice question, following two types of studies were considered:

1. Studies comparing SIB with (SIB + PEEP) and without PEEP valve
2. Studies comparing T-piece resuscitator (TPR, that has inbuilt provision to provide PEEP) with an SIB without a PEEP valve.

Two RCTs have compared PPV with and without PEEP during resuscitation. In an RCT conducted in Tanzania, Holte et al. compared use of SIB with and without a PEEP valve.[5] Midwives trained in the Helping Babies Breathe (HBB) program conducted the resuscitation. No difference was observed in the heart rate pattern (primary outcome), Apgar score or mortality. In a multicentric RCT, Szyld et al. enrolled neonates born at >26 weeks of gestation needing PPV at birth.[6] Neonates received PPV with either a TPR or an SIB. The TPR was used with a PEEP valve set at a pressure of 5 cmH_2O. Each center participating in the study was also randomized to use SIB with and without a PEEP valve with a pressure of 5 cmH_2O. On comparison of neonates receiving PPV with TPR and neonate receiving PPV with SIB without PEEP valve, the former had lower need of intubation in the delivery room and received a lower peak inspiratory pressure (PIP). After resuscitation, neonates who received PPV with PEEP needed mechanical ventilation and CPAP for fewer days. Similar beneficial effects were also observed in the subgroup of neonates in which TPR was compared with SIB + PEEP valve. Therefore, some of the benefits observed may be associated with use of TPR rather than the use of PEEP.

A systematic review published in 2021 included the above-mentioned RCTs (n = 933).[7] No difference was observed in the duration of PPV, need for intubation, chest compression, medications; incidence of air leaks, and bronchopulmonary dysplasia (BPD) and, mortality before hospital discharge. Neonates in the SIB + PEEP group had a longer duration of hospitalization (mean difference: 0.14 days; 95% CI: 0.01–0.27), although the difference does not seem to be clinically significant. The following outcomes were not reported— need and duration of any respiratory support (including noninvasive and invasive ventilation), need and duration of invasive ventilation, need for surfactant, and incidence of severe intraventricular hemorrhage.

Sufficient studies were not available to evaluate the effect of use of PEEP in extremely preterm neonates.

Level of Evidence

Overall, evidence of very low to low certainty was available on the use of PEEP while providing PPV to neonates needing resuscitation at birth **(Table 16.1)**.[7] Therefore, no recommendation can be made about the use of PEEP with PPV during resuscitation of neonates in the delivery room. There is a need to conduct well planned and adequately powered RCTs with clinically important outcomes. However the International Liaison Committee on Resuscitation (ILCOR) in its 2020 guidelines has suggested using PEEP for the initial ventilation of premature newborn infants during delivery room resuscitation (weak recommendation, low-quality evidence).

TABLE 16.1: Outcomes in Comparison of Positive Pressure Ventilation with and without Positive End-expiratory Pressure

Outcome	Number of studies (number of neonates)	Relative risk or mean difference with 95%CI	Certainty of evidence
Duration of PPV (seconds)	1 (516)	−3.85 (−29.5 to +21.8)	Very low
Intubation during resuscitation	1 (516)	2.30 (0.48–9.67)	Moderate
Chest compression or medications	1 (516)	1.43 (0.54–3.80)	Very low
Air leaks	1 (516)	2.30 (0.48–9.67)	Very low
Bronchopulmonary dysplasia	1 (516)	1.03 (0.58–1.81)	Low
Mortality before hospital discharge	2 (933)	0.99 (0.59–1.67)	Very low

(PPV: positive pressure ventilation)

■ 2. T-PIECE VERSUS SELF-INFLATING BAG

Practice Question

Does use of TPR in comparison to the use of SIB improve the resuscitation and respiratory outcomes in neonates needing PPV at birth?

The *subgroups of interest* were (i) Full term and late preterm neonates and (ii) Extremely preterm neonates.
The *outcomes* were:

1. *Resuscitation outcomes:*
   a. Duration of positive pressure ventilation
   b. Need of intubation
   c. Need of advanced steps of resuscitation

2. *Respiratory outcomes:*
   a. Need and duration of any respiratory support (including non-invasive and invasive ventilation)
   b. Need and duration of invasive ventilation
   c. Incidence of BPD
   d. Incidence of pulmonary air leaks

3. *Other outcomes:*
   a. Incidence of hypoxic ischemic encephalopathy (HIE)
   b. Neonatal mortality

Evidence Summary

Use of a T-piece resuscitator allows the resuscitation personnel to set peak inspiratory pressure and positive end-expiratory pressure during PPV. Mannequin studies have shown that TPR provides a more consistent PIP and tidal volume during PPV.[8,9] TPR has been compared with SIB in four RCTs enrolling a total of 1,247 patients.[6,10-12] Of these in three RCTs,[6,11,12] the majority of neonates enrolled were born at term gestation while one RCT[10] included neonates born at <29 weeks of gestation.

Dawson et al. randomized neonates born at <29 weeks of gestation to receive PPV, if needed during resuscitation by TPR (n = 41) or SIB (without a PEEP valve, n = 39).[10] In both the groups, room air was used to initiate PPV. The primary outcome of oxygen saturation at 5 minutes after birth was comparable in the two groups. Although, need for 100% oxygen and use of continuous positive airway pressure (CPAP) was higher in the TPR group, the difference was not significant. Of neonates who left the delivery room on CPAP, a lesser proportion of neonates in the TPR group (7% vs. 23%; P = 0.05) were intubated in the next 24 hours. No difference was observed in the need of surfactant or incidences of BPD, air leaks, or death. The study did not report the need and duration of different types of respiratory support.

In a quasi-randomized trial conducted in India, Thakur et al. allocated neonates born at >26 weeks of gestation to receive PPV, if needed during resuscitation, with TPR (n = 40) or SIB (without PEEP valve, n = 50) by date of birth (even or odd).[12] Of the 90 neonates enrolled in the study 37 were born at <34 weeks of gestation. Resuscitation was initiated with room air. Duration of PPV, which was the primary outcome of the study, was significantly shorter in the TPR group. Also, a significantly greater proportion of neonates in the TPR group needed only room air for resuscitation (72.5% vs. 38%) and a lesser proportion needed intubation (15% vs. 34%). No difference was observed in the need of CPAP or invasive ventilation, maximum inspired oxygen concentration (FiO_2) or mean airway pressure, duration of mechanical ventilation, surfactant administration or mortality. In the subgroup of neonates born at <34 weeks of gestation, a significantly lesser proportion of neonates in the TPR group needed invasive ventilation (31.6% vs. 77.8%, P = 0.008).

In another trial from India, Kookna et al. allocated neonates born at ≥28 weeks of gestation to receive PPV, if needed at 30 seconds after birth, with TPR (n = 25) or SIB (without PEEP valve, n = 25).[11] Of the 50 neonates enrolled in the study 7 (14%) were born preterm. Resuscitation was initiated with room air. Duration of PPV, which was the primary outcome of the study, was significantly shorter in the TPR group. No difference was reported in the oxygen saturation, need of chest compression, need of intubation, incidence of HIE, air leaks, or death before hospital discharge.

In a multicentric RCT, Szyld et al. enrolled neonates born at >26 weeks of gestation needing PPV at birth.[6] Neonates received PPV with either a TPR (n = 511) or an SIB (n = 516). The TPR was used with a PEEP valve set at a pressure of 5 cmH$_2$O. Each center participating in the study was also randomized to use SIB with and without a PEEP valve with a pressure of 5 cmH$_2$O. No significant difference was observed in the proportion of neonates who reached an HR >100 at 2 minutes (93.7% vs. 90.3%) which was the primary outcome of the study.

TABLE 16.2: OUTCOMES IN COMPARISONS OF T-PIECE RESUSCITATOR WITH SELF-INFLATING BAG FOR POSITIVE PRESSURE VENTILATION DURING RESUSCITATION

Outcome	Number of studies (number of neonates)	Relative risk or mean difference with 95%CI	Certainty of evidence
Duration of PPV (seconds)	3 (1,088)	−19.8 (−27.7 to −12)	Moderate
Intubation during resuscitation	4 (1,266)	0.89 (0.76–1.05)	Very low
Chest compression or medications	4 (1,247)	0.58 (0.28–1.23)	Very low
Air leaks	4 (1,247)	1.29 (0.60–2.77)	Very low
Bronchopulmonary dysplasia	4 (1,247)	0.64 (0.43–0.95)	Very low
Mortality before hospital discharge	4 (1,247)	0.74 (0.40–1.34)	Very low

(PPV: positive pressure ventilation)

Neonates in the TPR group were significantly less likely to be intubated in the delivery room (17% vs. 26%) and were given lower PIP and FiO_2. Among neonatal outcomes, days on mechanical ventilation and duration of oxygen therapy were lower in the TPR group while no difference was observed in the incidence of HIE, air leaks, need of mechanical ventilation, or death before hospital discharge. In the subset of very low birth weight (VLBW) neonates (85 in TPR and 110 in SIB group), those in the TPR group had lower need of intubation for ventilation, lower incidence of BPD and shorter duration of oxygen therapy.

In a systematic review of the above four studies, no effect of the intervention was observed on neonatal mortality, intubation, chest compression or medications during resuscitation; admission to the neonatal intensive care unit (NICU), air leak, intraventricular hemorrhage, or duration of hospitalization **(Table 16.2)**.[7] Neonates resuscitated with TPR received shorter duration of PPV and had a lower incidence of BPD.

Level of Evidence

Overall, evidence of very low to low certainty was available on the use of TPR in preference to SIB for providing PPV to neonates needing resuscitation at birth.[7] Three of the four studies included in the above-mentioned systematic review were small in size and a high risk of bias. Another important factor to consider is cost associated with the use of TPR as it has a higher initial acquisition cost, recurring cost of disposable ventilation circuits, and need of pressurized gas source (SIB can be used without a pressurized gas source). In addition, some of the benefits of TPR can be because of the use of PEEP and studies are needed to evaluate the benefit of TPR over SIB when both are used with provision of PEEP.

Due to very low certainty of evidence, well planned and adequately powered RCTs with clinically important outcomes are required to compare TPR and SIB, especially in preterm neonates at risk of lung injury.

3. MONITORING OXYGEN THERAPY IN TERM AND PRETERM NEONATES

Practice Questions

i. *Does monitoring of oxygen therapy with a pulse oximeter versus relying only on color (central cyanosis) improve the resuscitation, respiratory, and other outcomes in neonates needing resuscitation at birth?*

ii. *Does use of signal extraction technology versus use of nonsignal extraction technology improve the resuscitation and respiratory outcomes in neonates needing resuscitation at birth?*

iii. *What is the best method of application of pulse oximeter probe in neonates needing resuscitation to achieve a reliable and early signal?*

iv. *What oxygen saturation targets should be used in term and preterm neonates during resuscitation?*

The *subgroups of interest* were (i) Full term and late preterm neonates and (ii) Extremely preterm neonates
The *outcomes* were:

1. *Resuscitation outcomes:*
   a. Duration of positive pressure ventilation/time to onset of spontaneous breathing
   b. Need of intubation
   c. Need of advanced steps of resuscitation
2. *Respiratory outcomes:*
   a. Need and duration of any respiratory support (including non-invasive and invasive ventilation)
   b. Need and duration of invasive ventilation
   c. Incidence of bronchopulmonary dysplasia
3. *Other outcomes:*
   a. Incidence of HIE
   b. Neonatal mortality

Evidence Summary

i. *Does monitoring of oxygen therapy with a pulse oximeter versus relying only on color (central cyanosis) improve the resuscitation, respiratory and other outcomes in neonates needing resuscitation at birth?*

Till the turn of this century, the assessment of the baby at birth and response to resuscitative measures was assessed by clinical examination—oxygenation by color of the baby and heart rate by palpation of pulse or precordial auscultation. Use of pulse oximetry was first evaluated for rapid, objective, and continuous assessment of heart rate and oxygen saturation. Subsequently, recognition of the harmful effects of hyperoxia and publication of "normal" oxygen saturation values in neonates not needing any resuscitation led to the recommendations about the use of room air for initiating PPV, monitoring oxygen saturation by pulse oximetry during resuscitation and titrating the oxygen fraction in the inspired air based on time since birth and oxygen saturation value. Thereafter, assessment of oxygen saturation by pulse oximeter has become an integral part of the neonatal resuscitation, even if heart rate is monitored by more accurate and objective methods like electrocardiography.

Studies have evaluated the ability of pulse oximetry to assess oxygen saturation during resuscitation and have published normative values.[13-16] No RCTs have directly compared assessment of oxygenation by color and pulse oximetry. In a small study enrolling 20 neonates, a high degree of variability was noted among 27 observers in judging whether a baby appears "pink".[17]

The addition of pulse oximeters to the resuscitation equipment adds a substantial cost and needs training of the care providers. HBB program, an international neonatal resuscitation program customized for use in resource-limited settings and targeted at training of midwives and the Navjat Shishu Suraksha Karyakram (NSSK), a program by National Health Mission, aimed to train health personnel in basic newborn care and resuscitation, do not include assessment of oxygenation by any method and the resuscitative steps are guided by breathing efforts and heart rate.[18,19] Although these simplified resuscitation algorithms have been shown to be effective (in comparison to no objective training), evidence about the effect of adding assessment of oxygenation by pulse oximetry is not available.[20] This is especially relevant for neonates born after prolonged fetal hypoxia or at preterm gestation.

ii. *Does use of signal extraction technology versus use of nonsignal extraction technology improve the resuscitation and respiratory outcomes in neonates needing resuscitation at birth?*

Performance of a pulse oximeter during resuscitation can be measured by time taken to acquire signal and display values and the reliability of the values. Bright light, motion of the baby, and low systemic circulation may downgrade the performance of a pulse oximeter at the resuscitation table. Signal extraction technology (SET) has been claimed to overcome the interference due to motion or low circulation. The practice question of the use of SET was addressed in the National Neonatology Forum Clinical Practice Guidelines (CPG) on oxygen therapy in neonates released in December 2021.[21] The Guideline Writing Group identified seven observational studies that have compared SET-based and non-SET-based pulse oximeters. Time taken to display data was reported by two studies (n = 380) and the pooled mean difference (0.65 seconds; –1.91 lower to +0.61) was not significantly different with the two types of pulse oximeters. Rates of true (OR: 0.99; 95% CI: 0.68–1.45) and false alarms (OR: 0.95; 95% CI: 0.64–1.42) were also not significantly different. Incidence of the drop-out alarms was lower in the SET group. No evidence is available whether the lower incidence of signal drop out is associated with change in use of various resuscitation interventions or other clinical outcomes. The Guideline Writing Group concluded that "in neonates on respiratory support pulse oximeters with or without signal extraction technology may be used for monitoring of oxygen saturation; however, the benefit of reduced dropout rate with the SET group pulse oximeters may make them preferable in neonates with hemodynamic instability, movement artifacts, transport as well as in the delivery room." This recommendation should be interpreted in light of higher cost of acquisition and maintenance of SET-based pulse oximeters and lack of evidence on the benefit in the clinical outcomes.

iii. *What is the best method of application of pulse oximeter probe in neonates needing resuscitation to achieve a reliable and early signal?*

To save time at the time of resuscitation, the pulse oximeter is switched on before the delivery of the infant. After the infant is born the sensor can be applied on the baby by two methods: applying the sensor to infant first (STIF) followed by the cable to the pulse oximeter second or applying the cable to the pulse oximeter first followed by sensor to infant second (STIS). Idea is to get a reliable signal as fast as possible. Reliability of oxygenation needs assessment against the measurement done on an arterial blood gas sample and no study has evaluated this invasive method. Reliability of heart rate can be assessed relatively more easily by comparing the heart rate acquired from an ECG signal. Three RCTs have evaluated the different methods of the application of pulse oximeter sensor on the infant.[22-24] Two studies, one each with SET-based and non-SET-based pulse oximeters, have used ECG to check the reliability of the signal.[22,24] Both the studies reported that the STIF method provides a reliable signal more quickly. One study that used "stable display of heart rate and saturation without blinking" as indicator of the reliable signal concluded that the STIS provides a reliable signal more quickly.[23] It has been proposed that with the STIS method with the cable attached to the pulse oximeter and sensor in air, the pulse oximeter may obtain erroneous signals and despite displaying on the screen first, the values may not be accurate. The study that found STIS to be a better approach did not use an objective method to label the reliability of the signal. Based on the evidence available, application of the sensor to the infant first followed by attachment of the cable to the pulse oximeter second may provide a reliable signal more quickly.

iv. *What oxygen saturation targets should be used in term and preterm neonates during resuscitation?*

In 2010, for the first time, the International Liaison Committee on Resuscitation recommended use of pulse oximetry for titrating the oxygen administration during neonatal resuscitation.[25] The recommendations were based on a number of studies that reported that term and preterm neonates breathing at birth and not needing any resuscitation may take up to 10 minutes to achieve an oxygen saturation value considered normal in the neonatal period.[25] The guidelines provided target oxygen saturation from 1–10 minutes after birth based on the interquartile range of values obtained in healthy term babies following vaginal birth at sea level. Neonates born preterm or by cesarean section have been reported to have lower SpO_2 values during the first 10 minutes and may take longer to reach an SpO_2 of >90%.[16] Neonates born with lung immaturity or intrapartum asphyxia may need oxygen administration, PPV, or surfactant administration to achieve "normal" oxygen saturation. Further, the presently recommended cut-offs are based on neonates resuscitated with immediate cord clamping. Studies have suggested that neonates with or without need of resuscitation if managed with delayed cord clamping are likely to have higher oxygen saturation values.[26,27]

Level of Evidence

The four practice questions identified under the scope of oxygen monitoring during resuscitation have been answered by observational studies or small RCTs (OECBM Level 2 evidence). None of the studies have reported important outcomes identified *a-priori* in this review. Implementation research is also needed to incorporate optimum oxygen management in neonatal resuscitation algorithms recommended for resource-limited settings.

■ 4. LARYNGEAL MASK AIRWAY VERSUS INTUBATION

Practice Question

Is the use of laryngeal mask airway (LMA) noninferior to intubation in neonates needing PPV during resuscitation at birth?

The *subgroups of interest* were neonates of different gestation or birth weight categories.

The *outcomes* were:

1. *Resuscitation outcomes:*
   a. Duration of PPV/time to onset of spontaneous breathing
   b. Need of intubation
   c. Need of advanced steps of resuscitation
2. *Respiratory outcomes:*
   a. Need and duration of any respiratory support (including non-invasive and invasive ventilation)
   b. Need and duration of invasive ventilation
3. *Other outcomes:*
   a. Incidence of HIE
   b. Neonatal mortality

Evidence Summary

Effective PPV is the most important intervention in neonatal resuscitation. PPV is initiated with a T-piece resuscitator or SIB attached to a mask. However, PPV with a mask may be ineffective due to improper technique to obtain a good seal between mask and face or due to airway obstruction. In such cases, intubation is needed to obtain a secure access to the airway. However, a rapid and successful intubation is a highly skilled activity, and a high incidence of delay or failure of intubation has been reported.[28] LMA consisting of an inflatable cuff attached to a silicone airway tube, is inserted orally using the provider's index finger without laryngoscopy. LMA can be used as an alternative to the mask, as a primary device to provide PPV or as an alternative to endotracheal tube. A Cochrane review updated in 2018 included eight RCTs—five comparing face mask with LMA and three comparing endotracheal intubation with LMA.[29] These RCTs included neonates born at late preterm or term gestation (minimum gestation of 34 weeks) and weighing >1,500 or 2,000 g.

Face Mask Versus Laryngeal Mask Airway (As Primary Device for Positive Pressure Ventilation)

In the five trials that reported the outcome, use of LMA was associated with a significant reduction in the need of intubation during resuscitation (RR: 0.24; 0.12–0.47, moderate certainty of evidence). Neonates randomized to the LMA group needed PPV for a significantly shorter duration **(Table 16.3)** and had lower probability of an Apgar score of ≤7 at 5 minutes (RR: 0.34, 95% CI: 0.16–0.74) and NICU admission (RR 0.6; 95% CI: 0.4–0.9). No difference was reported in the incidence of death or HIE **(Table 16.3)**. The need of epinephrine during resuscitation or incidence of adverse effects have been reported by one study each and no difference was observed.

TABLE 16.3: OUTCOMES IN COMPARISONS OF VENTILATION WITH LARYNGEAL MASK AIRWAY OR BAG AND MASK DURING RESUSCITATION

Outcome	Number of studies (number of neonates)	Relative risk or mean difference with 95%CI	Certainty of evidence
Duration of PPV (seconds)	4 (325)	−18.9 (−24.35 to −13.44)	-
Intubation during resuscitation	5 (660)	0.24 (0.12–0.47)	Moderate
NICU admission	2 (191)	0.6 (0.4–0.9)	Moderate
Death or HIE	2 (191)	0.65 (0.17–2.43)	Moderate

(HIE: hypoxic ischemic encephalopathy; NICU: neonatal intensive care unit; PPV: positive pressure ventilation)

TABLE 16.4: OUTCOMES IN COMPARISONS OF VENTILATION WITH LARYNGEAL MASK AIRWAY OR INTUBATION DURING RESUSCITATION

Outcome	Number of studies (number of neonates)	Relative risk or mean difference with 95%CI	Certainty of evidence
Failure to insert device	3 (158)	0.95 (0.17–5.42)	Very low
Death or HIE	1 (68)	0.59 (0.11–3.32)	Low

(HIE: hypoxic ischemic encephalopathy)

After the 2018 Cochrane Review was published, a large RCT has been conducted in Uganda enrolling a total of 1,154 neonates.[30] In neonates with an estimated gestation of >34 weeks and estimated weight >2,000 g and needing PPV at birth, midwives used a bag with a face mask or LMA. No difference (RR: 1.16; 95% CI: 0.90–1.51) was observed in the primary outcome which was a composite of death within 7 days or admission to NICU with moderate-to-severe HIE. Also, no difference was observed in the need of advanced steps of resuscitation or adverse events.

Intubation versus Laryngeal Mask Airway

Three studies were included in the systematic review. No difference was observed in time to insert the device, failure to insert device, successful insertion during first attempt, duration of PPV, Apgar score and death or HIE **(Table 16.4)**.

Level of Evidence

Overall, evidence of moderate certainty is available that in comparison to face mask, use of LMA is associated with lower need of intubation and NICU admission without any difference in the incidence of death or HIE. Low or very low-quality evidence indicates that no difference is observed when comparing LMA with intubation. The 2020 version of the neonatal resuscitation program by American Academy of Pediatrics has moved LMA from the section on intubation to the section on PPV and has included LMA insertion in the Neonatal Resuscitation Program (NRP) essentials course.[31]

5. CARDIOPULMONARY RESUSCITATION RATIOS AND TECHNIQUE

Practice Questions

i. *Which technique for chest compression in neonates undergoing resuscitation at birth is the preferred method—thumb or two-finger technique?*

ii. *What ratio of chest compression and ventilation is most appropriate in neonates undergoing resuscitation at birth?*

The *subgroups of interest* were: (i) Full term and late preterm neonates and (ii) Extremely preterm neonates.
The *outcomes* were:

1. *Resuscitation outcomes:*
   a. Time to return of spontaneous circulation
   b. Duration of chest compression
   c. Need of epinephrine
   d. Incidence of resuscitation failure resulting in death of neonate in the delivery room or within one hour of birth
   e. Incidence of soft-tissue or bony injury causally associated with resuscitation

2. *Other outcomes:*
   a. Incidence of HIE
   b. Neonatal mortality

Evidence Summary

Prolonged fetal hypoxia or asphyxia can lead to myocardial depression and bradycardia. In this state, the heart may not be able to pump sufficient blood to the vital organs and chest compression is needed to generate sufficient stroke volume. To ensure oxygenation and ventilation, chest compressions need to be combined with delivery of effective PPV. Efficiency of chest compression to maintain circulation depends on the depth of the compression, technique of chest compression, and the frequency of compression in coordination with ongoing PPV.

i. *Which technique for chest compression in neonates undergoing resuscitation at birth is the preferred method—thumb or two-finger technique?*

Current neonatal resuscitation guidelines recommend use of two-thumb technique to provide chest compression if heart rate is <60 after 30 seconds of effective PPV.[32] A number of manikin-based studies have compared two-thumb (TT) and two-finger (TF) techniques of chest compression.[33-45] Observations from most of the studies favor the TT technique as it was able to generate a greater depth of chest compression, lesser variability of chest compression, smaller fatigue score, higher systolic and diastolic blood pressure and more frequent correct positioning of the hand on chest.[33-43] However, all these studies have been conducted in manikins (except one on an animal model and another for checking positioning on healthy neonates). None of the studies have been conducted in neonates actually needing chest compression and therefore important outcomes including duration of chest compression, time to return of spontaneous circulation, need for administration of epinephrine, rate of resuscitation failure, incidence of HIE, and mortality have not been reported. Chest compression can also lead to bone and soft tissue injury. No evidence is available on the incidence of injuries with different techniques of chest compression.

ii. *What ratio of chest compression and ventilation is most appropriate in neonates undergoing resuscitation at birth?*

Current neonatal resuscitation guidelines recommend a 3:1 ratio of chest compression to ventilation with a total of 120 events in a minute has been recommended in the NRP.[32] In adult resuscitation a higher ratio of chest compression is provided. However, in neonates, the primary aim of the resuscitation is aeration of the lungs and therefore, a higher rate of breaths is recommended. Similar to studies on the technique of chest compression, studies evaluating different ratios of chest compressions and ventilation have been conducted in manikins or animal models. Manikin-based studies have shown that in comparison to other ratios of chest compression and ventilation that have higher events of chest compression (5:1) and/or less interruptions in the events (10:2 or 15:2), the usually practiced ratio of 3:1 is associated with more consistent depth of chest compression without any difference in the provider fatigue.[46,47] Animal studies have shown similar time to return of spontaneous circulation and similar levels of the bio-markers of brain or lung injury.[48-51] None of the studies have been conducted in neonates actually needing chest compression and therefore important outcomes including duration of chest compression, time to return of spontaneous circulation, need for administration of epinephrine, rate of resuscitation failure, incidence of HIE, and mortality have not been reported.

Level of Evidence

The two practice questions identified under the scope of chest compression have been answered by manikin or animal studies (OECBM Level 5 evidence). None of the studies have reported important outcomes identified a priori in this review. Human studies are needed to evaluate the effect of different depths of chest compression or different ratios of chest compression and ventilation. Such studies will be difficult to conduct due to rarity of the event, emergent situation of resuscitation, and ethical issues.

6. EPINEPHRINE DOSE AND ROUTE

Practice Question

What dose of epinephrine is most appropriate by endotracheal or intravascular route in neonates undergoing resuscitation at birth?

The *subgroups of interest* were: (i) Full term and late preterm neonates and (ii) Extremely preterm neonates born at <28 completed weeks of gestation or with birth weight <1000 g.
The *outcomes* were:

1. *Resuscitation outcomes:*
   a. Time to return of spontaneous circulation
   b. Number of doses of epinephrine
   c. Cumulative dose of epinephrine
   d. Incidence of resuscitation failure resulting in death of neonate in the delivery room or within one hour of birth
   e. Incidence of severe intraventricular hemorrhage
2. *Other outcomes:*
   a. Incidence of HIE
   b. Neonatal mortality

Evidence Summary

Use of epinephrine is recommended if heart rate does not increase to >60 bpm despite effective and coordinated positive pressure ventilation and chest compressions. The neonatal resuscitation program recommends a dose of 0.01–0.03 mg/kg intravenously at intervals of every 3–5 minutes. If intravenous access is not available, epinephrine may be administered via endotracheal route using a dose in the higher end of the recommended range. Epinephrine is used infrequently in neonatal resuscitation and its need indicates prolonged and severe fetal hypoxia and/or asphyxia. Resuscitation failure and incidence of HIE is high in neonates who need epinephrine. International Liaison Committee on Resuscitation (ILCOR) updated its systematic review on dose and frequency of administration of epinephrine in April 2021.[52] The review could find only two observational studies comparing intravenous and endotracheal routes.[53,54] No difference was observed in the mortality before hospital discharge, failure to achieve return to spontaneous circulation (ROSC), time to ROSC and need of an additional dose of epinephrine (certainty of evidence very low for all the outcomes, **Table 16.5**). Other important outcomes including rates of HIE and intraventricular hemorrhage (IVH) were not reported. The review could not identify studies reporting different doses or intervals of epinephrine administration.

TABLE 16.5: OUTCOMES IN COMPARISONS OF EPINEPHRINE ADMINISTRATION BY ENDOTRACHEAL AND INTRAVENOUS ROUTES

Outcome	Number of studies (number of neonates)	Relative risk or mean difference with 95%CI	Certainty of evidence
Death before discharge	1* (50)	1.03 (0.62–1.71)	Very low
Failure to achieve return of spontaneous circulation	2* (97)	0.97 (0.38–2.48)	Very low
Time to return of spontaneous circulation (minutes)	1* (50)	+2.0 (−0.6 to +4.6)	Very low
Need of an additional dose of epinephrine	2* (97)	1.94 (0.18–20.96)	Very low

*All the studies included are observational.

Level of Evidence

Evidence of very low certainty is available to inform the choice of different doses and routes of epinephrine administration. No studies are available to evaluate this practice question in different gestation age groups.

7. INTRAOSSEOUS VERSUS UMBILICAL VEIN FOR EMERGENCY INFUSION

Practice Question

Which route—intraosseous or umbilical vein cannulation—for administration of volume bolus in neonates undergoing resuscitation at birth is the preferred one?

The *subgroups of interest* were: (i) Full term and late preterm neonates and (ii) Extremely preterm neonates.
The *outcomes* were:

1. *Resuscitation outcomes:*
   a. Time to return of spontaneous circulation
   b. Incidence of resuscitation failure resulting in death of neonate in the delivery room or within one hour of birth
   c. Incidence of soft-tissue or bony injury causally associated with resuscitation
2. *Other outcomes:*
   a. Incidence of HIE
   b. Neonatal mortality

Evidence Summary

A systematic review conducted to answer this research question did not find any eligible study.[55] Current NRP guidelines recommend the use of epinephrine in case of severe bradycardia unresponsive to chest compression and of a volume expander if there is evidence of hypovolemia and the baby is not responding to resuscitation.[56] Epinephrine can be administered by intravenous or endotracheal route. A bolus of volume expander if indicated must be administered intravenously. The guidelines further recommend that "outside of the delivery room setting, and when umbilical venous catheterization is not feasible, vascular access may be secured with the intraosseous route."[56] Use of the intraosseous route has been associated with local complications.[57-59] Due to lack of supporting evidence for intraosseous route, the intravenous route remains the primary route of choice for administering volume bolus during neonatal resuscitation.

Level of Evidence

No RCTs or observational studies have been conducted to answer this research question. Use of intraosseous route for vascular access if intravenous access cannot be obtained is based on expert opinion (Level 5 evidence) only.

8. SODIUM BICARBONATE FOR RESUSCITATION

Practice Question

Does administration of sodium bicarbonate or no sodium bicarbonate administration in neonates undergoing resuscitation at birth impact the resuscitation outcomes?

The *subgroups of interest* were: (i) Full term and late preterm neonates and (ii) Extremely preterm neonates.
The *outcomes* were:

1. *Resuscitation outcomes:*
   a. Duration of PPV/time to onset of spontaneous breathing
   b. Time to return of spontaneous circulation
   c. Incidence of resuscitation failure resulting in death of neonate in the delivery room or within one hour of birth
2. *Other outcomes:*
   a. Incidence of HIE
   b. Neonatal mortality
   c. Incidence of severe IVH in preterm neonates

Evidence Summary

Prolonged fetal hypoxia and ischemia can lead to anaerobic metabolism and accumulation of lactic acid in tissues. Acidosis can lead to poor myocardial contractility and poor response to epinephrine. Administration of sodium bicarbonate has been proposed to reverse acidosis and improve the myocardial function. Only one small RCT (n = 55) has been conducted to evaluate the role of sodium bicarbonate during resuscitation.[60] The trial did not show any effect on death before discharge (RR: 1.04, 95% CI: 0.49–2.21), abnormal neurological examination at discharge (RR: 0.86, 95% CI: 0.30–2.50), incidence of HIE (RR: 1.30, 95% CI: 0.88–1.92), and incidence of IVH (RR: 1.04, 95% CI: 0.23–4.70).

Level of Evidence

Evidence from a single small RCT does not support the use of sodium bicarbonate during neonatal resuscitation (Level 2 evidence). Evidence is not available to access role of sodium bicarbonate in specific subgroup population of neonates, e.g., extremely low birth weight neonates.

CONCLUSION

The evidence-base for several practices that are part of neonatal resuscitation guidelines are clearly based on very low quality of evidence or expert opinion. This chapter reviewed evidence for several neonatal resuscitation practice guidelines in the delivery room namely, use of PEEP during PPV, use of T-piece instead of SIB, use of pulse oximetry for monitoring oxygen therapy in term and preterm neonates, use of LMA instead of intubation, most appropriate method for chest compression, optimal epinephrine dose and route, use of intraosseous route compared to umbilical venous route for emergency infusion, and use of sodium bicarbonate. For all the above practices currently incorporated in neonatal resuscitation guidelines, the level of evidence currently available is low to very low. There is clearly a need for well-designed and robust RCTs to answer the questions that have been addressed in this chapter.

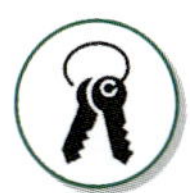 **KEY POINTS**

1. No recommendation can be made on the use of PEEP in neonates needing positive pressure ventilation (PPV) for resuscitation in the delivery room due to low to very low quality of evidence.

2. The evidence available on the use of T-piece resuscitator in preference to self-inflating bag for providing PPV to neonates needing resuscitation at birth is of very low to low certainty.

3. There is insufficient evidence that use of pulse oximeter compared to assessing color has improved resuscitation outcomes. Nor is there sufficient evidence to recommend signal extraction technology over other technologies for improving neonatal resuscitation outcomes.

4. Low or very low-quality evidence indicates that no difference is observed when comparing laryngeal mask airway (LMA) with intubation.

5. Current guidelines for chest compression technique are based on studies in animals/manikins. Human studies are required to assess their impact on meaningful resuscitation outcomes.

6. Evidence of very low certainty is available to inform the choice of different doses and routes of epinephrine administration.

7. Use of intraosseous route for vascular access if intravenous access cannot be obtained is based on expert opinion as there are no randomized controlled studies on this subject.

8. The current recommendations not to use of sodium bicarbonate during neonatal resuscitation are based on results from a single small randomized controlled trial (RCT).

■ REFERENCES

1. Wyckoff MH, Wyllie J, Aziz K, Almeida MF de, Fabres J, Fawke J, et al. Neonatal Life Support: 2020 International Consensus on Cardiopulmonary Resuscitation and Emergency Cardiovascular Care Science with Treatment Recommendations. Circulation. 2020;142:S185-221.

2. Alonso-Coello P, Schünemann HJ, Moberg J, Brignardello-Petersen R, Akl EA, Davoli M, et al. GRADE Evidence to Decision (EtD) frameworks: a systematic and transparent approach to making well-informed healthcare choices. 1: Introduction. BMJ. 2016;353:i2016.

3. Alonso-Coello P, Oxman AD, Moberg J, Brignardello-Petersen R, Akl EA, Davoli M, et al. GRADE Evidence to Decision (EtD) frameworks: a systematic and transparent approach to making well-informed healthcare choices. 2: Clinical practice guidelines. BMJ. 2016;353:i2089.

4. Centre for Evidence-Based Medicine (CEBM), University of Oxford. (2010). OCEBM Levels of Evidence. [online] Available from https://www.cebm.ox.ac.uk/resources/levels-of-evidence/ocebm-levels-of-evidence [Last accessed January, 2023].

5. Holte K, Ersdal H, Eilevstjønn J, Gomo Ø, Klingenberg C, Thallinger M, et al. Positive end-expiratory pressure in newborn resuscitation around term: a randomized controlled trial. Pediatrics. 2020;146:e20200494.

6. Szyld E, Aguilar A, Musante GA, Vain N, Prudent L, Fabres J, et al. Comparison of devices for newborn ventilation in the delivery room. J Pediatrics. 2014;165:234-9.e3.

7. Trevisanuto D, Roehr CC, Davis PG, Schmölzer GM, Wyckoff MH, Liley HG, et al. Devices for administering ventilation at birth: a systematic review. Pediatrics. 2021;148:e2021050174.

8. Bennett S, Finer NN, Rich W, Vaucher Y. A comparison of three neonatal resuscitation devices. Resuscitation. 2005;67:113-8.

9. Roehr CC, Kelm M, Fischer HS, Bührer C, Schmalisch G, Proquitté H. Manual ventilation devices in neonatal resuscitation: Tidal volume and positive pressure-provision. Resuscitation. 2010;81:202-5.

10. Dawson JA, Schmölzer GM, Kamlin COF, Pas AB te, O'Donnell CPF, Donath SM, et al. Oxygenation with T-piece versus self-inflating bag for ventilation of extremely preterm infants at birth: a randomized controlled trial. J Pediatrics. 2011;158:912-918.e2.

11. Kookna S, Singh AK, Pandit S, Dhawan N. T-piece resuscitator or self inflating bag for positive pressure ventilation during neonatal resuscitation: a randomized controlled trial. J Dent Med Sci. 2019;18:66-74.

12. Thakur A, Saluja S, Modi M, Kler N, Garg P, Soni A, et al. T-piece or self inflating bag for positive pressure ventilation during delivery room resuscitation: an RCT. Resuscitation. 2015;90:21-4.

13. O'Donnell CPF, Kamlin COF, Davis PG, Morley CJ. Feasibility of and delay in obtaining pulse oximetry during neonatal resuscitation. J Pediatrics. 2005;147:698-9.

14. Rao R, Ramji S. Pulse oximetry in asphyxiated newborns in the delivery room. Indian Pediatr. 2001;38:762-6.

15. Gandhi B, Rich W, Finer N. Time to achieve stable pulse oximetry values in VLBW infants in the delivery room. Resuscitation. 2013;84:970-3.

16. Dawson JA, Kamlin COF, Vento M, Wong C, Cole TJ, Donath SM, et al. Defining the reference range for oxygen saturation for infants after birth. Pediatrics. 2010;125:e1340-7.

17. O'Donnell CPF, Kamlin COF, Davis PG, Carlin JB, Morley CJ. Clinical assessment of infant colour at delivery. Archives Dis Child-Fetal Neonatal Ed. 2007;92:F465.

18. Singhal N, Lockyer J, Fidler H, Keenan W, Little G, Bucher S, et al. Helping babies breathe: global neonatal resuscitation program development and formative educational evaluation. Resuscitation. 2012;83:90-6.

19. Child Health Division, Ministry of Health and Family Welfare (GOI). (2020). Navjaat Shishu Suraksha Karyakram (NSSK). Resuscitation and Essential Newborn Care Resource Manual. [online] Available from https://www.nhm.gov.in/images/pdf/programmes/child-health/guidelines/NSSK/NSSK-Resource-Manual.pdf [Last accessed January, 2023].

20. Versantvoort JMD, Kleinhout MY, Ockhuijsen HDL, Bloemenkamp K, Vries WB de, Hoogen A van den. Helping babies breathe and its effects on intrapartum-related stillbirths and neonatal mortality in low-resource settings: a systematic review. Arch Dis Child. 2020;105:127.

21. Agrawal G, Dalal SS, Garg AK, Kumar R, Shah S, Singh D. Clinical practice guidelines: oxygen therapy in neonates. National Neonatology Forum of India, New Delhi, India. 2021. Available from https://www.nnfi.org/assests/upload/usefull-links-pdf/Oxygen_therapy_in_neonates_NNFI_CPG_Dec2021.pdf [Last accessed March, 2023]

22. Saraswat A, Simionato L, Dawson J, Thio M, Kamlin C, Owen L, et al. Determining the best method of Nellcor pulse oximeter sensor application in neonates. Acta Paediatr. 2012;101:484-7.

23. Louis D, Sundaram V, Kumar P. Pulse oximeter sensor application during neonatal resuscitation: a randomized controlled trial. Pediatrics. 2014;133:476-82.

24. O'Donnell CPF, Kamlin COF, Davis PG, Morley CJ. Obtaining pulse oximetry data in neonates: a randomised crossover study of sensor application techniques. Archives Dis Child-Fetal Neonatal Ed. 2005;90:F84.

25. Kattwinkel J, Perlman JM, Aziz K, Colby C, Fairchild K, Gallagher J, et al. Part 15: Neonatal Resuscitation. Circulation. 2010;122:S909-19.

26. Lara-Cantón I, Badurdeen S, Dekker J, Davis P, Roberts C, Pas A te, et al. Oxygen saturation and heart rate in healthy term and late preterm infants with delayed cord clamping. Pediatr Res. 2022;1-6.

27. Andersson O, Rana N, Ewald U, Målqvist M, Stripple G, Basnet O, et al. Intact cord resuscitation versus early cord clamping in the treatment of depressed newborn infants during the first 10 minutes of birth (Nepcord III): a randomized clinical trial. Maternal Heal Neonatol Perinatology. 2019;5:15.

28. Falck AJ, Escobedo MB, Baillargeon JG, Villard LG, Gunkel JH. Proficiency of pediatric residents in performing neonatal endotracheal intubation. Pediatrics. 2003;112:1242-7.

29. Qureshi MJ, Kumar M. Laryngeal mask airway versus bag-mask ventilation or endotracheal intubation for neonatal resuscitation. Cochrane Db Syst Rev. 2018;3:CD003314.

30. Pejovic NJ, Höök SM, Byamugisha J, Alfvén T, Lubulwa C, Cavallin F, et al. A randomized trial of laryngeal mask airway in neonatal resuscitation. New Engl J Med. 2020;383:2138-47.

31. Mani S, Pinheiro JMB, Rawat M. Laryngeal masks in neonatal resuscitation: a narrative review of updates 2022. Children. 2022;9:733.

32. Aziz K, Lee HC, Escobedo MB, Hoover AV, Kamath-Rayne BD, Kapadia VS, et al. Part 5: Neonatal Resuscitation: 2020 American Heart Association Guidelines for Cardiopulmonary Resuscitation and Emergency Cardiovascular Care. Circulation. 2020;142:S524-50.

33. Saini SS, Gupta N, Kumar P, Bhalla AK, Kaur H. A comparison of two-fingers technique and two-thumbs encircling hands technique of chest compression in neonates. J Perinatol. 2012;32:690-4.

34. Dorfsman ML, Menegazzi JJ, Wadas RJ, Auble TE. Two-thumb vs two-finger chest compression in an infant model of prolonged cardiopulmonary resuscitation. Acad Emerg Med. 2000;7:1077-82.

35. Lee SY, Hong JY, Oh JH, Son SH. The superiority of the two-thumb over the two-finger technique for single-rescuer infant cardiopulmonary resuscitation. Eur J Emerg Med. 2018;25:372-6.

36. Huynh TK, Hemway RJ, Perlman JM. The two-thumb technique using an elevated surface is preferable for teaching infant cardiopulmonary resuscitation. J Pediatrics. 2012;161:658-61.

37. Udassi S, Udassi JP, Lamb MA, Theriaque DW, Shuster JJ, Zaritsky AL, et al. Two-thumb technique is superior to two-finger technique during lone rescuer infant manikin CPR. Resuscitation. 2010;81:712-7.

38. Jiang J, Zou Y, Shi W, Zhu Y, Tao R, Jiang Y, et al. Two-thumb encircling hands technique is more advisable than 2-finger technique when lone rescuer performs cardiopulmonary resuscitation on infant manikin. Am J Emerg Medicine. 2015;33:531-4.

39. Jo CH, Cho GC, Lee CH. Two-thumb encircling technique over the head of patients in the setting of lone rescuer infant CPR occurred during ambulance transfer. Pediatr Emerg Care. 2017;33:462-6.

40. Jo CH, Jung HS, Cho GC, Oh YJ. Over-the-head two-thumb encircling technique as an alternative to the two-finger technique in the in-hospital infant cardiac arrest setting: a randomised crossover simulation study. Emerg Med J. 2015;32:703.

41. Christman C, Hemway RJ, Wyckoff MH, Perlman JM. The two-thumb is superior to the two-finger method for administering chest compressions in a manikin model of neonatal resuscitation. Archives Dis Child-Fetal Neonatal Ed. 2011;96:F99.

42. Reynolds C, Cox J, Livingstone V, Dempsey EM. Rescuer exertion and fatigue using two-thumb vs. two-finger method during simulated neonatal cardiopulmonary resuscitation. Front Pediatr. 2020;8:133.

43. Martin PS, Kemp AM, Theobald PS, Maguire SA, Jones MD. Do chest compressions during simulated infant CPR comply with international recommendations? Arch Dis Child. 2013;98:576.

44. Whitelaw CC, Slywka B, Goldsmith LJ. Comparison of a two-finger versus two-thumb method for chest compressions by healthcare providers in an infant mechanical model. Resuscitation. 2000;43:213-6.

45. Bruckner M, O'Reilly M, Lee TF, Neset M, Cheung PY, Schmölzer GM. Effects of varying chest compression depths on carotid blood flow and blood pressure in asphyxiated piglets. Archives Dis Child-Fetal Neonatal Ed. 2021;106:553-6.

46. Srikantan SK, Berg RA, Cox T, Tice L, Nadkarni VM. Effect of one-rescuer compression/ventilation ratios on cardiopulmonary resuscitation in infant, pediatric, and adult manikins. Pediatr Crit Care Me. 2005;6:293-7.

47. Hemway RJ, Christman C, Perlman J. The 3:1 is superior to a 15:2 ratio in a newborn manikin model in terms of quality of chest compressions and number of ventilations. Archives Dis Child-Fetal Neonatal Ed. 2013;98:F42.

48. Dannevig I, Solevag AL, Saugstad OD, Nakstad B. Lung injury in asphyxiated newborn pigs resuscitated from cardiac arrest: the impact of supplementary oxygen, longer ventilation intervals and chest compressions at different compression-to-ventilation ratios. Open Respir Medicine J. 2012;6:89-96.

49. Dannevig I, Solevåg AL, Sonerud T, Saugstad OD, Nakstad B. Brain inflammation induced by severe asphyxia in newborn pigs and the impact of alternative resuscitation strategies on the newborn central nervous system. Pediatr Res. 2013;73:163-70.

50. Solevåg AL, Dannevig I, Wyckoff M, Saugstad OD, Nakstad B. Return of spontaneous circulation with a compression:ventilation ratio of 15:2 versus 3:1 in newborn pigs with cardiac arrest due to asphyxia. Archives Dis Child-Fetal Neonatal Ed. 2011;96:F417.

51. Solevåg AL, Dannevig I, Wyckoff M, Saugstad OD, Nakstad B. Extended series of cardiac compressions during CPR in a swine model of perinatal asphyxia. Resuscitation. 2010;81:1571-6.

52. Liley HG, Kim H-S, Mildenhall L, Schmölzer GM, Rabi Y, Ziegler C, et al. Dose, route and interval of epinephrine (adrenaline) for neonatal resuscitation; Consensus on Science with Treatment Recommendations [URL]: International Liaison Committee on Resuscitation (ILCOR) Advanced Life Support Task Force. [online] Available from http://ilcor.org [Last accessed January, 2023].

53. Halling C, Sparks JE, Christie L, Wyckoff MH. Efficacy of intravenous and endotracheal epinephrine during neonatal cardiopulmonary resuscitation in the delivery room. J Pediatrics. 2017;185:232-6.

54. Barber CA, Wyckoff MH. Use and efficacy of endotracheal versus intravenous epinephrine during neonatal cardiopulmonary resuscitation in the delivery room. Pediatrics. 2006;118:1028-34.

55. Granfeldt A, Avis SR, Lind PC, Holmberg MJ, Kleinman M, Maconochie I, et al. Intravenous vs. intraosseous administration of drugs during cardiac arrest: a systematic review. Resuscitation. 2020;149:150-7.

56. Aziz K, Lee CHC, Escobedo MB, Hoover AV, Kamath-Rayne BD, Kapadia VS, et al. Part 5: Neonatal Resuscitation 2020 American Heart Association Guidelines for Cardiopulmonary Resuscitation and Emergency Cardiovascular Care. Pediatrics. 2021;147:e2020038505E.

57. Ellemunter H, Simma B, Trawöger R, Maurer H. Intraosseous lines in preterm and full term neonates. Archives Dis Child-Fetal Neonatal Ed. 1999;80:F74.

58. Oesterlie GE, Petersen KK, Knudsen L, Henriksen TB. Crural amputation of a newborn as a consequence of intraosseous needle insertion and calcium infusion. Pediatr Emerg Care. 2014;30:413-4.

59. Suominen PK, Nurmi E, Lauerma K. Intraosseous access in neonates and infants: risk of severe complications: a case report. Acta Anaesth Scand. 2015;59:1389-93.

60. Lokesh L, Kumar P, Murki S, Narang A. A randomized controlled trial of sodium bicarbonate in neonatal resuscitation: effect on immediate outcome. Resuscitation. 2004;60:219-23.

Self Assessment

1. In comparison to self-inflating bag, the use of T-piece resuscitator has been shown to be associated with which benefits?
   a. Shorter duration of positive pressure ventilation
   b. Lower incidence of hypoxic-ischemic encephalopathy
   c. Lower incidence of pneumothorax
   d. All of the above

2. While coordinating chest compression and positive pressure ventilation, what is the advantage of using 3:1 ratio instead of 5:1, 10:2 or 15:2 ratio?
   a. Earlier return of spontaneous circulation
   b. More consistent depth of chest compression
   c. Lower neonatal mortality
   d. Less fatigue

3. What quality of evidence is available for the advanced steps in neonatal resuscitation?

Answers

For answers, go to the end of the Book, Page no. 323

Evolution of Neonatal Resuscitation Practices

17. **International Guidelines: Evolution and Current Status**
   Aparna C

International Guidelines: Evolution and Current Status

Aparna C

Lessons to Learn

- ○ Evolution of neonatal resuscitation guidelines
- ○ Systematic reviews and grading of recommendations, assessment, development, and evaluation (GRADE) process
- ○ Evidence to decision framework
- ○ Scoping reviews and evidence updates

EVOLUTION OF NEONATAL RESUSCITATION GUIDELINES

The recognition that there would be a proportion of babies at birth who would need help to transit from fetal life for establishing effective breathing is not new and has been known for eons. A range of practices (much different from what is currently practiced) evolved over time, but none were "evidence-based" as there was limited to no data for neonatal resuscitation practices even up to the 1960s or 1970s. There were no formal guidelines for neonatal resuscitation until the emergence of its felt need with the inception and growth of neonatal care as a subspecialty in and around the 1970s.

In the 1970s, the National Institutes for Health, USA funded projects to improve neonatal education which resulted in development of several educational resources known as the Neonatal Educational Program (NEP). This in a way formed the basis for the subsequent Neonatal Resuscitation Program (NRP).[1] In the 1980s, the Committee of the Fetus and Newborn of the American Academy of Pediatrics (AAP) created a Task Force for Neonatal Resuscitation. After extensive consultations with the American Heart Association (AHA) and other organizations, the NRP was formally launched in 1987 and the first NRP training course was conducted at New Orleans, USA. The training program aimed to teach the principles of neonatal resuscitation with the goal of providing *"a skilled provider for every delivery and a skilled team for every resuscitation".*

From its inception, it was evident that NRP had to be flexible and adaptive to keep pace with emerging evidence and be able to provide for the different types of skill sets required by different levels of healthcare providers. An important guiding principle of NRP has been to provide practice recommendations based on best available evidence. Due to paucity of data, several of the recommendations were based on consensus of experts in the field. During the initial years, these were informal, but over the years a more systematic evaluation of evidence started to become the basis of developing recommendations and the process of consultation became global with the founding of the International Liaison Committee on Resuscitation (ILCOR) in 1992. The modular nature of NRP has allowed it to adapt to provide the skill sets required by different types of trainees and healthcare providers.

It was during the AHA's Fourth National Conference on Cardiopulmonary Resuscitation and Emergency Cardiovascular Care in 1992 that the seeds for international cooperation were sown. ILCOR was constituted in 1992 after the European Resuscitation Council (ERC) meeting in UK attended by ERC, AHA, Australian Resuscitation Council (ARC), Heart and Stroke Foundation of Canada (HSFC), and the Resuscitation Council of Southern Africa (RCSA). The original mission statement of ILCOR issued in 1993 stated as follows "*To provide a consensus mechanism by which the international science and knowledge relevant to emergency cardiac care can be identified and reviewed. This consensus mechanism will be used to provide consistent international guidelines on emergency cardiac care for basic life support (BLS), pediatric life support (PLS), and advanced life support (ALS). While the major focus will be upon treatment guidelines, ILCOR will also address the effectiveness of educational and training approaches and topics related to the organization and implementation of emergency cardiac care. ILCOR will also encourage coordination of dates for guidelines development and conferences by various national resuscitation councils. These international guidelines will aim for a commonality supported by science for BLS, PLS, and ALS.*"[2] Over the years ILCOR has worked in keeping with its original mission statement. Over the years, evidence evaluation has shifted from a 5-year cycle to a continuous process. It has since adopted a strategy to disseminate, promote, and implement the results of the scientific evidence for resuscitation.[3]

Over time resuscitation councils and organizations in various countries have adapted the core international guidelines for their regions. Recognizing that the NRP may be challenging to implement in resource constrained settings the AAP in 2009, in collaboration with the World Health Organization (WHO) and several other partners, initiated a program "Helping Babies Breathe" (HBB) targeted at nurses, midwives, and traditional birth attendants in developing countries. In 2012, the WHO released its guidelines on basic newborn resuscitation for use at first level and higher facilities in low-and-middle income countries. Over the years, resuscitation guidelines have begun to address issues of training and resource material, communication skills, and team behavior and also evaluation of the implementation of the guidelines.

GUIDELINE DEVELOPMENT PROCESS

The ILCOR task forces as well as other member councils have been partnering along with AHA for the process of evidence review for neonatal resuscitation guidelines. The methodological experts of ILCOR have used three types of evidence reviews for developing the current guidelines—systematic reviews, scoping reviews, and evidence updates.[4]

Systematic Reviews

Each ILCOR task force identifies the most important research questions in that area mentioning the questions in the PICOST format (population, intervention, control, outcome, study design and time) using Delphi survey or by discussion within the expert group. Relevant outcomes for the questions are also determined and classified as: (1) critical, (2) important, and (3) not important. Search for relevant studies is performed in standard databases such as the MEDLINE, Embase, and Cochrane library using selected search terms.

The methodology experts in the group then evaluate the quality of evidence using the Cochrane risk-of-bias tool[5] or using the grading of recommendations, assessment, development, and evaluation (GRADE) approach.[6] The GRADE approach is used to categorize the quality of evidence for each critical outcome as "high", "moderate", "low", or "very low". Evidence from randomized controlled trial (RCT) was of "high" quality while evidence from observational studies was considered to be of "low" quality. Quality of evidence is downgraded based on the consideration of five criteria—risk of bias, inconsistency, imprecision, indirectness, and publication bias **(Tables 17.1 and 17.2)**. The GRADE system's evaluation of RCTs is depicted in **Table 17.1** and is described in greater detail in following section:

Risk of Bias

The risk of bias within a RCT is determined by analyzing the following limitations within each study: (1) *Selection bias* is assessed by evaluating the technique used for *randomization* and the appropriateness of *allocation concealment*; (2) *Measurement bias* can be minimized by *blinding* the participants—the family, clinicians involved as well as research team to the intervention. Whenever blinding is not possible, e.g., in an RCT comparing masks versus prongs for delivering positive pressure ventilation (PPV), the outcome assessors must be blinded to the intervention. Measurement bias due to open label nature of the

TABLE 17.1: GRADE APPROACH TO ASSESS QUALITY OF EVIDENCE FROM RANDOMIZED CONTROL TRIALS (RCTs)

Factor	Assessment criteria	Serious	Very serious
Risk of bias	Five parameters: 1. Allocation concealment 2. Blinding of parents/clinicians/trial investigators 3. Blinding of outcome assessors 4. Intention-to-treat (ITT) analysis or postrandomization exclusions (if active exclusions) 5. Loss to follow-up (downgrade if >20% or if greater than event rate in control arm)	Risk in any one of the five parameters In studies involving an intervention that cannot be blinded (e.g., PPV using masks vs. prongs), do not consider the parameter "blinding of parents/clinicians/trial investigators" for downgrading	Risk in two or more of the five parameters
Inconsistency	I^2 and P for heterogeneity Number of studies	$I^2 \geq 60\%$ or P for heterogeneity <0.05 OR Single study	–
Indirectness	Indirect nature of available evidence In four parameters: 1. Population 2. Setting (LMIC/HIC) 3. Intervention 4. Outcome	Serious risk in any one of the four parameters	Serious risk in two or more of the four parameters
Imprecision	1. Optimal information size (OIS)/number of events (number of subjects in the systematic review is lower than the sample size calculated conventionally for an RCT with standard assumptions for control event rate and clinically plausible effect size) 2. 95% CI crossing the clinical decision threshold between recommending and not recommending treatment—the clinical threshold is usually taken as 10% relative risk reduction for critical outcomes and 25% relative risk reduction for noncritical outcomes	1. OIS not met OR 2. Imprecise as per the confidence intervals crossing the clinical decision threshold *NB:* Do not consider the OIS, if only one study is included (because we would have already downgraded for inconsistency)	When both the criteria (OIS *and* "imprecise" results) are met
Publication bias	1. Funnel plot suggestive of publication bias 2. Check international and national trial registries and published protocols that suggest non-publication of results of the completed trials	Risk in one of the two parameters	–

(CI: confidence interval; GRADE: grading of recommendations, assessment, development, and evaluation; HIC: high-income country; LMIC: low- and middle-income country; PPV: positive pressure ventilation)

TABLE 17.2: ASSESSMENT CRITERIA FOR CERTAINTY OF EVIDENCE

Study design	Certainty of evidence begins at this level	Lower if	Higher if
Randomized control trials	High or moderate	Risk of bias	Large effect
		Inconsistency	Dose response seen
Observational studies	Low or very low	Indirectness	All plausible confounding would reduce demonstrated effect or would suggest a spurious effect when results show no effect
		Imprecision	
		Publication bias	

study is not likely when the outcome is *"objective"* (e.g., mortality); (3) *Appropriateness of analysis*: Analysis by intention-to-treat is considered to be associated with least risk of bias. The authors look for "active" exclusions due to any reason, including incorrect random allocation, not received allocated treatment, received the "other" treatment, and refusal to take treatment after randomization. Downgrade the evidence, if there are any. Exclusions due to death, referral, withdrawal of consent after randomization, or loss to follow-up need not be used for downgrading; (4) *Loss to follow-up*: Evidence is downgraded for loss to follow-up if follow-up attrition is more than an arbitrary cut-off of 20% or if there is differential loss to follow-up in both groups after ruling out other reasons.

Inconsistency

Inconsistency for a given outcome is assessed by exploring the differences in the *direction* as well as *size* of the effects observed across studies. The quality of evidence is not downgraded if the direction of the effect is similar across studies and confidence limits overlapped, whereas quality is downgraded if the direction of the effect is conflicting across studies and confidence limits do not overlap.

Indirectness

The evidence is downgraded for lack of directness when there are substantial differences in the context where the research was conducted and the context where it was intended to be applied—with respect to the *population* (preterm versus term newborns), *setting* (low-middle income versus high-income setting), *intervention,* or the *outcome.*

Imprecision

The degree of certainty of the effect estimate is assessed as a function of the *sample size* and number of *events*—studies with relatively few participants or events (and thus wide confidence intervals around effect estimates) are downgraded for imprecision.

Publication Bias

Considering that the perceived statistical significance of an intervention may be affected by the selective publication of studies based on study results, the quality of evidence is downgraded, if publication bias is strongly suspected based on a *funnel plot* to assess the same or based on evaluation of national and international *registries* of published studies or protocols of unpublished studies.

In addition to the above, the Cochrane risk of bias assessment considers potential sources of funding and conflicts of interest of authors of the study.

Formulating recommendations after ascertaining quality of evidence—from evidence to decision: After ascertaining the certainty of evidence, the strength of a recommendation reflects the extent to which the guideline panel is confident that desirable effects of an intervention outweigh undesirable effects, or vice versa, across the range of patients for whom the recommendation is intended. Each recommendation is graded as *"strong"*, when the guideline panel clearly feels that benefits outweigh harms or vice versa, as *"weak"* when benefits seem to outweigh the harms but there are trade-offs or areas of uncertainty and as *"context specific"* if benefits outweigh harms, or vice versa in some situations.

When an intervention is endorsed with a *strong* recommendation, most patient families would prefer the same, the clinicians are likely to ensure that patients receive the recommended management strategy and may use it as a quality indicator for ensuring the appropriateness of a process and policymakers would adapt the same into their policies and performance indicators. When an intervention is supported by a *weak* recommendation on the other hand, some families may not prefer the course of action, clinicians will recognize that decision to use or not use the treatment modality may need to be individualized and may seek decision making aids, while policymakers may discuss the action plan with other stakeholders. The key factors that help in assessing the strength of a recommendation are listed in **Table 17.3**.

TABLE 17.3: Parameters Determining the Strength of a Recommendation	
Parameter	**Comment**
Certainty/quality of evidence for critical outcomes	The higher the certainty of the evidence, the more likely a strong recommendation is warranted
Balance between desirable and undesirable outcomes	The larger the differences between the desirable and undesirable consequences, the more likely a strong recommendation is warranted
Values and preferences	The greater the variability in values and preferences, or uncertainty about typical values and preferences, the more likely a weak recommendation is warranted
Resource use	The higher the costs of an intervention (the more resources consumed), the less likely a strong recommendation is warranted

Assessment of quality of observational studies, studies of diagnostic accuracy: Similar to the GRADE tool for RCTs, Quality Assessment of Diagnostic Accuracy Studies (QUADAS)-2 is used for studies of diagnostic accuracy and GRADE criteria for observational studies is used to evaluate observational studies.

Scoping Reviews

In this second type of review, the guideline group determines the available research evidence relevant to the research question and to determine whether this is sufficient to perform a systematic review. Hence scoping reviews may address much broader questions (unlike specified research questions addressed in a systematic review) and may not be able to provide treatment or an intervention-related guideline.

Like for systematic reviews, the task force begins by defining relevant research questions in the PICOST format, does a systematic literature search using online databases and constructs evidence tables. The final output is in the form of a narrative review of existing literature with the analysis and insights of the taskforce members. The recommendation from scoping reviews is written based on the format of Preferred Reporting Items for Systematic Reviews and Meta-analyses (PRISMA).[7] The narrative summary as well as task force insights to the research question are then presented for public review on the ILCOR website and final version incorporated in the relevant international consensus on cardiopulmonary resuscitation and emergency Cardiac Care Science with Treatment Recommendations (CoSTR) publication.

Evidence Update

Unlike the systematic and scoping reviews, evidence updates consist of tabular compilation of research questions, search strategy used, and a list of recent literature in the form of guidelines, systematic reviews, and recent original articles. The search is limited to English language articles on MEDLINE and is generally compiled and published as an appendix of the CoSTR main guideline. Evidence updates are typically included within the main recommendation with a note on whether they may mandate a systematic review in subsequent editions of the guideline.

PROCESS OF IDENTIFICATION OF TOPICS FOR UPDATE

The content experts of neonatal task force which includes neonatologists and nursing professionals review the prior set of research questions and categorize them into three groups: questions that can be retired, questions that remain relevant but require additional scientific evidence, and questions that have sufficient evidence to justify a systematic review. New research topics are also identified and added to the list. The list is then posted for public review, amended based on feedback and finalized. The CoSTR members meet over virtual meetings regularly and physically annually to discuss the progress on allotted systematic reviews. Some examples of topics that were chosen for review for the 2020 update include prediction of need for respiratory support in the labor room (evidence update), effect of briefing/debriefing of team members on neonatal resuscitation (scoping review), and tracheal intubation and suctioning in nonvigorous neonates delivered through meconium-stained amniotic fluid (systematic review).

■ THE WAY FORWARD

The ILCOR has largely standardized the approach to the process of guideline development so as to ensure that updated and evidence-based recommendations are made for every step in resuscitation. However, there are still some areas where the guidelines remain consensus based or historical assessment based. Areas of research gaps are being identified within each research topic (e.g., the influence of tracheal intubation and suctioning within select subgroup of nonvigorous neonates born through meconium-stained amniotic fluid, such as, gestational age, thickness of meconium, and operator experience).

In view of the pragmatic reasons, it is necessary to have a uniform standardized approach to resuscitation ensuring that every step complies with the highest quality of scientific evidence.

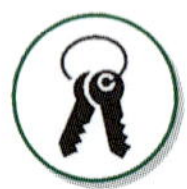

KEY POINTS

1. Development of resuscitation guidelines is a continuous process.
2. Evidence generation process includes systematic reviews and scoping reviews.
3. GRADE process/Cochrane risk of bias is used for ascertaining quality of evidence.
4. Evidence to decision framework is used for formulating guidelines.

■ REFERENCES

1. Halamek LP. The Genesis, Adaptation, and Evolution of the Neonatal Resuscitation Program. NeoReviews. 2008;9;e142-9.

2. Perkins GD, Neumar R, Monsieurs KG, Lim SH, Castren M, Nolan JP, et al. International Liaison Committee on Resuscitation. The International Liaison Committee on Resuscitation: review of the last 25 years and vision for the future. Resuscitation. 2017;121:104-16.

3. International Liaison Committee on Resuscitation. (2020). Continuous evidence evaluation guidance and templates. [online] Available from

https://www.ilcor.org/documents/continuous-evidence-evaluation-guidance-and-templates. [Last accessed January. 2023].

4. Morley PT, Atkins DL, Finn JC, Maconochie I, Nolan JP, Rabi Y, et al. Evidence Evaluation Process and Management of Potential Conflicts of Interest: 2020 International Consensus on Cardiopulmonary Resuscitation and Emergency Cardiovascular Care Science with Treatment Recommendations. Circulation. 2020;142(16_suppl_1):S28-40.

5. O'Connor D, Higgins J, Green S. (2011). Cochrane Handbook for Systematic Reviews of Interventions. [online] Available from https://handbook-5-1.cochrane.org/chapter_5/5_defining_the_review_question_and_developing_criteria_for.htm. [Last accessed January, 2023].

6. Schünemann H, Brozek J, Guyatt G, Oxman A. (2013). Handbook for Grading the Quality of Evidence and the Strength of Recommendations Using the GRADE Approach. [online] Available from https://gdt.gradepro.org/app/handbook/handbook.html. [Last accessed January, 2023].

7. PRISMA. (2021). PRISMA for scoping reviews. [online] Available from http://www.prisma-statement.org/Extensions/ScopingReviews. [Last accessed January, 2023].

Ethical Issues and Research in Neonatal Resuscitation

Termination and Non-initiation of Resuscitation

Tejo Pratap Oleti

Lessons to Learn

- Ethical principles for decision making for terminating/non-initiation of resuscitation
- Current guidelines for termination/non-initiation of resuscitation in neonates
- Evidence to support the decision-making process for termination of resuscitation
- Translating evidence and decision making into practice

The decision to terminate resuscitation or not to initiate resuscitation in a newborn infant at birth is a challenging ethical issue. The decision-making process is compounded by paucity of data, lack of uniformity in the standards and quality of appropriate health care, demographic profile, and sociocultural and religious beliefs of a region. These variables make it hard to generalize guidelines across the globe. Besides, ethical issues are also governed by local legal framework and judgements.

In countries like India, most of compounding factors alluded to earlier exist in large measure—heterogeneous population background, high level of medical illiteracy, non-availability of appropriate medical assistance, varied religious and local beliefs, and practices. The birth of a baby is a very significant event for all families, as is also death which is an emotional issue. The medical provider's dilemma is to balance evidence and family's emotions when faced with a situation of terminating resuscitation or not to initiate resuscitation in a newborn infant at birth. This chapter will attempt to provide practice guidelines that may facilitate crossing the threshold of decision making by the medical provider.

■ LEGAL AND ETHICAL ISSUES

There is to the best of our understanding no legal framework that addresses the issue of termination of resuscitation (TOR) in newborns. Even though there has been a continuous debate on end-of-life decisions amongst critically ill neonates in intensive care units, there is no framework to support such decisions, even though they have been in practice across the world. The Groningen Protocol[1] in the Netherlands is the closest that comes to a formal document addressing the end-of-life decisions amongst newborn infants. As a norm, in most of the situations the family and healthcare providers take the decision largely based on the clinical condition of the neonate. It is important to understand that the ethical principles applicable to adults and older children would also apply to newborn infants.

The parents' *autonomy* to choose the treatment for their newborn infant (as guardians of the infant) must be respected. However, the decision on clinical interventions should be based in the best interest of baby (*beneficence*) and the healthcare provider must ensure that this decision does no harm to the infant (*non-maleficence*). The decisions on end-of-life care must not be influenced by the family background. These decisions must be based on clear communication between the care provider and the family in a transparent manner. The parents are surrogates in neonates' decisions, and hence need to be given sufficient time for informed decision making. Often, it places the family at a disadvantaged situation when they are expected to take a decision as in an emergency resuscitation situation at birth, Wherever information is available like fetus with lethal malformation/syndrome or getting born at periviable period, one should try to counsel and provide information during the antenatal period to give sufficient time for the family to arrive at an informed decision.

The CEASE (Clinical features, Effectiveness, Ask, Stop, Explain) framework, proposed by Torke et al., is ready-reckoner guide for care providers to use in these difficult situations **(Box 18.1)**.[2]

DECISION MAKING FOR TERMINATION OF RESUSCITATION

The situations where care providers are likely to experience dilemma of TOR include a neonate born limp and not responding to cardiopulmonary resuscitative efforts, neonate born at periviable gestations or neonates born with lethal malformations. The following illustrative cases will highlight the process involved in decision making in such scenarios as described above.

Case 1: A 32-year-old third gravida is admitted to the delivery room at 38^{+2} weeks of gestation with decreased fetal movements. Cardiotocography (CTG) showed sinusoidal pattern. She delivered a baby boy by emergency lower segment cesarean section (LSCS). The neonate was limp at birth. CPR was initiated and administered effectively as per standard resuscitation protocol. In spite of the neonatal team's best efforts, the baby's heart rate remained <60 bpm, pulses were not palpable, and no

---

BOX 18.1: CEASE (CLINICAL FEATURES, EFFECTIVENESS, ASK, STOP, EXPLAIN) FRAMEWORK

1. *Clinical features that predict survival:*
   a. Team leader (clinician) should know the background of the neonate which includes antenatal and perinatal events.
   b. Clinician should look at all events during pregnancy and should review the investigations available including ultrasound scan reports.
2. *Effectiveness of resuscitation efforts:*
   a. Clinicians should strictly adhere to cardiopulmonary resuscitation (CPR) algorithm.
   b. The qualitative assessment must include optimal PPV rate, proper choice of equipment, saturation targeting, chest compression rate, depth of compression, and sufficient time for chest recoil.
3. *Ask the other clinicians for input:*
   a. It is essential for team leader to take inputs from all the team members before taking decision.
   b. Non-hierarchical information gathering is proven to be safe, effective and beneficial.
4. *Stop resuscitation efforts:*
   a. Once team feels resuscitative efforts have not achieved restoration of spontaneous circulation (ROSC) or the interventions needed to sustain circulation are unsustainable, the decision to withdraw the supports should be initiated.
   b. The decision might become complex due to advanced interventions use, family, and hospital factors.
   c. Family presence during resuscitation has been shown to help in decision making on TOR. However, many clinicians are not comfortable with the family presence during resuscitation as it might put undue pressure on team's performance.
   d. Increasingly evidence is showing NOT to take the family members consent before stopping/withhold resuscitation. It should be based on clinical status of the neonates and hospital protocols.
5. *Explain what has happened to family:*
   a. The clinical team led by senior member should explain: what has happened, answer queries of the family, and provide emotional support.
   b. Team members can be trained on the communication aspects by using SPIKES (setting up the interview, patient's perception, invitation, knowledge, emotions) protocol.
   c. Role play and other active learning methodologies have been shown to help to build good communication culture.

---

reliable pulse oximetry recordings were seen. Should resuscitation be continued or aborted?

What Does the Evidence Say?

Effective CPR should help in reappearance of spontaneous circulation (ROSC). However, we may not be able to achieve the same on every attempt. There are no good quality studies on the timing of TOR. Data and studies from adults and pediatric population indicate that practicing definite criteria will help in taking decision. However, the results depend on the site of incident and quality of care provided.

An International Liaison Committee on Resuscitation (ILCOR) systematic review,[3] noted that neonates requiring prolonged CPR beyond 10 minutes, had less chances of survival ($\approx$ 69%) and only few survived without moderate-to-severe neurodevelopmental outcomes ($\approx$11%). However, the data is limited and based on just 470 neonates from 15 studies. In an another recent systematic review Foglia et al.,[4] analyzed data from 16 studies and 577 neonates. Survival and lost to follow-up varied among studies (2–100%). Only 10.8% of the neonates survived without moderate-to-severe neurodevelopmental impairment (NDI) and 69% of the neonates died either before discharge or at the time of follow-up. In most of the studies follow-up was at 15–24 months. They concluded that neonates requiring CPR beyond 10 minutes are at high risk of mortality and moderate-to-severe NDI, but survival without NDI is also possible. Exposure to specific duration of CPR is unlikely to predict abnormal outcomes. The results were similar across the subgroup of gestations (<36 or ≥36 weeks), type of study (population based), interventions (initiation of therapeutic hypothermia) and restoration of heart rate after 20 minutes of life. Haines et al.[5] looked at the outcomes in apparent stillborn babies born at extreme premature gestations (22+0 to 27+6 weeks). Majority of these neonates (97%) died on day 1. None of the neonates with undetectable heart rate at 5 minutes of life survived till discharge.

Before considering TOR, the care providers should ensure the quality of resuscitative efforts as mentioned in CEASE algorithm. One should check for adherence to algorithm and dosages of drugs, carefully review the history, and other clinical findings. One should also look for reversible causes such as tension pneumothorax, cardiac tamponade, hypothermia, hypoglycemia, severe metabolic acidosis, drugs toxicity (look at drugs administered to mother during birthing process), pulseless arrhythmia, etc.

Family Considerations

As mentioned earlier, it is still a dilemma whether to allow the family members to stay on during resuscitation or not. Their presence might help them to understand the management, might have a positive psychological effect on them and provide them a sense of satisfaction that they did the best possible for their baby. Aborting the resuscitative efforts does not solely depend on the patient's clinical status and benefits of continuing the resuscitative measures, but also on the family's wishes. Healthcare providers should help them understand the rationale behind the decision for TOR. The final decision must be one of consensus.

Practice Points

The current recommendation states *"In newly born babies receiving resuscitation, if there is no heart rate and all the steps of resuscitation have been performed, cessation of resuscitation efforts should be discussed with the team and the family. A reasonable time frame for this change in goals of care is around 20 minutes after birth"* (strong recommendation, weak evidence with limited data).[3] The care providers should look at all reversible causes before deciding about TOR. Using ECG and other techniques will help to detect any pulseless arrhythmias. A proper debriefing session with the team and effective communication with the family will help the clinical team to work efficiently.

Case 2: A 36-year-old woman delivers a baby girl with a birth weight of 680 g at a gestational age 23^{+0} weeks by emergency LSCS. She has had multiple abortions in the past. The present pregnancy was complicated by severe preeclampsia and antepartum hemorrhage. Her first trimester screen for trisomy, targeted fetal anomalies scan, and other investigations were reported as normal. The baby is limp at birth. The family has not been counselled before birth. Should resuscitation be done to help the neonate survive? Will the neonate have a good long-term outcome if she survived?

What Does Evidence Say?

The outcome of the neonates born at 22–28 weeks of gestation has improved remarkably over the last few decades. The improvement is more in the high-income countries. Bell et al.[6] reported the survival and long-term outcome in extremely preterm neonates born in 19 academic centers in the USA. The overall survival rate was 78%. However, survival rates among actively treated neonates at 22 and 23 weeks were 30% and 55.8% respectively. At 22–26 months corrected age neonates born at 22 weeks with a Bayley III cognitive composite scores <70 was 25.8% whereas it was 8.3% at 26 weeks. The incidence of cerebral palsy was 48.4% and 32.1% at 22 and 23 weeks respectively. Brumbaugh et al.[7] reported survival and neurodevelopment outcomes at 18–22 months in neonates born with birth weight <400 g and gestation between 22–26 weeks. The overall survival till discharge was 12.7% and among the actively treated neonates who survived, 74% of the neonates had moderate-to-severe neurodevelopment impairment.

A systematic review by Ramaswamy et al.[8] analyzed mortality trends in neonates born at extremely low gestational ages (ELGAN) and those born with extremely low birth weight (ELBW) in low- and middle-income countries. The survival rates were 34% (95% CI: 31–37%) and 39% (34–44%) for ELBW and ELGAN neonates respectively. It was as low as 18% in lower income countries. Sahoo et al.[9] in a study from India amongst 231 ELBW neonates reported a survival rate was 62% and it was below 30% for neonates born before 26 weeks of gestation. The survival rates significantly decreased in neonates with birth weights below 600 g (<30%). In another study from India, Gupta et al.[10] reported a 28% survival amongst ELBW babies and none survived with birth weight <750 g. Mukhopadhyay et al.[11] while reporting the neurodevelopment outcomes of ELBW neonates at corrected age of

2 years from North India observed that 54% of neonates had an overall Motor DQ >85, whereas only 17% had Mental DQ score >85.

Outcomes in neonates at very low gestations also depend on good quality antenatal care, perinatal interventions such as antenatal steroid coverage and $MgSO_4$ administration practices apart from the golden hour and quality neonatal intensive care unit (NICU) management. European guidelines advise to initiate resuscitation in all neonates born after 24 weeks of gestation.[12] ILCOR guidelines propose that resuscitation can be withheld for neonates born before 22 weeks of gestation. They also advise to discuss the option of resuscitation with parents before initiation for neonates born between 22–24 weeks of gestation. The discussion should include outcomes at respective units and the baby's best interests.

Practice Points

In the Indian setting, it may be reasonable to resuscitate all the neonates who are born after 25 weeks of gestation or born with a birth weight of >600 g. For neonates born between 23–25 weeks of gestation, care providers need to discuss the options with parents and decide based on available local data. Accurate gestational age measurement is key before taking a decision. Even with first trimester scan, dating may vary from ±1–2 weeks and ultrasound scan-based estimations of fetal weight measurement may vary between ±10 and 15%.

Whenever it is possible, consent should be obtained from parents for initiation/non-initiation of resuscitation before delivery. When the consent is not available for neonates born at periviable periods, it is reasonable to initiate resuscitation which allows parents time to decide about further continuation of care.

Case 3: A 32-year-old woman is admitted in labor with a gestation of 39^{+6} weeks. She had irregular antenatal visits. A recent scan showed oligohydramnios and bilateral renal agenesis. Parents were explained about the prognosis. Parents opted for non-aggressive management. Later CTG became suspicious and meconium-stained liquor was detected. The neonate was born limp and the neonatal team did not initiate resuscitation.

Evidence and Practice Points

It is often difficult to prognosticate with certainty which malformation will have bad prognosis. With the advancement in medical care, there are new treatment options available for several of these malformations which have resulted in significant improvement in the functionality of the child. Factors that can help in decision making include success rate of available therapies, risks involved with the therapy, increment in quality of life with the therapy, duration of life gained with the therapy and pain, discomfort, and cost associated with the therapy.

In case of lethal malformations such as anencephaly where there is enough evidence to say that the neonate will not survive, one can withhold resuscitation. If a lethal malformation/genetic syndrome is suspected in the neonate and parents are in dilemma regarding an end-of-life decision, it is reasonable to support the infant till definitive diagnosis is available. It will also give time for parents to take the decision. Bereavement and genetic counseling should be offered to all these families to overcome the stress and prevent recurrence of the condition.

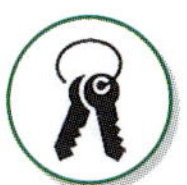

KEY POINTS

1. Termination of resuscitation (TOR)/non-initiation of resuscitation is an important ethical challenge in neonatal resuscitation.
2. TOR decisions must abide by the ethical principles and legal statutes that exist in a country.
3. The common situations where these decisions have to be taken are a baby not responding to effective cardiopulmonary resuscitation (CPR), babies born at periviable gestation and those born with lethal malformations.
4. It is reasonable to stop resuscitation in a neonate after 20 minutes if there are no signs of reappearance of spontaneous circulation (ROSC).
5. Decision to withhold resuscitation in periviable gestation should be based on best interest of the neonate and the family.
6. TOR decisions should be based on review of available evidence and local data and respect family's decisions following communication with the family in an honest and transparent manner.

■ REFERENCES

1. Verhagen E, Sauer PJ. The Groningen protocol: euthanasia in severely ill newborns. N Engl J Med. 2005;352(10):959-62.

2. Torke AM, Bledsoe P, Wocial LD, Bosslet GT, Helft PR. CEASE: a guide for clinicians on how to stop resuscitation efforts. Ann Am Thorac Soc. 2015;12(3):440-5.

3. Wyckoff MH, Wyllie J, Aziz K, de Almeida MF, Fabres JW, Fawke J, et al. Neonatal Life Support 2020 International Consensus on Cardio-pulmonary Resuscitation and Emergency Cardiovascular Care Science with Treatment Recommendations. Resuscitation. 2020;156: A156-87.

4. Foglia EE, Weiner G, de Almeida MFB, Wyllie J, Wyckoff MH, Rabi Y, et al. Duration of resuscitation at birth, mortality, and neurodevelopment: a systematic review. Pediatrics. 2020;146(3):e20201449.

5. Haines M, Wright IM, Bajuk B, Abdel-Latif ME, Hilder L, Challis D, et al. Population-based study shows that resuscitating apparently stillborn extremely preterm babies is associated with poor outcomes. Acta Paediatr. 2016;105(11):1305-11.

6. Bell EF, Hintz SR, Hansen NI, Bann CM, Wyckoff MH, DeMauro SB, et al. Mortality, in-hospital morbidity, care practices, and 2-year outcomes for extremely preterm infants in the US, 2013–2018. JAMA. 2022;327(3):248-63.

7. Brumbaugh JE, Hansen NI, Bell EF, Sridhar A, Carlo WA, Hintz SR, et al. Outcomes of extremely preterm infants with birth weight less than 400 g. JAMA Pediatr. 2019;173(5):434-45.

8. Ramaswamy VV, Abiramalatha T, Bandyopadhyay T, Shaik NB, Bandiya P, Nanda D, et al. ELBW and ELGAN outcomes in developing nations: systematic review and meta-analysis. PLoS One. 2021;16(8):e0255352.

9. Sahoo T, Anand P, Verma A, Saksena M, Sankar MJ, Thukral A, et al. Outcome of extremely low birth weight (ELBW) infants from a birth cohort (2013-2018) in a tertiary care unit in North India. J Perinatol. 2020;40(5):743-49.

10. Gupta S, Adhisivam B, Bhat BV, Plakkal N, Amala R. Short-term outcome and predictors of mortality among very low birth weight infants: a descriptive study. Indian J Pediatr. 2021;88(4):351-7.

11. Mukhopadhyay K, Mahajan R, Malhi P, Kumar A. Neurodevelopmental outcome of extremely low birth weight children at corrected age of two years. Indian Pediatr. 2016;53(5):391-3.

12. Madar J, Roehr CC, Ainsworth S, Ersdal H, Morley C, Rüdiger M, et al. European Resuscitation Council Guidelines 2021: newborn resuscitation and support of transition of infants at birth. Resuscitation. 2021;161:291-326.

 # Self Assessment

1. Identify following statements whether they are True or False:
   a. Ethical guidelines for neonates are much better framed compared to adults
   b. Euthanasia is permitted under Indian laws
   c. Parents are surrogates for making decisions regarding their neonates

2. What are the 6 ethical principles, one should follow while caring neonates?

3. Expand CEASE algorithm.

4. Following can be considered as lethal malformations where we can withhold resuscitation?
   a. Bilateral renal agenesis
   b. Anencephaly
   c. Thanatophoric dysplasia
   d. All the above

5. What are the driving criteria while offering available therapies to parents for the neonate with malformation?

6. A 28-year-old pregnant women gave birth to a neonate at gestational age of 25 weeks at a SNCU with a birth weight of 580 g. Mother did not receive antenatal steroids. Baby cried immediately after birth. How will you guide the parents to take decision on continuation/withdrawal of care?

Answers

For answers, go to the end of the Book, Page no. 324

End-of-life Care

Rashna Dass Hazarika

Lessons to Learn

- Defining end-of-life care or palliative care
- Components of end-of-life/palliative care in newborn
- Care after death of baby

The previous chapter discussed issues related to termination or non-initiation of resuscitation. After discussion with the parents about the prognosis, treatment options, the healthcare provider may provide the option of palliative care for their baby. Parents act as surrogate decision makers for newborns. Hence, they need to be given relevant, accurate, and honest information regarding their baby's condition so that they can participate in the decision-making process. The parents, keeping in mind the best interest of the baby, may opt for palliative care. In situations where it has been decided not to continue with resuscitation of the baby, and the baby has breathing efforts, it may take time before the breathing efforts cease and the heartbeat stops. This chapter deals with issues related to provision of palliative care when parents opt for it rather than continuing with resuscitative efforts.

■ WHAT IS PALLIATIVE CARE?

World Health Organization (WHO) describes palliative care as an approach that improves the quality of life of patients (adult and children) and their families who are facing problems associated with life-threatening illness.[1] The focus is on early identification, assessment, and treatment of pain and other problems whether physical, psychosocial, or spiritual for prevention and relief of suffering. This is done through a series of steps[2]—deciding eligibility for end-of-life/palliative care **(Table 19.1)**, sharing information with parents/family, plan of action, and providing palliative care.

■ PROVIDING END-OF-LIFE/PALLIATIVE CARE

The most important principle is to minimize suffering to the baby.[3]

TABLE 19.1: CONDITIONS ELIGIBLE FOR END OF LIFE CARE IN THE DELIVERY ROOM

Category	Criteria	Example(s)
1	Antenatal or postnatal diagnosis not compatible with life	Bilateral renal agenesis, anencephaly
2	Antenatal or postnatal diagnosis with high risk of morbidity or death	Bilateral hydronephrosis with impaired renal function. Spina bifida with paraparesis
3	Babies born at the margins of viability	Gestational age ≤23 weeks ($\pm$ with bilateral cerebral hemorrhage)

Preparing Parents

Parents should be prepared for what to expect—intermittent breathing efforts/gasping breathing, color change in the baby, some movements, and even continued presence of heart beats during this period. In babies who have malformations/deformities, the parents/family must be explained about them.

Providing Families Private Time with their Baby

When the baby is dying, it may be desirable to provide the family with private time with the baby. If the baby has ECG leads or vascular lines or endotracheal tubes, they must be removed, and the baby covered in a clean and warm sheet before handing the baby to the parents and family to hold the baby. Where possible the families may be provided with a separate, quiet room. During this time, the nurse must intermittently auscultate to check for heartbeat of the baby till it completely stops.

Providing Pain Relief

In some babies the heartbeat may continue for several hours. To decrease suffering, the healthcare team may provide oral opiate to the baby to reduce pain and discomfort, but ensuring it causes no harm.

Feeding

Some babies who are extremely preterm or those with severe malformations may live for several hours/days. In such cases, it would be unethical not to provide feeds or fluids to the baby. Where feasible oral feeds may be provided via a nasogastric tube. Where oral feeding is not possible, the baby may be provided intravenous fluids. In all such situations, the baby is provided minimum fluids to maintain hydration and not augmented as in growing babies. Investigations are avoided, except those that would help in establishing a diagnosis of the condition. Parents should be allowed to spend time with the baby if they desire. Requests for spiritual help should be allowed as per the culture of the region.

■ CARE AFTER DEATH

Parents should be comforted and allowed to grieve in private once death occurs. Hospital procedures should be completed with minimum fuss for the parents. Counseling of parents is to be done and wherever possible called for a follow-up meeting to discuss about the cause of death of the baby and its impact on future pregnancies.

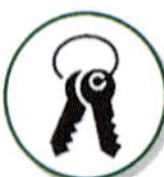 **KEY POINTS**

1. Parents remain the best surrogate decision makers for the baby and sharing their decisions with the healthcare provider (HCP) is the norm.

2. End-of-life care includes preparing the parents and providing private time for them with their dying baby, pain relief, and fluid/feeds.

3. The ultimate goal of end-of-life care is to provide a death of dignity.

■ REFERENCES

1. World Health Organization. (2020). Palliative care. [online] Available from https://www.who.int/news-room/fact-sheets/detail/palliative-care [Last accessed January, 2023].

2. Akyempon AN, Aladangady N. Neonatal and perinatal palliative care pathway: a tertiary neonatal unit approach. BMJ Pediatrics Open. 2021;5:e000820.

3. American Academy of Pediatrics and American Heart Association. In: Weiner GM, Zaichkin J (Eds). Textbook of Neonatal Resuscitation, 8th edition. IL, USA: American Academy of Pediatrics; 2021.

Self Assessment

1. A 32 week baby is delivered by emergency LSCS for abruptio placentae. The baby is limp, pale without respiratory efforts. Baby is intubated and shifted to the NICU and put on mechanical ventilator. An USG of the cranium reveals extensive intracranial hemorrhage. What will be your approach for further management of this baby?

2. In babies, who qualify for end-of-life care, parents have/do not have *(choose correct option)* a role in decision making for the further plan of therapy.

Answers

For answers, go to the end of the Book, Page no. 325

Research Priorities in Neonatal Resuscitation

Suksham Jain

Lessons to Learn

- Importance of evidence in neonatal resuscitation
- Research priorities for evidence generations for steps of neonatal resuscitation
- Research areas related to training in neonatal resuscitation
- Implementation and innovation research for neonatal resuscitation

Neonatal resuscitation has been practiced for a very long time but most of it was not evidence based. It was only in the 1970s that training for neonatal resuscitation was systematized. During the initial years of the neonatal resuscitation program (NRP), the recommendations were largely based on expert opinion and consensus due to paucity of data. However, with the initiation of international collaboration for resuscitation guidelines by the establishment of the International Liaison Committee on Resuscitation (ILCOR) in 1992, evidence generation began to gain momentum. Over the past three decades several of the neonatal resuscitation recommendations are supported by moderate to high quality evidence. However, there are still recommendations that have not changed over time and lack robust evidence to support them. It is not sufficient that we have interventions based on good evidence, but for the practices to have an impact on neonatal outcomes, the ability to implement them effectively across levels of health care and ensure skill acquisition of healthcare providers at all delivery points is equally important.[1] It is therefore important that implementation research also needs to be addressed and prioritized as we move toward improved neonatal and child survival. The challenge of implementing neonatal resuscitation guidelines in low-middle-income countries (LMIC) where almost 80% of the neonatal deaths occur is even greater.[2] Retention of skills is a challenge when event rates for asphyxia experienced by each healthcare provider could be low, especially in health facilities at the primary and secondary levels. This is supported by data from Helping Babies Breathe (HBB) study which observed that skilled birth attendants used positive pressure ventilation (PPV) 1–3 three times in a year as it was needed in 3–6% of babies and chest compressions in 1% of the babies only.[3]

RESEARCH PRIORITIES

The research priorities in neonatal resuscitation can be categorized into the following groups:

- Issues relevant to the existing neonatal resuscitation guidelines
- Issues related to training
- Implementation research
- New ideas and innovations

NEONATAL RESUSCITATION GUIDELINES

Table 20.1 provides a list of current recommendations which need validation and more data because they have been based on limited data or expert opinion due to lack of data.[4,5]

TABLE 20.1: Research Areas Related to Current Resuscitation Guidelines

S. no.	Current recommendations needing more evidence	Evidence on which recommendation is based
1.	Efficacy of skin-to-skin care on mother's abdomen compared to use of radiant warmer in delivery room to prevent hypothermia in preterm babies of varying gestations	Limited data
2.	Efficacy of swaddling newborn babies after birth in food-grade plastic bag up to the level of the neck to prevent hypothermia in resource-limited settings	Limited data
3.	Use of early or delayed cord clamping in term and preterm babies in need of resuscitation	Expert opinion
4.	Appropriate sequence of initial steps during newborn resuscitation	Expert opinion
5.	Use of tracheal suction in nonvigorous babies born through meconium-stained amniotic fluid who need positive pressure ventilation (PPV)	Expert opinion
6.	Use of positive end-expiratory pressure in newborn infants needing PPV	Limited data
7.	Use of laryngeal mask airway for PPV in nonvigorous newborns born through meconium-stained liquor	Limited data
8.	Use of electrocardiography (ECG) for the rapid and accurate measurement of the newborn's heart in-term and preterm babies	Limited data
9.	During chest compressions, use of ECG for the rapid and accurate assessment of heart rate	Expert opinion
10.	The benefit of using 100% oxygen for ventilation during chest compressions	Expert opinion
11.	The use of chest compression to ventilation in a ratio of 3:1 during neonatal resuscitation	Expert opinion
12.	The efficacy of intraosseous route for infusions during neonatal resuscitation	Expert opinion

Contd...

Contd...

S. no.	Current recommendations needing more evidence	Evidence on which recommendation is based
13.	Efficacy of intratracheal epinephrine during neonatal resuscitation at higher dose compared to intravenous dose	Limited data
14.	Optimal (heart rate) threshold, dose, and intervals. Route for the administration of epinephrine (adrenaline) during neonatal resuscitation	Limited data
15.	Benefits and harm (short- and long-term) of single versus multiple dose of epinephrine (adrenaline) during neonatal resuscitation	Limited data

Training in Neonatal Resuscitation

Training is an important component for skill building. Neonatal resuscitation skills acquisition and retention requires multimodal approach of education and training so that provider performance is maximized with better patient outcome. Data pertaining to various modes of training in isolation and as a part of 'care bundle' is available but its impact on neonatal outcome is limited. Deliberate practice (with discrete goal to achieve, immediate feedback on the performance and ample time for repetition to improve performance) and mastery learning (set criteria for passing using deliberate practice that implies mastery in the tasks being learnt) is the preferred approach but it lacks assessment at frequent intervals with conventional retraining every 1–2 years. Delinking of frequency of booster training with type of observer trained and the results of repeat assessment can result in poor performance in real-life scenario and poor economic return of expenditure on training. **Table 20.2** lists some of the training issues related to neonatal resuscitation that needs more evidence generation.

IMPLEMENTATION RESEARCH

In regions of the world with high burden of asphyxia and neonatal mortality, availability of trained human resource is a challenge. Complex guidelines are often difficult to comprehend and implement in these situations. There are also health system challenges related to equipment and supplies. **Box 20.1** lists some of the implementation research issues related to neonatal resuscitation that needs to be addressed.

INNOVATIONS AND DISCOVERY

There have been several innovations as newer evidence for guidelines have come up. However, their implementation is challenging in low resource settings[6] due to their cost and complexity which needs to be addressed. **Box 20.2** lists some of the possible areas where innovative research in neonatal resuscitation should focus on.

TABLE 20.2: RESEARCH IN NEONATAL RESUSCITATION TRAINING AND TEACHING

Topic for research	Current available level of evidence
Role of visual display of algorithm in form of charts, pocket guide, and mobile Apps as a clinical decision tool in successful resuscitation (with outcome as number of successful resuscitations as per algorithm in terms of speed and accuracy)	Only for chart display
Peer-to-peer support as the communication between colleagues in form of information sharing, inquiry, assertion, shared intentions, and evaluation of plans and impact on decision-making during resuscitation, and individual stress (subject to confounder in form of level of individual training of peer group)	Limited data
Spaced learning versus massed learning approach for neonatal resuscitation for knowledge and skill retention at end of 3, 6, and 9 months among skilled birth attendants, nurses, and medical officers at different levels of healthcare facility (community, district, and tertiary center)	Limited data
Simulation-based individual versus team training and bedside performance	Limited data
In person expert coaching/mentorship and clinical outcome of neonatal resuscitation	Limited data
Role of video telemedicine in referral and outcome of neonatal resuscitation	Limited data
Role of autoguidance using audio-video prompts software to guide actions during Neonatal Resuscitation Program (NRP)	Limited data
Role of audio-visual or direct observation audits of neonatal resuscitation as a quality improvement initiative	Expert opinion
In-situ simulation training (in actual clinical scenario) vs. off-site simulation in a laboratory and successful resuscitation at birth	Expert opinion
Skill performance after training with high fidelity manikins (simulated physical features mimicking the resuscitation in patients) versus routine manikins	Limited data
Corrective feedback devices (visual display of depth of chest compressions, prompt audio devices, e.g., metronome) and patient outcome after resuscitation	Limited data
Cost benefit analysis of automated feedback devices used during resuscitation	Limited data
Gamified learning using leaderboards (competition among trainees) and serious games in knowledge, training, and skill retention of neonatal resuscitation	Limited data
Augmented/virtual reality (incorporates a computer-generated holographic image) for skill training and retention basic and advanced neonatal resuscitation	Limited data
Improving the time to corrective steps in neonates needing resuscitation (basic and or advanced) post-training	Limited data

BOX 20.1: IMPLEMENTATION RESEARCH IN NEONATAL RESUSCITATION

Research issues:
1. Impact of simplified neonatal resuscitation algorithms used by trained health workers on neonatal outcomes
2. Models for scaling up strategies for prevention of asphyxia and neonatal resuscitation
3. Strategies for retention of health worker skills in neonatal resuscitation in low-resource settings
4. Technologies for monitoring quality of neonatal resuscitation guidelines at different levels of health care

BOX 20.2: Innovations in Neonatal Resuscitation

Research issues:
1. Can neonatal resuscitation be performed with intact umbilical cord?
2. Can neonatal resuscitation be performed on the mother's abdomen?
3. Equipment for newborn resuscitation by mother's bedside with intact umbilical cord
4. Low-cost devices for positive pressure ventilation of neonates
5. Different types of automated and App-based monitoring devices for heart rate and respiratory mechanics during resuscitation
6. Low cost exhaled CO_2 monitors to assessing placement of endotracheal tubes
7. Use of AI for complex resuscitation situations—for training and monitoring
8. Low-cost neonatal resuscitation simulators

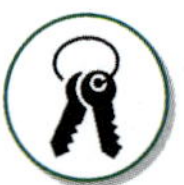

KEY POINTS

1. Data on unanticipated needs of resuscitation at various level of delivery point for successful resuscitation is needed.
2. Research in the field of neonatal resuscitation steps should be a continuum, as level of evidence is moderate-to-low quality in various domains.
3. Neonatal resuscitation skills of provider have a potential of change in clinical outcome, which needs to be assessed objectively.
4. Research priorities must address the challenges of implementing neonatal resuscitation programs in low- and middle-income countries (LMICs).

■ REFERENCES

1. Cheng A, Magid DJ, Auerbach M, Bhanji F, Bigham BL, Blewer AL, et al. Part 6: Resuscitation Education Science: 2020 American Heart Association Guidelines for Cardiopulmonary Resuscitation and Emergency Cardiovascular Care. Circulation. 2020;142(16_suppl_2):S551-9.

2. Bettinger K, Mafuta, E, Mackay A, Bose C, Myklebust H, Haug I, et al. Improving Newborn Resuscitation by Making Every Birth a Learning Event. Children. 2021;8(16):1194.

3. Morris SM, Fratt EM, Rodriguez J, Ruman A, Wibecan L, Nelson BD. Implementation of the Helping Babies Breathe Training Program: a systematic review. Pediatrics. 2020;146(3):e20193938.

4. Wyckoff MH, Wyllie J, Aziz K, de Almeida MF, Fabres JW, Fawke J, et al. Neonatal Life Support 2020 International Consensus on Cardiopulmonary Resuscitation and Emergency Cardiovascular Care Science with Treatment Recommendations. Resuscitation. 2020;156:A156-87.

5. Weiner GM, Zaichkin J. Updates for the Neonatal Resuscitation Program and Resuscitation Guidelines. Neoreviews. 2022;23(4):e238-49.

6. Garvey AA, Dempsey EM. Simulation in Neonatal Resuscitation. Front Pediatr. 2020;8:59.

Beyond Resuscitation Issues

Resuscitation in Low-resource Settings

Abhishek S Aradhya

Lessons to Learn

- Challenges of implementing neonatal resuscitation in low resource settings
- Solutions to address the gap in delivery of neonatal resuscitation
- Simplified neonatal resuscitation algorithms
- Managing out-of-hospital deliveries needing resuscitation at birth

Despite advances in health care, there is gross disparity in survival of neonates between developed and low- and middle-income countries (LMICs). This is evident, as nearly 50 million babies die within the first month in Asian and African LMICs compared to 1 million deaths in developed countries.[1] Intrapartum events contribute to nearly one-fourth of neonatal mortality globally. As a result, an estimated 7 lakh neonates die every year.[2] Studies suggest that implementation of neonatal resuscitation training in low resource settings can avert nearly one-fourth of these intrapartum-related deaths every year.[3]

In the Indian scenario, birth asphyxia is the third leading cause of neonatal mortality after preterm births and infections. Birth asphyxia contributes to nearly one-fifth of neonatal mortality.[4] The institutional deliveries have increased between 2015–16 and 2019–21 from 79–89% as per the latest National family Health Survey (NFHS-5). Thus, skilled assistance at delivery has also improved from previous figure of 81–89%. The skilled assistance comprised of doctors (62%), nurses, midwives or auxiliary nurse and midwife (ANMs) (27%). There is limited data available on the presence of personnel with neonatal airway skills at delivery. Neonatal mortality rate (NMR) has improved from previous figure of 30–25/1,000 live births in the recently concluded NFHS-5;[5] and further to 20/1,000 livebirths as per latest sample registration survey (SRS) data. But India is still far behind the target of single digit NMR as per the Sustainable Developmental Goal by 2030. The impact of scaling up basic neonatal resuscitation at all delivery sites has been estimated by mathematical modeling with Maternal and Neonate Directed Assessment of Technology

(MANDATE) and has found to decrease neonatal mortality from 6.6/1,000 live births to 4.3/1,000 live births in India.[6] There is a greater need to close the equity gaps to in terms of skilled human resource to equipment irrespective of the setting of the deliveries, whether they occur in urban, rural, public sectors, or a private sector or home delivery.

CHALLENGES AND SOLUTIONS

There are numerous challenges for quality care immediately after birth. They range from lack of skilled personnel to availability of appropriate equipment to poor compliance to the resuscitation algorithm. This section outlines a few of the challenges in low-resource settings and their potential solutions **(Table 21.1)**.

Skilled Personnel at Delivery

As mentioned earlier, there is an improvement in institutional deliveries. However, there is limited information on the availability of skilled attendant to handle neonates immediately after birth. Many deliveries, especially vaginal and elective lower segment cesarean section are perceived as low-risk deliveries. This perception leads to poor preparation, and a pediatrician or a nurse trained in neonatal airway management may not be available at all times, especially when needed.

Approaches include basic resuscitation training for the available nurses, trained birth attendants, and community midwives. Although

TABLE 21.1: CHALLENGES AND SOLUTIONS OF NEONATAL RESUSCITATION IN RESOURCE-LIMITED SETTINGS

Challenges	Solutions
Skilled personnel at delivery	Basic resuscitation training to first-line staff, and periodic refresher trainings
Temperature maintenance at delivery	Promoting skin-to-skin contact in delivery room on mother's abdomen, food-grade polyethylene wrap for preterm babies
Umbilical cord management	Delayed cord clamping needs to be ensured while on mother's abdomen
Airway clearance devices	Bulb suction, mucus extractor, and clean cloth
Devices to provide PPV	Self-inflating bag is preferred. Mouth to tube and mask, mouth to mask are alternatives if self-inflating bag is not available
Use of oxygen during resuscitation	Use room air for term babies. Oxygen concentrators can be used in neonates needing additional O_2
Advanced airway	Laryngeal mask airway in neonates >34 weeks after failed BMV if no expertise for intubation available
Maintenance of resuscitation equipment	Disinfection guidelines need to be customized. Sodium hypochlorite can be used for disinfection.
NRP algorithm	HBB action plan
Data documentation	Monitor data on a register

(BMV: bag and mask ventilation; HBB: helping babies breathe; PPV: positive pressure ventilation)

a structured approach to training them exists, the evidence of its effect on neonatal morality is of low quality. However, this approach of training needs to be explored in remote settings where access to basic health care and transportation is scarce.

In places where trained personnel are available, the optimal frequency of training is not defined. Studies have shown that skills, especially that of using bag and mask and behavioral skills wane with time.[7] The integrations of skills into clinical practice may not happen after training without additional practice and mentoring. There is a need for booster training or refresher training. The American Academy of Pediatrics recommends frequent booster training at a frequency that supports retention of knowledge, skills, and behavior.[8] Studies have attempted weekly or monthly refresher training and have found better retention of skills. Simulation using low fidelity mannequin can be utilized for retention of skills. Regular debriefing after each neonatal resuscitation event also helps continued learning and creates a safe environment for learning. Digital interventions such as playing resuscitation video or using Apps with mobile-based virtual reality on neonatal resuscitation can also be utilized for retention of skills in the current smart phone era.[9]

Temperature Maintenance at the Time of Delivery

Hypothermia in delivery room needs to be avoided as much as possible as it has a dose response relationship with mortality and increases morbidities such as respiratory distress, hypoglycemia, infections, etc. Maintenance of environment temperature by avoiding convective loss by ensuring closure of doors, windows, switching off fans is similar across all the settings. After an uncomplicated vaginal delivery, placing the baby on mother's abdomen with skin-to-skin contact is the best way to prevent hypothermia across all settings and this practice in particular should be encouraged in all low-resource settings. Though, use of head caps and covering the baby after drying and use of food-grade polyethylene wraps have been recommended to prevent hypothermia, these can be challenging to implement in scarce-resource settings due to cost and supply-related issues.[10]

Umbilical Cord Management

As per NFHS-5 data, nearly two-thirds of <5-year-old children and 57% of women have anemia.[5] Anemia is a major nutritional problem in India. Delayed cord clamping while on mother's abdomen needs to be practiced irrespective of the setting to reduce the risk of anemia. Delayed cord clamping becomes a critical intervention as incidence of anemia is even more prevalent in low-resource settings. Training and regular audits can help ensure compliance with this practice.

Airway Clearance Devices

Routine airway suctioning is no longer recommended in a baby who is crying and/or breathing well even if there is meconium-stained liquor. Unnecessary suctioning is to be avoided to reduce the risk of bradycardia or trauma. Even in babies born with meconium-stained liquor and are non-vigorous, they need positive pressure ventilation (PPV) first rather than routine endotracheal suctioning. Central suction or electric/pedal-based pressure-regulated suction pumps are preferred. When not available, bulb suction, mucus extractor, and clean gauze/cloth are alternatives. All these alternatives can pose additional risk of infection, if reused or improperly cleaned.

Devices to Provide Positive Pressure Ventilation

Self-inflating resuscitation bag with mask ventilation (BMV) is the preferred mode to deliver PPV even in low-resource settings. Various high quality affordable bags and mask are available at costs of between INR 500–1,000. Alternatives to BMV that have been used include mouth to tube and mask, mouth to mask, mouth to mouth. However, all these alternatives have safety concerns with their use and are best avoided.

Resuscitation with Room Air

It is currently recommended that in all term and late preterm babies, PPV should be initiated with room air.[8] If the baby is preterm or needs additional supplemental oxygen, it can be delivered using either piped line oxygen source or oxygen concentrators using blenders. However, administration of blended oxygen may be a challenge in most delivery rooms in low-resource settings and there is a need to develop low-cost technology for delivering blended oxygen.

Advanced Airway

Less than 1% of babies require advanced resuscitation in the form of intubation, chest compressions, or medication. Although endotracheal intubation is the preferred mode of advanced airway but it demands greater technical skill by the provider. Laryngeal mask airway (LMA) is a simpler and technically less demanding alternative to endotracheal intubation. While studies using LMA in babies >34 weeks gestation have observed shorter resuscitation and need for intubation compared to BMV,[11] its implementation in low-resource settings needs more evidence.

Maintenance of Resuscitation Equipment and Disinfection

Reusable equipment such as self-inflating resuscitation bag, laryngo-scopes, etc., need to be thoroughly disinfected. Common challenges encountered are inappropriate disassembly, improper disinfection, and inadequate rinse after disinfection. PATH has developed neonatal equipment reprocessing recommendations for resource-limited settings.[12] For example, the resuscitation bag needs to be disassembled, washed with soap and water and after drying undergoes either autoclave or ethylene oxide sterilization or chemical sterilization (soaking in 0.5% hypochlorite or 2% glutaraldehyde). The frequency of disinfection must be customized depending upon the load of the unit and feasibility. After each use, the tip of the resuscitation bag can be cleaned with gauze soaked in alcohol/0.5% hypochlorite.

Data Documentation

The resuscitation data is essential to understand the load of the unit, performance, gaps, and for planning strategies for improvement. Data has several challenges ranging from completeness, accuracy, missing data especially deaths/referral data, etc. With the expansion of National Digital Health Mission, the inequities are expected to improve. Until then, the units can continue to maintain and monitor data on a printed register.

■ NEONATAL RESUSCITATION ALGORITHM

The flow of resuscitation is updated on a regular basis by the International Liaison Committee on Resuscitation (ILCOR). The latest flow is suitable for facilities in settings with adequate resources. Although, the flow has been made on evidence-based practices, the availability of equipment such as pulse oximeter, ECG, continuous positive airway pressure (CPAP), etc., are a major limitation in resource-limited settings. World Health Organization (WHO) in its second edition of essential newborn care has proposed to include the simpler algorithm from Helping Babies Breathe (HBB) algorithm.

Helping Babies Breathe

The HBB (Helping Babies Breathe) action plan is largely graphical with simpler text including assessment, airway clearance, stimulation, and assisted ventilation within the golden minute but does not address issues of oxygen use, advanced ventilation, chest compressions, etc. Most neonates requiring resuscitation respond to simple measures such as drying, suction, stimulation, and bag and mask ventilation. The HBB 2nd edition has incorporated recommendations from the 2015 ILCOR Consensus on Science with Treatment Recommendations.[13,14] Systematic review has shown implementing HBB in low-resource settings has moderate evidence of reducing intrapartum-related stillbirths and first day neonatal mortality.[15] The development of HBB as an education tool was recently reviewed by Singhal et al.[16]

Médecins Sans Frontières Mid-Level Neonatal Resuscitation Algorithm

Médecins Sans Frontières (MSF)/Doctors Without Borders is an international medical-humanitarian organization which has been working in low-resource settings and has been using the HBB guidelines for providing neonatal resuscitation. Over time, they became aware of increased capacity of their field teams for providing more advanced neonatal resuscitation interventions. In the absence of an intermediate-level algorithm, MSF adapted and developed a mid-level neonatal resuscitation algorithm for their field teams in 2017 incorporating the available international recommendations.[17]

Navjaat Shishu Suraksha Karyakram

To reduce asphyxia-related morbidity and mortality, the Indian government launched the Navjaat Shishu Suraksha Karyakram (NSSK) training program which focused on essential newborn care and neonatal resuscitation in 2009. The intended trainees were physicians and nurses working at primary and secondary levels of health care. The updated neonatal resuscitation algorithm launched in 2020 has been harmonized with the current available evidence and guidelines.[18] *Figure* **21.1** is the updated NSSK neonatal resuscitation algorithm.

◼ OUT-OF-HOSPITAL DELIVERY

The out-of-hospital delivery can be planned or unplanned. Around 11% of deliveries in India happen outside the hospital settings.[5] Planned deliveries at home usually happen in remote areas where access to basic health facility is lacking and should have a trained birth attendant wherever possible. Unplanned deliveries usually happen in travel settings like while on ambulance (on the way to hospital), train or occasionally while on a plane. Usually, unplanned deliveries are near-term deliveries and are precipitous births. Although the out-of-hospital delivery presents different set of challenges to the provider, the physiologic principles and flow of resuscitation are based on ensuring stabilization using TABC (Temperature, clear Airway, Breathing, Circulation) principles. The perinatal outcomes of out-of-hospital delivery are generally worse (2–3-fold higher mortality) than in hospital deliveries. This section provides some strategies for resuscitation in out-of-hospital settings.[14]

- *Temperature management:* Maintaining normothermia becomes a challenge in the absence of external source of heat. One should try increasing the room temperature to above 25°C by adjusting a heat source. The environment should be free from convective air currents (closed door/windows, switch off fans, etc.). Dry the baby with clean towels and providing skin-to-skin contact at birth should be encouraged. Using food-grade polyethylene to wrap the infant can also be considered. Covering the baby's head with a cotton cap would provide additional help.

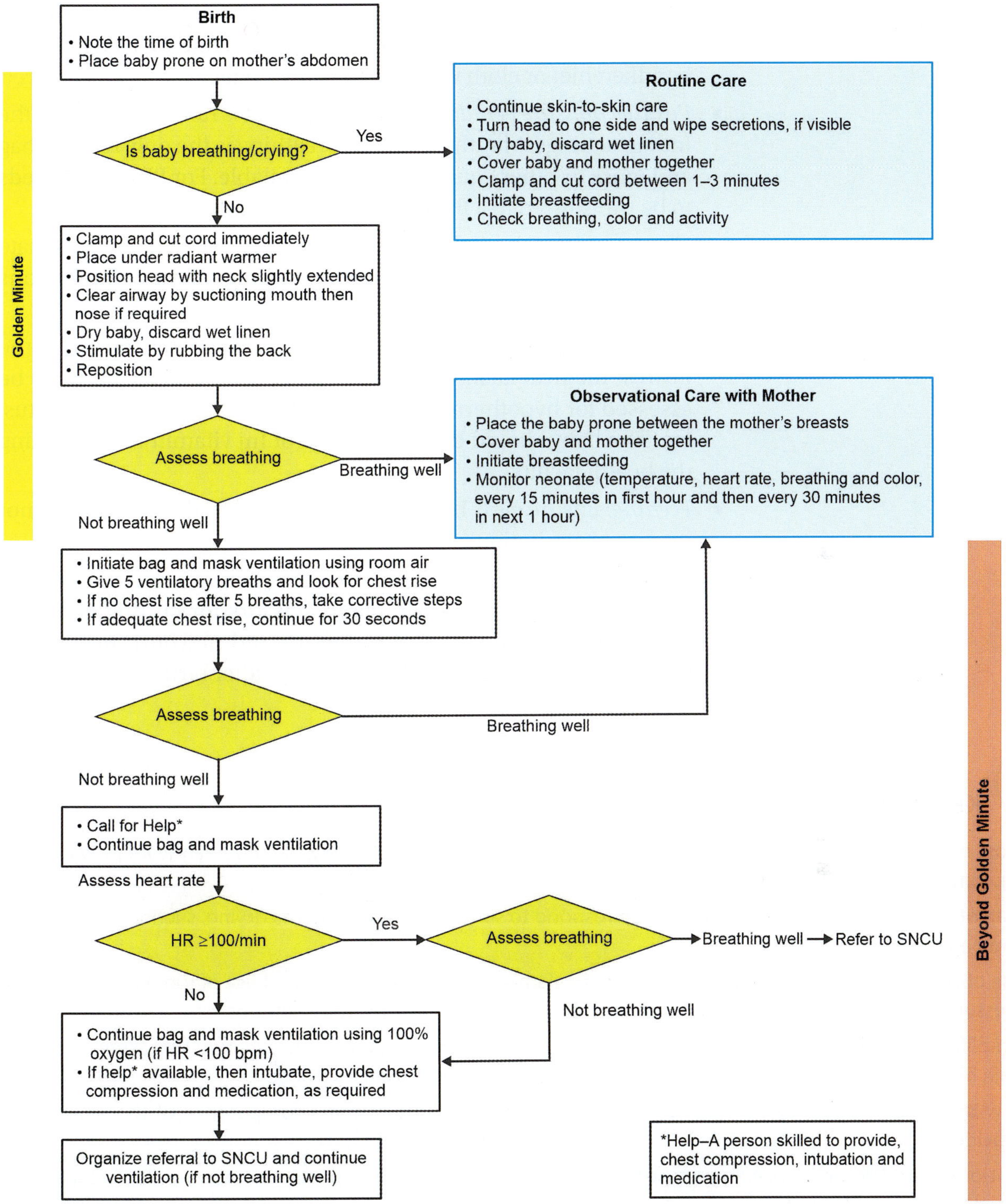

FIG. 21.1 NSSK neonatal resuscitation algorithm (SNCU: special newborn care unit).
Source: Reproduced with permission, Child Health Division, Ministry of Health and Family Welfare, Government of India.

- *Clearing secretions:* If the secretions are obstructing the airway, turn the newborn to one side. Clear the secretions using a clean handkerchief or cloth wrapped in index finger.
- *Positive pressure ventilation:* Emergency kit is rarely available in the Indian settings. Mouth-to-mouth breathing is the only resort if bag and mask or other equipment is not available. For PPV, baby needs to be transferred to a firm surface and needs to be covered.
- *Chest compressions:* If the heart rate remains <60 even after adequate chest rise from mouth-to-mouth breathing, chest compressions can be considered.
- *Transport:* The newborn and mother need to be transported to the nearest medical facility as soon as possible. The baby needs to be assessed for hypothermia, respiratory distress, neurological status, etc. The baby should be given a dose of Inj vitamin K on reaching the health facility.
- *Feeding:* Ensure early breastfeeding initiation if the neonate did not require resuscitation.
- *Infection control:* Ensure hand washing prior to resuscitation with soap and water. Use sterile blade/scissors for cutting cord and a clean tie for the cord. Both mother and newborn need to be monitored for infection in the first 3 days after birth.

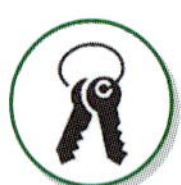 **KEY POINTS**

1. Most of the healthcare facilities in low-resource settings have inadequately trained healthcare providers or equipment for neonatal resuscitation.
2. Majority of neonates requiring resuscitation respond to simple measures such as drying, suction, stimulation, and bag and mask ventilation.
3. Use of skin-to-skin care for warmth, delayed cord clamping, avoiding suction, and use of room air for positive pressure ventilation are interventions that must be promoted in low-resource settings.
4. Simplified algorithms as in Helping Babies Breathe program and *Navjaat Shishu Suraksha Karyakram* can help train healthcare providers to improve asphyxia outcomes in low-resource settings.
5. Low-dose high-frequency training sessions or simulation ensure optimal competency of the healthcare providers.
6. Out-of-hospital deliveries needing resuscitation require use of most appropriate resources available, especially when they are unplanned.

REFERENCES

1. Oestergaard MZ, Inoue M, Yoshida S, Mahanani WR, Gore FM, Cousens S, et al. Neonatal mortality levels for 193 countries in 2009 with trends since 1990: a systematic analysis of progress, projections, and priorities. PLoS Med. 2011;8(8):e1001080.

2. Liu L, Johnson HL, Cousens S, Perin J, Scott S, Lawn JE, et al. Global, regional, and national causes of child mortality: an updated systematic analysis for 2010 with time trends since 2000. Lancet. 2012;379(9832):2151-61.

3. Lee AC, Cousens S, Wall SN, Niermeyer S, Darmstadt GL, Carlo WA, et al. Neonatal resuscitation and immediate newborn assessment and stimulation for the prevention of neonatal deaths: a systematic review, meta-analysis and Delphi estimation of mortality effect. BMC Public Health. 2011;11(Suppl 3):S12.

4. Sankar MJ, Neogi SB, Sharma J, Chauhan M, Srivastava R, Prabhakar PK, et al. State of newborn health in India. J Perinatol. 2016;36(s3):S3-8.

5. International Institute for Population Sciences (IIPS) and ICF. (2021). National Family Health Survey 5 (NFHS-5), 2019-2021: India: Volume I. [online] Available from http://rchiips.org/nfhs/NFHS-5Reports/NFHS-5_INDIA_REPORT.pdf [Last accessed January, 2022].

6. Kamath-Rayne BD, Griffn JB, Moran K, Jones B, Downs A, McClure EM, et al. Resuscitation and obstetrical care to reduce intrapartum-related neonatal deaths: a MANDATE study. Matern Child Health J. 2015;19:1853-63.

7. Reisman J, Arlington L, Jensen L, Louis H, Suarez-Rebling D, Nelson BD. Newborn resuscitation training in resource-limited settings: a systematic literature review. Pediatrics. 2016; 138:e20154490.

8. Aziz K, Lee CHC, Escobedo MB, Hoover AV, Kamath-Rayne BD, Kapadia VS, et al. Part 5: Neonatal Resuscitation 2020 American Heart Association Guidelines for Cardiopulmonary Resuscitation and Emergency Cardiovascular Care. Pediatrics. 2021;147(Suppl 1):e2020038505E.

9. Umoren R, Bucher S, Hippe DS, Ezenwa BN, Fajolu IB, Okwako FM, et al. eHBB: a randomised controlled trial of virtual reality or video for neonatal resuscitation refresher training in healthcare workers in resource-scarce settings. BMJ Open. 2021;11(8):e048506.

10. Belsches TC, Tilly AE, Miller TR, Kambeyanda RH, Leadford A, Manasyan A, et al. Randomized trial of plastic bags to prevent term neonatal hypothermia in a resource-poor setting. Pediatrics. 2013;132:e656-61.

11. Qureshi MJ, Kumar M. Laryngeal mask airway versus bag-mask ventilation or endotracheal intubation for neonatal resuscitation. Cochrane Database Syst Rev. 2018;3(3):CD003314.

12. PATH. (2016). Reprocessing Guidelines for Basic Neonatal Resuscitation Equipment in Resource-limited Settings. [online] Available from https://www.path.org/resources/reprocessing-guidelines-for-basic-neonatal-resuscitation-equipment-in-resource-limited-settings/ [Last accessed January, 2023].

13. Helping Babies Breathe, 2nd Edition Update Guide. (2010). [online] Available from https://www.healthynewbornnetwork.org/hnn-content/uploads/HBB_Overview-of-changes-to-HBB-2nd-Edition_2016-1.pdf. [Last accessed January, 2023].

14. Versantvoort JMD, Kleinhout MY, Ockhuijsen HDL, Bloemenkamp K, de Vries WB, van den Hoogen A. Helping Babies Breathe and its effects on intrapartum-related stillbirths and neonatal mortality in low-resource settings: a systematic review. Arch Dis Child. 2020;105(2):127-33.

15. Watterberg K; Committee on Fetus and Newborn. Providing Care for Infants Born at Home. Pediatrics. 2020;145(5):e20200626.

16. Singhal N, McMillan DD, Savich R, Matovelo D, Santorino D, Kamath-Rayne BD. Development and impact of helping babies breathe educational methodology. Pediatrics. 2020;146(Suppl 2):S123-33.

17. Umphrey L, Breindahl M, Brown A, Saugstad OD, Thio M, Trevisanuto D, et al. When Helping Babies Breathe is not enough: designing a novel, mid-level neonatal resuscitation algorithm for Médecins Sans Frontières field teams working in low-resource hospital settings. Neonatology. 2018;114(2):112-23.

18. NHM. (2020). Navjaat Shishu Suraksha Karyakram 2020. Resuscitation and Essential Newborn Care Resource Manual. [online] Available from: https://nhm.gov.in/images/pdf/programmes/child-health/guidelines/NSSK/NSSK-Resource-Manual.pdf [Last accessed January, 2023].

Self Assessment

1. Implementation of neonatal resuscitation training in low-resource settings can avert nearly .... of these intrapartum-related deaths every year.

2. Birth asphyxia contributes to nearly .... of neonatal mortality.

3. One of the important aim of Sustainable Development Goal 2030 is to reduce NMR to ....

4. The best way to ensure low intensity high frequency trainings in NRP is by:
   a. Two yearly NRP certification
   b. NSSK training
   c. Simulation sessions monthly
   d. All the above

5. The best way to reduce hypothermia after an uncomplicated vaginal delivery irrespective of the setting is:
   a. Use of head cap
   b. Use of polythelene wrap
   c. Maintaining ambient delivery room temperature >25°C
   d. Skin-to-skin contact with mother's abdomen

6. Laryngeal mask airway can be used as an alternative to intubation for PPV in above:
   a. 30 weeks
   b. 32 weeks
   c. 34 weeks
   d. 38 weeks

7. The following are ways to disinfect self inflating resuscitation bag:
   a. Clean the tip with gauze soaked in spirit after each use
   b. Disassemble bag, wash with soap and water, ethylene oxide sterilization monthly
   c. Chemical disinfection by soaking in 0.5% hypochlorite
   d. All the above

8. The following statement is TRUE with regard to neonatal resuscitation algorithm:
   a. Availability of pulse oximeter, CPAP, ECG is a major limitation to use ILCOR 2020 recommended neonatal resuscitation algorithm in resource-limited settings
   b. WHO endorses Helping Babies Breathe (HBB) algorithm

   c. India has developed NSSK resuscitation guidelines harmonized with ILCOR 2020 guidelines
   d. All the above

9. Even in 21st century, out-of-hospital delivery in India occurs in more than.......% of cases.
   a. 10%
   b. 15%
   c. 20%
   d. 25%

10. The following is a useful strategy to ensure compliance of delayed cord clamping:
   a. Training
   b. Regular audits
   c. Issue notice from hospital head to ensure DCC
   d. Both a and b

Answers

For answers, go to the end of the Book, Page no. 325

Communication and Counseling for Neonatal Survival

Chandrakala BS

Lessons to Learn

- Importance of communication in team performance, before and after resuscitation.
- Key behavioral skills to be followed during resuscitation.
- General aspects and points to ponder while communicating to parents.
- Antenatal counseling in periviable condition.

Communication is essential part of resuscitation (either before, during, or after the resuscitation), be it with other specialties, within the team or with the parents. Ineffective communication is one of the major causes for preventable infant deaths.[1]

The key behavioral skills to be followed during resuscitation for effective teamwork are adapted from Centers of Advanced and Perinatology Education (CAPE), Lucile Packard Children's Hospital at Stanford University.[2]

KEY BEHAVIORAL SKILLS DURING RESUSCITATION

1. *Know your environment:* Location, equipment, personnel to be called for help.
2. *Use all available information and resources:* Collect prenatal/medical problems in mother, intrapartum history.
3. *Anticipate the problem:* Brief team members, discuss plan of action, assign clear roles, and responsibilities.
4. *Identify a team leader:* Effective leadership qualities.
5. *Clear communication:* Calm and direct manner, closed loop communication, it is a three-step process for conveying orders. Communication should be of bidirectional (leader to member and vice versa) for knowledge-sharing and corrective action when necessary.
6. *Maintain professional behavior:* Work together in congenial, supportive manner.

7. *Delegate workload optimally* to team members knowing their capabilities and limitations.

8. *Situational awareness:* Re-evaluate the baby's status frequently and communicate within the group.

9. *Call for help early:* It is not a sign of weakness or incompetence.

THE TEAM LEADER

- Team leader with excellent leadership qualities, organizes the team and ensures the preparation is done at right time and in the right way, knows the risks and complications, counsels the family and brief the team members on the plan of action.

- Teams should routinely follow closed-loop communication to ensure that messages are properly received.

- The communication should be bidirectional to facilitate knowledge-sharing and inquiry.

- Team leader briefs the members about the event that is yet to happen to prepare them to reduce the risk of failure or harm.[3]

- Team members should aim to be assertive yet respectful when communicating and call each other by name, maintaining eye contact to get attention.

Tools for Leadership

Leader may use SBAR (situation, background, assessment, recommendation) tool,[4] callouts, check-backs, and hand-off techniques to communicate effectively with team members. An example of communication by SBAR tool is shown in *Figure* **22.1**.

COUNSELING

Clinical scenarios for counseling regarding newborn resuscitation issues can be created at multiple levels:

- *Antenatal counseling:* When a major fetal problem is detected in the scan or anticipating a preterm delivery or resuscitation of sick baby.

  - *Postresuscitation counseling:* At admission to neonatal intensive care unit (NICU).

  - *Postnatal counseling:* For parents whose baby is being cared in NICU; or dealing with distressed parents who are yet to take decisions on resuscitation/management of the periviable newborn.

Prepare the Parents

Need of resuscitation at birth is frequent with preterm babies, more so with extreme preterm infants or those with high maternal or fetal risk factors. The degree of resuscitation varies depending on the specific condition.

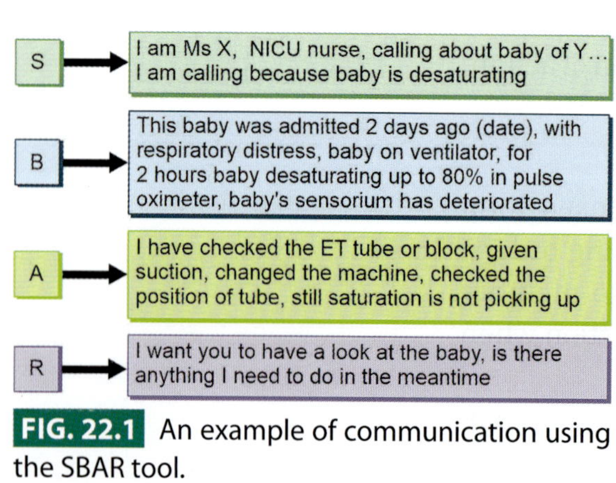

FIG. 22.1 An example of communication using the SBAR tool.

Parents often encounter deeply distressing situations when informed about the need for resuscitation or admission to NICU as they may not be mentally prepared to face the situation. The parent-infant separation is one of the factors to cause anxiety and depression.[4]

- The communication should be open and honest.
- Information given should be consistent and accurate, appropriately tailored to the situation.
- Information should be straightforward, and prepare the parents for what is to come
- Parents need to feel "empowered" and "involved" and not feel alone in developing a plan for care for their newborn.

General points to follow for counseling are listed in **Table 22.1**. Various strategies that may be employed for effective parental communication are summarized in **Table 22.2**.

Antenatal Counseling

Every high-risk family should have an antenatal consultation before the baby is delivered. Providing antenatal counseling is important to: (i) build a rapport, caring relation between baby, parent, and hospital staff; (ii) create possibilities for open and genuine conversations between parents and health team; (iii) convey understanding and empathy; and (iv) foster the building of respect, confidence, and trust.

Antenatal Counseling for Parents Whose Baby Needs NICU Admission[6]

- Neonatologists are often called for counseling for impending premature/high risk delivery or complex congenital anomalies. It is important to provide anticipatory information to parents on the care of their baby.
- Obtain complete family history, pregnancy details, any risk for neurodevelopmental problems, and inform them that their involvement is essential for taking decision[7,8] on baby care.
- Relieve parental anxiety, obtain consent, facilitate multidisciplinary approach if needed, discuss medical problems and treatment plans and support breastfeeding and milk expression.[9,10]

TABLE 22.1: VERBAL AND NONVERBAL COUNSELING—KEY POINTS

Verbal communication	**Nonverbal communication**
1. Posture—head level	1. Asking open questions (how, what, when, where, why?) Not using close question (Are you? Did you? Has he/she? Does she/he?)
2. Distance—appropriate distance	
3. Eye contact—pay attention as they speak	
4. Remove the barriers—block between both	2. Use responses and gestures which show interest
5. Taking time—sitting, without hurry, quietly smiling	3. Reflect back what the person says
6. Touch—appropriate (which give assurance)	4. Empathize (getting into the feeling of the person)
	5. Avoid words which sound judgment

TABLE 22.2: STRATEGIES FOR COMMUNICATING EFFECTIVELY WITH PARENTS

Consultation phases	Key points
To prepare for consultation	
Preparation and setting	• Speak with the mother's healthcare provider, obtain all relevant information regarding maternal and fetal health • Ensure use of interpretive services by a professional translator, if required
Create a comfortable environment	• Make sure to talk with both parents, if feasible • Make sure the consultation is not disturbed (e.g., turn pager to vibrate mode, close the door or curtains, let the nurse know) • Sit down, shake hands (if appropriate) and introduce yourself first, slowly and clearly • Demonstrate openness to communication with and involvement of parents • Ask about participants (e.g., use names, including the infant's name, if known, and if parents agree you can use it)
Assess parental knowledge of concerned issues, along with perspectives, concerns, expectations, needs and preferences	• Ask what they know about the concerned issue for which consultation is being offered • Make sure you understand and acknowledge their values, perspectives and concerns (e.g., cultural/social background, religious beliefs, family structure) • Adjust ways of communicating information to respect their values and preferences • Support their involvement in decision making with inclusive wording (e.g., *'How can I support you?'; 'We can make this decision together'*)
During consultation	

• Ensure factors that are important to parents are discussed (e.g., Ask what is important to them)
• Discuss different choices or options
• Share weighted and balanced information
	Typically, parents want to know about likelihood of survival, risk of neurodevelopmental outcomes (with related challenges and opportunities), what medical problems might be encountered, possible treatments, what a preterm baby looks like, what it is like to be in the NICU, what happens after birth, how to manage breastfeeding, and their own role in the NICU (with explanations)
	• Present parents with the choices they need to make, clearly and accurately
	• Offer appropriate management options based on the clinical situation
	• Include both positive and negative aspects of care, pros and cons of the options, treatable and untreatable conditions
	• Disclose potential outcomes *according to parental preferences*:
	  – Use grading words *(majority, most, significant, some, a minority)* and numbers when possible *(6 out of 10, rather than 60%)*
	  – Use a consistent denominator when presenting different options, outcomes or event rates, to make the information easier to understand, interpret or compare *(XX out of 10, 100 or 1000)*. For example, saying *'Out of 100 babies, 20 will die, 20 will survive with neurodevelopment delay (NDD), and 60 will survive with no NDD,'* is better than saying 20 out of 100 for one outcome, then 1 out of 5 for another.
	• Disclose uncertainty (i.e., the limits of statistics when applied to a particular baby)

Additional strategies to build trust	Allow parents to lead the conversation: • Use their verbal, nonverbal cues to pace discussion • Ask how you can support them • Invite them to share how they see the situation • Use open-ended questions (*'How … ?', 'Could you tell me more?', 'Can you describe .. ?'*) • Always ask whether parents have questions or need clarification

Contd...

Contd...

Consultation phases	Key points
	Listen for concerns and emotions, and be empathetic and supportive: • Validate the difficulty of their situation • Use a soft voice, allow silences, use appropriate touch • Acknowledge and be sensitive to emotional reactions and concerns • Support parental needs and values Answer questions and be sure parents have received and understand the information to the extent they want to Maintain eye contact with both parents Offer time to think and reflect Avoid interrupting. Be quiet as parents describe perspectives, values or preferences *Note:* Obtaining informed consent for a management plan requires—at a minimum-sharing accurate information tailored to the parents' needs regarding the risk of death and NDD, and the opportunity of having a surviving child with or without NDD
Show compassion and acknowledge parental distress	• Reassure parents that they did not do anything to cause preterm birth • Confirm the uniqueness of their family and of the unborn baby • Acknowledge their baby as a being, not a GA • Provide value-neutral information (i.e., by including the positives of having an infant they can love and cherish) • Be honest
Concluding the consultation	
Provide support and give parents realistic hope	• Validate their situation as very difficult and their reactions as understandable • Tell them that every hour, day and week that the pregnancy continues (with baby and mom in stable condition) has positive effects • Make sure they know that they are not alone • Make sure they understand that you are there to provide more information and answer new questions • Invite them to write their questions down as they think of them, for next time • Meet with parents the following day, if possible, or at any time after the initial consultation

Reproduced with permission from: Daboval T, Ferretti E, Rohde K, Muirhead P, Moore G. Neonatal ethics teaching program—scenario-oriented learning in ethics: antenatal consultation at the limit of viability. MedEdPORTAL. 2015;11(1).[5]

Counseling Parents Whose Baby is in NICU

Follow the GALPAC approach.

- **G**reet and introduce yourself.
- **A**sk them to share how they share the situation and how you can support them.
- **L**isten for concerns and emotions and understand what they are undergoing.
- **P**raise them for the concern they have on their baby.
- **A**dvice in a clear understandable language, communicate on the baby's condition effectively.

- **C**heck whether they have understood what you shared with them and whether they have any questions.

For further reading on Recommendations about Prenatal Counseling in Policy Statement, refer to American Academy of Pediatrics (AAP) and American College of Obstetricians and Gynecologists (ACOG) recommendations.[11,12]

PERIVIABLE PERIOD: COMMUNICATION FOR DECISION MAKING

Definition

Periviable period is defined as delivery from $20^{0/7}$ weeks to $25^{6/7}$ of gestation.[13] The survival rate in the developed economies varies from: 23–27% for 23 weeks, 42–59% for 24 weeks, and 67–76% at 25 weeks.[14-16]

Counseling Parents for Periviable Neonates

Table 22.3 provides an overview of recommendations on "when to resuscitate" and "when to consider resuscitation" for periviable period in different countries.[14-16]

The data from India is highly variable across the country and not uniform. Decisions should be based on the best available evidence for that baby in that geographic area/institution.

The decision to resuscitate should be guided by the ethical principles of beneficence (doing good), nonmaleficence (doing no harm), autonomy (respecting individual preferences), and justice. In centers where facilities are unavailable, in-utero transfer to tertiary care centers is ideal to reduce the mortality and morbidity of periviable newborns. Currently, there is no evidence to support routine cesarean section to improve the neonatal outcome in extremely low birth weight infants.[17]

Communication with parents for births in the periviable period and its outcome needs training. It is important to investigate the socio-environmental and family status, which influence their decision. Following points need to be obtained before counseling:

- Accurate gestational age (number of days into the week of gestation).
- Estimation of risk of neurodevelopmental delay, mortality, quality of later life, data of survival in the local area based on gestation, gender, history of antenatal corticosteroids, and clinical course in NICU.

Different centers have different data on survival. Whether to initiate resuscitation or not, should be based on the information that is provided.

TABLE 22.3: Gestational Age for Considering "Full Resuscitation" and "Consider Resuscitation" Followed in Different Countries

	ACOG	*Australia/ New Zealand*	*Japan*	*Sweden*	*Canada*	*BAPM (UK)*	*Sri Lanka*
Full resuscitation	$\geq24^{+0}$ weeks	$\geq25^{+0}$ weeks	$\geq22^{+1}$ weeks	$\geq23^{+1}$ weeks	$\geq24^{+0}-25^{+0}$ weeks	$\geq24^{+0}$ weeks	≥26 weeks
Consider resuscitation	$\geq22^{+0}-23^{+6}$ weeks	$\geq23^{+0}-24^{+6}$ weeks	Not stated	$\geq22^{+1}$ weeks	$\geq23^{+0}-24^{+0}$ weeks	$\geq22^{+1}-23^{+6}$ weeks	$\geq24^{+0}-25^{+6}$ weeks

(ACOG: American College of Obstetricians and Gynecologists; BAPM: British Association of Perinatal Medicine)

Ethical Challenges

Antenatal counseling of parents of extreme gestation at 22^{+0} to 25^{+6} poses ethical challenges, as there is no clear-cut evidence for recommending a particular option. It varies with different care settings as shown in **Table 22.3**. Shared decision-making is advocated for decision-making, where parents with their families along with healthcare providers make decision together about optimal care. Personalization is the most effective strategy in prenatal counseling practices.

Personalized Counseling

The three essential components of personalized counseling are listed here:

1. Providing, clear, accurate, and unbiased medical evidence about reasonable alternatives—including no intervention—and the risks and benefits of each.

2. Expertise of the healthcare professional in communication and tailoring the evidence to individual parents/patients.

3. Understanding of patient values, goals, informed preferences, and concerns, which may include treatment burdens.

Almost all guidelines have concluded that personalization is ideal. However, research is needed on how the counseling needs to be adjusted to suit the unborn infant.[18-22] There are many factors which influence parents' decision—including grief, emotions, intensive care environment, and nature of the information they receive.[23] Parents are usually handicapped by the lack of information and are confused by the medical terminology. They find it difficult to understand and retain complex information:

- Parents expect to be provided with culturally sensitive and relevant, comprehensive information in a compassionate and sensitive manner.

- The information should be given calmly without rushing through and engaging parents in decision making.

- Provide informational material and avoid giving information by multiple healthcare workers.

■ GUIDING PRINCIPLES DURING UNCERTAINITY

There are situations where it is difficult to decide one way or the other, both for parents and the neonatologist, and mostly concerned with periviable fetus/newborn.

Multidisciplinary neonatal palliative care should be initiated, while taking decision to withdraw or withhold care. If both parents and the healthcare professionals do not reach a consensus, second opinion should be taken either from a colleague or Ethical Committee. In such situations, understand the parental view on optimizing survival or minimizing suffering in advance (antenatal counseling). Whether to go for palliative care or not, is by stepwise approach based on newborn condition and parental wishes. Care being given should be regularly re-evaluated and redirected, keeping in mind the institutional policies and local laws. A simple guide to follow is:

- When physician thinks it is clearly beneficial to infant—provide treatment even if parents prefer to forego.

- When physician thinks it is ambiguous or uncertain—treat if parents prefer treatment; withhold/withdraw if parents want to forego.

- If physician feels it is futile—parents prefer treatment then provide treatment and withhold or withdraw, if parents prefer to forego treatment.

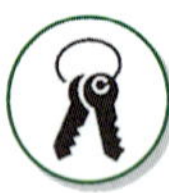

KEY POINTS

1. Communication is an important requirement for teamwork during neonatal resuscitation. It has shown to decrease medical errors, minimizes delay for action and increases patient safety. It creates work efficiency within the team leading to job satisfaction and reduced burnout.

2. Communication (both verbal and nonverbal) should be complete, clear, brief, and timely. The key behavioral skills should be followed during resuscitation for effective teamwork.

3. Prenatal counseling is important when the infant is born at the limit of viability because it poses prognostic uncertainty.

4. Antenatal counseling opens opportunities to connect and support baby, parents, and hospital staff for conversation, understanding, empathies, and to build respect, confidence, and trust.

■ REFERENCES

1. American Academy of Pediatrics and American Heart Association. In: Weiner GM, Zaichkin J (Eds). Textbook of Neonatal Resuscitation, 8th edition. 2020.

2. Halamek LP. Educational Perspectives: The Genesis, Adaptation, and Evolution of the Neonatal Resuscitation Program, NeoReviews. 2008;9;e142-9. DOI: 10.1542/neo.9-4-e142

3. Brogaard L, Hvidman L, Esberg G, Finer N, Hjorth-Hansen KR, Manser T, et al. Teamwork and adherence to guideline on newborn resuscitation: video review of neonatal interdisciplinary teams. Front Pediatr. 2022;10:828297.

4. Flacking R, Lehtonen L, Thomson G, Axelin A, Ahlqvist S, Moran VH, et al. Closeness and separation in neonatal intensive care. Acta Paediatr. 2012;101:1032-7.

5. Daboval T, Ferretti E, Rohde K, Muirhead P, Moore G. Neonatal ethics teaching program—scenario-oriented learning in ethics: antenatal consultation at the limit of viability. MedEdPORTAL. 2015;11(1).

6. Hauff PV, Long K, Taylor B, van Manen MA. Antenatal consultation for parents whose child may require admission to neonatal intensive care: a focus group study for media design. BMC Pregnancy Childbirth. 2016;16:103.

7. Boss RD, Hutton N, Sulpar LJ, West AM, Donohue PK. Values parents apply to decision-making regarding delivery room resuscitation in high-risk newborns. Pediatrics. 2008;122:583-9.

8. Côté-Arsenault D, Denney-Koelsch E. "My baby is a person": parents' experiences with life-threatening fetal diagnosis. J Palliat Med. 2011;14:1302-8.

9. Paul DA, Epps S, Leef KH, Stefano JL. Prenatal consultation with a neonatologist prior to preterm delivery. J Perinatol. 2001;21:431-7.

10. Griswold KJ, Fanaroff JM. An evidence-based overview of prenatal consultation with a focus on infants born at the limits of viability. Pediatrics. 2010;125:e931-7.

11. Cummings J, Committee on Fetus and Newborn. Antenatal counseling regarding resuscitation and intensive care before 25 weeks of gestation. Pediatrics. 2015;136(3):588-95.

12. Obstetric Care Consensus No. 4: Periviable Birth. Obstet Gynecol. 2016;127(6):e157-69.

13. Raju TN, Mercer BM, Burchfield DJ, Joseph GF Jr. Periviable birth: executive summary of a joint workshop by the Eunice Kennedy Shriver National Institute of Child Health and Human Development, Society for Maternal Fetal Medicine, American Academy of Pediatrics, and American College of Obstetricians and Gynecologists. Obstet Gynecol. 2014;123(5):1083-96.

14. Stoll BJ, Hansen NI, Bell EF, Shankaran S, Laptook AR, Walsh MC, et al. Eunice Kennedy Shriver National Institute of Child Health and Human Development Neonatal Research Network. Neonatal outcomes of extremely preterm infants from the NICHD Neonatal Research Network. Pediatrics. 2010;126:443-56.

15. Costeloe KL, Hennessy EM, Haider S, Stacey F, Marlow N, Draper ES. Short-term outcomes after extreme preterm birth in England: comparison of two birth cohorts in 1995 and 2006 (the EPICure studies). BMJ. 2012;345:7976.

16. Bolisetty S, Legge N, Bajuk B, Lui K. Preterm infant outcomes in New South Wales and the Australian Capital Territory. New South Wales and the Australian Capital Territory Neonatal Intensive Care Units' Data Collection. J Paediatr Child Health. 2015;51:713-21.

17. Lemyre B, Moore G. Counselling and management for anticipated extremely preterm birth. Paediatr Child Health. 2017;22(6): 334-41.

18. Arzuaga BH, Cummings CL. Deliveries at extreme prematurity: outcomes, approaches, institutional variation, and uncertainty. Curr Opin Pediatr. 2019;31(2):182-7.

19. Geurtzen R, van Heijst AFJ, Draaisma JMT, Kuijpers LJMK, Woiski M, Scheepers HCJ, et al. Development of nationwide recommendations to support prenatal counseling in extreme prematurity. Pediatrics. 2019;143(6):e20183253.

20. British Association of Perinatal Medicine. Perinatal Management of Extreme Preterm Birth before 27 weeks of gestation. A Framework for Practice. 2019.

21. Raju TN, Mercer BM, Burchfield DJ, Joseph Jr. GF. Periviable birth: executive summary of a joint workshop by the Eunice Kennedy Shriver National Institute of Child Health and Human Development, Society for Maternal-Fetal Medicine, American Academy of Pediatrics, and American College of Obstetricians and Gynecologists. Am J Obstet Gynecol. 2014;210:406-17.

22. Gaucher N, Nadeau S, Barbier A, Janvier A, Payot A. Personalized antenatal consultations for preterm labor: responding to mothers' expectations. J Pediatr. 2016;178:130-4:e137.

23. Xafis V, Wilkinson D, Sullivan J. What information do parents need when facing end-of-life decisions for their child? A meta-synthesis of parental feedback. BMC Palliative Care. 2015;14:19.

Self Assessment

1. All are True regarding antenatal counseling EXCEPT:
   a. Opens up opportunity to support baby and family.
   b. Helps us to understand, empathize, and build trust.
   c. Suboptimal interaction of healthcare provider and family leads to improper decision making
   d. To present them the international data of survival for decision making on resuscitation at periviable stage at your hospital.

2. The three steps of closed loop communication on giving medication are:
   a. Team leader commands the name, dose, route of the drug, the team member acknowledges, repeats it back and member reports after order is completed.
   b. Team leader commands, understands, and gives the medication in the correct order.
   c. Team leader commands, name, dose, route of the drug, member calculates the drug and document in the chart.
   d. None of the above.

3. All are True regarding strategies to build parent trust during counseling EXCEPT:
   a. Create comfortable environment
   b. Allow the parents to lead the conversation
   c. Ensure factors that are important to them are discussed
   d. Healthcare provider decides the plan for the baby

Answers

For answers, go to the end of the Book, Page no. 325

Quality Improvement in Neonatal Resuscitation

Akash Bang

Lessons to Learn

- Importance of quality improvement in neonatal resuscitation
- Steps in successful quality improvement process
- Measuring the quality-of-care
- Quality improvement indicators in neonatal resuscitation

WHAT IS QUALITY IMPROVEMENT AND WHY IS IT NEEDED?

The Need

Reducing neonatal mortality to below 12 per 1,000 live births by 2030 is one of the targets under the Sustainable Development Goal-3. Close to 7 lac newborns die every year in India and birth asphyxia contributes to every one in four newborn deaths.[1] Despite widespread trainings of birth attendants in basic and advanced neonatal resuscitation (NR) by the government as well as Indian Academy of Pediatrics (IAP) and National Neonatology Forum (NNF), why we have not been able to bring down the neonatal mortality as much as we thought we could? This is a question that often haunts many of us NR providers and trainers.

Role of Quality

It is estimated that 60% of all deaths in low-and-middle-income countries from conditions amenable to health care are due to poor quality-of-care whereas only 40% are due to nonutilization of health care.[2] Hence, it is extremely crucial that the quality-of-care is improved, and low-quality health systems are transformed to high-quality ones if we want to reap the benefits of various evidence-based interventions including neonatal resuscitation.

But how do we improve the healthcare provider practices? Most of the healthcare providers are sensitive toward patients and intend to provide good quality-of-care. The common reasons for poor quality-of-care includes lack of resources, e.g., infrastructure, staff, equipment, and supplies; insufficient clinical knowledge and skills; and lack of organization of services at health facilities. A systematic review of the effectiveness of various strategies showed that technology-based interventions like using Apps or only providing printed information like manuals have median effect size of 1%—point change.[3] The median effect size was around 10% points for a one-time training like neonatal resuscitation training. It was the team problem-solving approach typically used in quality improvement methodology that has the highest effect size of 28–38% points.

Definition

Quality improvement (QI) is a systems management approach that health workers can use to re-organize patient care at their level to ensure that patients receive good quality health care.[4] QI is a shift from individual-based approach to a system-based approach; from fault finding to problem solving; and primarily focuses on reorganizing care within the existing resources through a process redesign. For the same reason, QI is largely contextual—an improvement strategy that works at one facility may not work in another.

In short, quality improvement is the ideal strategy for problems like birth asphyxia for which we already know what are the evidence-based solutions, we know how to perform the intervention, but we just do not know how to make it happen—how to implement what we know.

STEPS IN SUCCESSFUL QUALITY IMPROVEMENT PROCESS

Quality improvement process can be understood through a simple four-steps model as follows:[4]

Step 1: Identifying a problem, forming a team, and writing an aim statement

- *Identifying a problem:* The problem chosen to be addressed must be picked from the local data. The health facility data needs to be reviewed to identify gaps in the health care. At times there may be multiple problems that seem glaring and hence, worth addressing. However, it is always wise to start with addressing only one problem at a time. Choosing a problem that is simple to measure, is easy to address, yet is relevant and significant for patient outcomes, does not need lot of new resources and has short turn-around time increases the chances of successful improvement and thereby initial motivation for the team. A simple prioritization matrix **(Table 23.1)** can be used to prioritize the order of choosing the problem to be addressed first, based on scoring few parameters which are as follows:

TABLE 23.1: PRIORITIZATION MATRIX FOR PRIORITIZING PROBLEMS TO BE ADDRESSED

Potential problems	Important for patient outcomes	Affordable in terms of time and resources	Easy to measure	Under control of team members	Total score
Score range	1–5	1–5	1–5	1–5	4–20
Key	1 = not important 5 = highly important	1 = not affordable 5 = very affordable	1 = very difficult 5 = very easy	1 = not at all under control 5 = entirely under control	
Problem 1					
Problem 2					
Problem 3					

Source: World Health Organization, Regional Office for South-East Asia. (2017). Improving the quality-of-care for mothers and newborns in health facilities. POCQI: Point of Care Quality Improvement. [Online] Available from https://www.newbornwhocc.org/POCQI-Learner-Manual.pdf [Last accessed January, 2023].

- Importance for improving patient outcomes (ask how important it will be for outcomes. Typically, problems that increase mortality will be extremely important)
- Ease and affordability in fixing that problem (ask how much time and resources it will take to fix this problem)
- Ease of measurement (ask how easy it is to measure the problem. Typically, hard outcomes like deaths will be the easiest to measure while soft, subjective or abstract outcomes such as satisfaction and happiness will be the most difficult to measure)
- Under control of team members (ask will the team members be able to fix the problem or is it totally out of their control)

- *Forming a team:* Forming an appropriate team will go a long way in success of the QI efforts. Enthusiastic healthcare providers from all levels and all departments which are actually involved in the process of caregiving related to the problem will constitute a good team. An ideal team can have anywhere from 4 to 10 members—a team size big enough to introduce perspectives and facilitate division of work, but small enough to stay focused. Involvement of at least one influential senior employee (in-charge nurse or department head) will make things move faster. The stakeholders must also have representation, e.g., if the aim is to increase the proportion of deliveries delivered on abdomen, including a mother in the team will introduce the mothers' perspective. Team leader needs to be assigned, from the start and need not be the highest rank employee.

- *Writing an aim statement:* Writing a clear aim statement helps all the team members to stay focused on a shared vision, realistically review successes and failures and consequently creates opportunities to celebrate or review the process. The aim needs to be

SMART—Specific, Measurable, Achievable (but also challenging), Relevant, and Timely. The aim statement needs to include clear and specific information on what we intend to improve, in whom (the patient population), by how much we aim to improve and by when. Example of a good and a poor aim statement is given in **Table 23.2**.

Step 2: Analyzing the problem and measuring quality-of-care

- *Analyzing the problem:* A complete root cause analysis of the problem is essential because that helps us understand what is happening currently in the system, thereby generating ideas about what can be changed in the system and what are the opportunities of improvement. The exercise also increases the team participation as everyone gets to give their insights. A root cause analysis helps the team weed out causes that are beyond our control and instead focus on causes that are the low hanging fruits under our control. Following are some popular tools used for analyzing the problem.

  - *Fishbone diagram:* The team brainstorms about all the possible causes that could be contributing to the problem classifying them under broad groups such as policies, people, place, and procedures. This gives a visual representation of the complexity of the problem and helps the team pick changes that are easy and feasible. In general, the problems listed under "place" and "procedures" are easy to address whereas "people" and "policies" are usually harder to change. However, for some problems, it may be necessary to change policies first. An illustrative fishbone diagram analyzing the root causes of high antibiotic usage in neonatal intensive care unit (NICU) is depicted in *Figure* **23.1**.[5]

TABLE 23.2: EXAMPLES OF A GOOD AND A POOR AIM STATEMENT

	Poor aim statement	Good aim statement
What	We aim to promote delayed cord clamping	We aim to increase delayed cord clamping
Who	In newborns immediately after birth	In all crying newborns immediately after birth
How much	–	From current 30 to 100%
By when	–	In 4 weeks

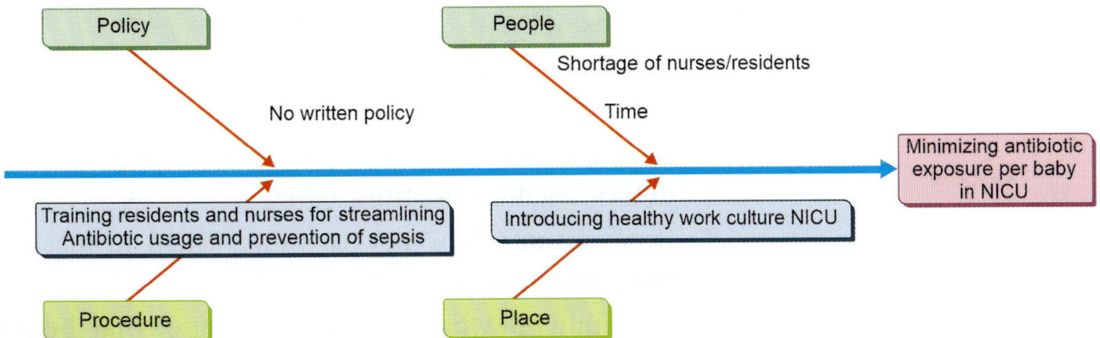

FIG. 23.1 An illustrative fishbone diagram analyzing the root causes of high antibiotic usage in a neonatal intensive care unit (NICU).[5]

- *Process flowchart:* This tool is especially useful in situations where there is a defined process through which each patient goes, and you want to analyze why certain outcomes are occurring. Examples of such processes would be screening in triage, admission and/or billing process, intrahospital shifting processes, resuscitations, etc.

  For creating a process flowchart, the team decides the start and the end points of the process that needs improvement, identifies, and draws the steps of the process as is being currently practiced, and then reviews it for two important questions: (1) Are some steps unnecessary and can be removed to make the process more efficient? and (2) Can some steps be reordered, redelegated or reorganized to make things easier/better for the teams?

  It is best for the team members to actually observe the whole process, and if needed draw their own version before reaching a consensus flowchart to obtain multiple perspectives. Process flowchart can be a very powerful tool as it brings the whole process in front of everyone's eyes and the whole team agrees to a version thereby putting down the problem on paper.

- *Five whys:* This tool helps the team to reach the root cause of a problem by trying to understand why something is the way it is. Here, the team identifies a problem to be fixed, keeps questioning "why," documents multiple alternative answers, and keeps repeating the "why" question till they reach an easily solvable step. Inevitably by fourth or fifth why, you would have reached to the bottom of the problem.

  To give an example from neonatal resuscitation, a team observes that many noncrying newborns are NOT getting effectively ventilated in the first golden minute, so they start asking five whys till they get a fixable problem as follows:

  1. *Why* effective ventilation is not getting established in first minute of life?
  2. Because doctors are spending a lot of time in corrective actions. *Why?*
  3. Because they are finding it tough to create a good seal with the masks. *Why?*
  4. Because they are holding the masks in a manner that is deforming the mask rims. *Why?*
  5. Because that is how they have always held the masks. Nobody taught them alternatives!

  Thus, within few whys, the team now knows that the solution of the seemingly complex problem (low proportion of noncrying newborns with effective ventilation established within first minute of life) lies in training the doctors in the skill of achieving a good seal with the mask.

- *Pareto chart:* Often there are multiple causes contributing to the same problem. Pareto principle states that 80% of the problem is due to only 20% of the causes. The team prepares a "Pareto chart" by charting all the possible contributory causes with their respective frequencies in a descending order. This helps them identify those few vital causes, which if fixed will lead to 80% improvement. Working on these vital causes will be more efficient than wasting time and resources on less frequent causes.

  Often more than one of the above tools can be used in combination. For example, first the team can brainstorm to create a *fishbone diagram* of all causes leading to the problem; then create a *Pareto chart* to pick up few most vital causes; and lastly, for each one of these vital causes, use *five whys* to reach a possible solution.

- *Measuring quality-of-care:* Measuring the quality-of-care through objective indicators is essential as it gives objective evidence of improvement; helps the team decide how they are progressing over time; and helps compare with other units. If we cannot or do not measure anything, we will not be able to improve it. Hence, the team needs to develop indicators and track them over time to document improvement.

  - *Process indicators* are those that measure the processes or actions taken by the team.

  - *Outcome indicators* are those that measure the results of the actions taken by the team.

In the above example, proportion of noncrying newborns receiving effective ventilation in first minute of life is a process indicator, whereas asphyxia specific early neonatal mortality may be the related outcome indicator. Thus, to measure how many newborns are receiving effective ventilation in first minute, and how it is affecting neonatal outcomes, we can develop two indicators as enumerated in **Box 23.1**.

For each indicator, it is essential to define who will collect the information, from which source and how frequently the information

---

BOX 23.1: Two Indicators to Measure How Many Newborns are Receiving Effective Ventilation in First Minute, and How it is Affecting Neonatal Outcomes

1. *Process indicator* = Number of noncrying newborns for whom effective ventilation is established in the first minute of life/Total number of noncrying newborns × 100.
2. *Outcome indicator* = Number of asphyxia-related deaths by 7 days of age/Total number of deaths by 7 days of age × 100.

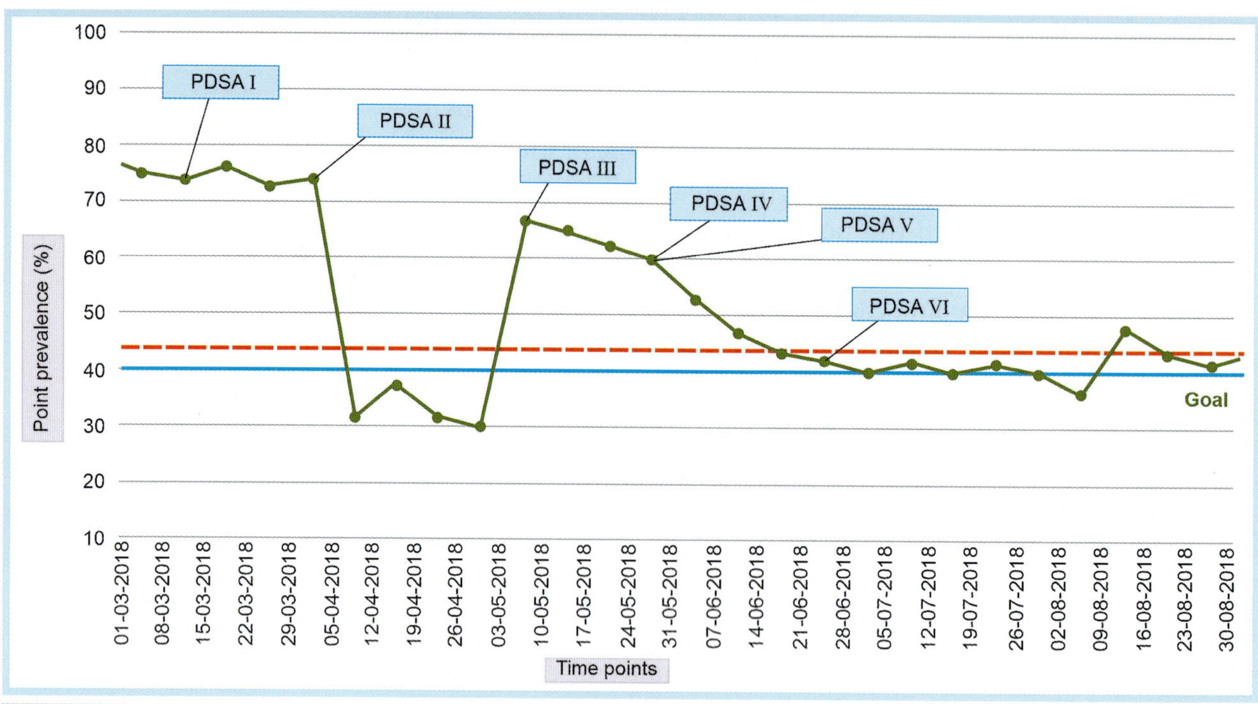

FIG. 23.2 Time series chart depicting the average antibiotic exposure rate in a neonatal intensive care unit (NICU) over time.[5]

will be collected. The team must not be overburdened with the task of collecting information that does not have direct bearing. It is better to have more frequent data collection within the limits of practical feasibility.

Next, the indicators generated periodically as per the predefined frequency are charted on Y-axis against time on X-axis to create a time series chart also called as a *run chart. Figure* **23.2** illustrates how a time series chart of average antibiotic exposure over time in an NICU looked like.[5]

Step 3: Developing and testing changes

- *Developing changes:* Once the root cause analysis is done, the team should brainstorm and list various change ideas that they feel will address the cause of the problem and will lead to improvement. These change ideas must be relevant to their own setting. The team together will need to review the complete list of change ideas and prioritize those that are effective (in terms of importance to the patient care) and feasible (in terms of practicality). Remember that for every problem, there will always be multiple possible solutions. The focus should be to identify solutions that are actionable within their spheres of influence in the short-term.

  Some common categories of changes are given in **Table 23.3**.[4]

- *Testing changes:* All the change ideas may not work in real life. Some may need modifications; some may be totally impractical. Hence, it is extremely important to test each change idea before permanently

TABLE 23.3: SOME COMMON GENERIC CATEGORIES OF CHANGES

Category	Description
Knowledge and skills improvement	Training
Eliminate waste	Stop doing useless or harmful things
Redelegation of tasks	Change who does what
Reorganization of tasks	Changing the order or location of tasks
Improve patient relationship	Listen to what patient or mother wants
Reduce variation	Make changes to bring uniformity of care

incorporating any of them into practice. Similarly, to understand what works and what does not, it is very important to test only one change at a time. Testing of each change idea is done using a PDSA cycle that stands for Plan, Do, Study, Act.

- *Plan:* Chalk out a detailed plan of what exact change idea will be tested, who will make the change, how and where will this be tested, when will the test start, over how many shifts or duration the testing will be done, and what do we expect learn from this test?

- *Do:* The assigned person actually tests the change idea as per the plan and documents what happened.

- *Study:* After the change idea has been tested, the team must study the learning points. Important issues to ponder upon include—was the change carried out as planned? If not why? Is this change feasible? If not, what needs to be modified to make it feasible? Is it acceptable to the stakeholders—the staff and the patients? Does it lead to some other important tasks being left out?

- *Act:* After studying the results as above, the team needs to decide to take one of the three actions—(1) *Adopt*: If the change worked well, leading to improvement and is feasible, it should be adopted, (i2) *Adapt*: If the change worked partially but needs some modifications, it should be modified, and (3) *Abandon*: If the change did not work at all, it needs to be discarded.

The plan-do-study-act (PDSA) cycle continues, and the team should pick up the next change idea for testing through another PDSA cycle. The common mistakes include continuing one PDSA cycle over a long duration and deciding the fate of the change tested in the PDSA cycle based on the outcome indicator. Remember that PDSA cycles are micro-level learning cycles and so are typically planned over one or few shifts or a few days. What we need to study is whether the change idea is feasible and acceptable, and NOT whether it is leading to improvement of indicators. It is only after you adopt or adapt a change idea and include it in the process that you start expecting the improvement and hence track the indicators.

Step 4: Sustaining improvement: Often the teams are enthusiastic while testing changes; the time and resources devoted to QI efforts are high initially and so we see a definite improvement. Over time, as the enthusiasm fades and the resources get diverted, there is a risk of losing the hard-earned improvement. To avoid this, the successful changes need to be hardwired in the system. Some specific actions to ensure this are—documenting the process, sharing the successes with the teams, educating the teams about the new way, bringing policymakers and administrators on board, addressing equipment, supplies related issues, getting changes in the policy, and handing over of the ownership to the team. Enthusiastic teams with an involved leader go a long way in sustaining the improvements.

SUGGESTED QUALITY IMPROVEMENT INDICATORS FOR NEONATAL RESUSCITATION

As already elaborated, the first step toward introducing QI in neonatal resuscitation will be defining and measuring some indicators to identify the problems. Various such indicators related to respective steps of neonatal resuscitation can include:

- Proportion of births with all equipment available
- Proportion of births with availability of at least one neonatal resuscitation program (NRP) trained personnel
- Proportion of newborns receiving immediate skin-to-skin care
- Proportion of breathing newborns receiving delayed cord clamping
- Proportion of nonbreathing newborns responding to initial steps of drying and stimulation
- Proportion of nonbreathing newborns that receive ventilation in the first minute of life
- Proportion of ventilated newborns showing signs of effective ventilation

Monitoring these indicators will help in identifying problem areas. Once the problems are identified, they can be listed and prioritized. The team will need to have nurses and doctors from neonatology, obstetrics, and anesthesia disciplines in addition to mothers. Since resuscitation is a well-defined algorithm, process flowchart will be a good analysis tool and can be complemented by other tools. Subsequently, developing change ideas and testing each one over a few shifts will help the teams decide whether to adopt, adapt or abandon each change. Tracking the indicators over time will help the team monitor the progress toward a shared vision.

CONCLUSION

Neonatal resuscitation is an evidence-based solution for birth asphyxia. However, it is imperative to ensure that the quality of neonatal resuscitation does not get lost while translating from guidelines to real-life practice because in low- and middle-income countries, more deaths occur due to suboptimal quality-of-care rather than lack of access to care. Quality Improvement (QI) is a system-based approach where teams focus on improving the quality-of-care through root cause analyses and process re-design. Using QI methods, teams need to develop and track process and outcome indicators related to resuscitation. Problems need to be identified, prioritized, analyzed and the change ideas need to tested one at a time. Tracking the indicators over time will help the team monitor the progress towards a shared vision. For bridging the gap between knowledge and quality-of-care, QI is the best and the most cost-effective strategy with the highest impact.

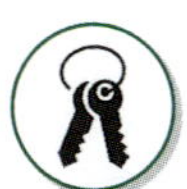 KEY POINTS

1. 60% of all deaths in low- and middle-income countries occur due to poor quality-of-care and not due to nonutilization of health care.

2. It is extremely crucial that the low-quality health systems are transformed to high-quality ones if we want to reap the benefits of an evidence-based intervention like neonatal resuscitation.

3. Quality improvement is a systems management approach that health workers can use to reorganize patient care at their level to ensure that quality does not get lost while translating from books and guidelines to the bedside point of care and patients receive good quality health care.

4. Quality improvement is the ideal strategy for problems like birth asphyxia for which we already know what are the evidence-based solutions; we know how to perform the intervention; but we just do not know how to make it happen—how to implement what we know.

5. Steps to quality improvement include identifying a problem, forming a team of stakeholders, analyzing the causes(s) of problems, measuring quality-of-care, developing change ideas, and testing these changes.

REFERENCES

1. Million Death Study Collaborators. Changes in cause-specific neonatal and 1-59-month child mortality in India from 2000 to 2015: a nationally representative survey. Lancet. 2017;390(10106):1972-80.

2. Kruk ME, Gage AD, Arsenault C, Jordan K, Leslie HH, Roder-DeWan S, et al. High-quality health systems in the sustainable development goals era: time for a revolution. Lancet Glob Health. 2018;6(11):e1196-252.

3. Rowe AK, Rowe SY, Peters DH, Holloway KA, Chalker J, Ross-Degnan D. Effectiveness of strategies to improve health-care provider practices in low-income and middle-income countries: a systematic review. Lancet Glob Health. 2018;6(11):e1163-75.

4. World Health Organization, Regional Office for South-East Asia. (2017). Improving the quality-of-care for mothers and newborns in health facilities. POCQI: Point of Care Quality Improvement. [Online] Available from https://www.newbornwhocc.org/POCQI-Learner-Manual.pdf [Last accessed January, 2023].

5. Jain M, Bang A, Meshram P, Gawande P, Kawhale K, Kamble P, et al. Institution of an Antibiotic Stewardship Programme for Rationalising Antibiotic Usage: a quality improvement project in the NICU of a public teaching hospital in rural central India. BMJ Open Qual. 2021;10(Suppl 1): e001456.

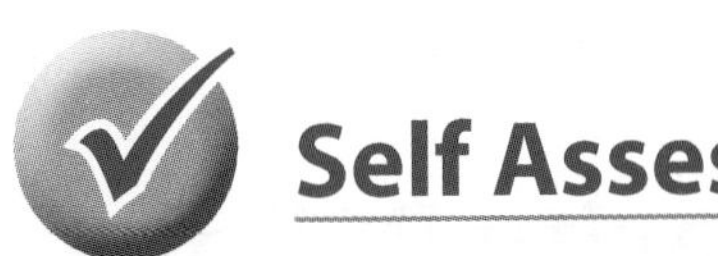

Self Assessment

1. What should be the qualities of an aim statement for a QI project?

2. Which one of the following is a WRONG match?
   a. Fishbone diagram—helps to understand multiple causes of a problem
   b. Process flowchart—helps to understand all the steps of a process
   c. Pareto chart—helps to track progress over time
   d. Five whys—helps to understand in depth the underlying causes of a problem

3. Proportion of newborns receiving delayed cord clamping is an outcome indicator—true or false?

4. What tool is used to track indicators?

5. To test a change idea, which cycle do we perform?

6. Why is it important to test the changes?
   a. To understand whether the change is working or not
   b. To increase acceptability among the health workers involved in the change
   c. To prevent large cost of failure
   d. All of the above

Answers

For answers, go to the end of the Book, Page no. 325

Training and Capacity Building

Vikas Goyal

Lessons to Learn

- Components of Neonatal Resuscitation Program (NRP) training course
- Levels of neonatal resuscitation courses
- Planning and conduct of the course
- Skills retention strategy
- Capacity development

The first structured Neonatal Resuscitation Program (NRP) course was launched by the American Academy of Pediatrics (AAP) in association with the American Heart Association (AHA) for the training of healthcare workers in 1987 in the USA. Soon thereafter in 1990 National Neonatology Forum (NNF) launched NRP in our country and within a few years, they created a pool of 150 instructors which eventually trained 12,000 healthcare workers in the skills of neonatal resuscitation.[1]

As we all know a trained healthcare worker in neonatal resuscitation is required to take care of a newborn baby at birth. In India every year around 27 million babies are born. As evident by the numbers, to have every birth attended by trained healthcare workers would require training on a large scale which can only be achieved by concentrated efforts of all the stakeholders concerned. Sensing the need, the Indian Academy of Pediatrics (IAP) launched the *"Neonatal Resuscitation Program First Golden Minute Project (IAPNRP FGM)"* in 2009 on a large scale. IAP also collaborated with the Government of India and helped them in creating a national pool of trainers for training in the public sector. In the private sector, provider courses in NRP were conducted across the country by IAP. Later, NNF joined hands with IAP and the project was renamed as *"IAP NNF NRP FGM"* Project. To date around 150,000 healthcare providers (physicians and other health professionals involved with delivery room care), both in the public and private sector, have been trained in neonatal resuscitation by IAP and NNF in India. Apart from this, the Government of India (and the state governments through its pool of trainers) is also conducting basic neonatal resuscitation courses for all the healthcare workers posted in delivery rooms in public hospitals using the *"Navjaat Shishu Surkasha Karyakram* (NSSK)" module.

NEONATAL RESUSCITATION PROGRAM IN INDIA

The training program provides an evidence-based approach to the care of the newborn baby at birth. It combines provision of relevant information (knowledge component) and skills for neonatal resuscitation. It also has a built-in assessment component.

Knowledge component: The first part of the training consists of providing participants with the latest evidence-based study material/video lectures followed by an assessment of knowledge by an online evaluation test. This step is a mandatory prerequisite for participants to be eligible for the skills part of the course.

Skill training: The second part consists of the skills training which are onsite workshops. During these sessions, skills are demonstrated on the manikin by the facilitators followed by hands-on practice by participants using a performance checklist. This is followed by evaluation of the participant's skills by the facilitators. The participants are expected to be able to demonstrate adequate skills required for neonatal resuscitation on a manikin under different simulated scenarios that are usual encountered in the delivery room. After successful completion of both components, the participant is awarded a certificate that is valid for 2 years.

LEVELS OF NEONATAL RESUSCITATION TRAINING

There are at present two levels of courses being provided for neonatal resuscitation in India.

Basic NRP Course

This course provides skills in neonatal resuscitation up to bag and mask ventilation. This course is best suited for all the healthcare workers directly related to newborn care at birth. The course at present is available for:

- Medical officers posted at birthing centers, 24 × 7 PHCs, maternity hospitals
- Nursing staff (auxiliary nurse midwives, nurses with GNM/bachelor's in nursing qualifications, and MSc nursing students) posted at birthing centers, 24 × 7 PHCs, maternity hospitals
- All obstetricians, pediatricians, anesthetists, postgraduate and medical interns directly involved in deliveries and emergency medicine
- AYUSH doctors posted at birthing centers/maternity hospitals
- Trained paramedics in private nursing homes

Basic NRP Course Curriculum

It has two components as alluded to above for the NRP training.

1. *Online module:* Participants are provided with an online module link where they have a pretest regarding their existing knowledge, attitude, and practice related to neonatal resuscitation. The next step is to watch video demonstrations and lectures on resuscitation. This is followed by a post-test to assess their knowledge of neonatal resuscitation. On successful completion of this part, the participant becomes eligible for the onsite skill training workshop.

2. *Skill training workshop:* Participants get hands-on training in resuscitation skills with the use of manikin, equipment, and supplies on workstations. Instructors demonstrate the skill followed by practice and evaluation using a performance checklist. Finally in the end, participants are evaluated using a performance evaluation test by the instructor. On successful demonstration of skills required for resuscitation on a manikin, the participants are certified to be trained in the basic NRP course.

Advanced NRP Course

This course covers all the required skills for neonatal resuscitation including advanced procedures such as intubation, chest compression, and medication. Besides this resuscitation in special conditions and care of the preterm baby at birth are also included in the course. It is appropriate for those who attend births and are responsible for anticipated resuscitation of a newborn with known risk factors, and for those who participate in neonatal resuscitation beyond positive-pressure ventilation.

Advanced NRP Course Curriculum

This too has two components as the basic NRP course.

1. *Knowledge component:* The participants are provided with a textbook of neonatal resuscitation followed by an online assessment of knowledge through multiple choice questions. Participants must obtain the minimum required marks to become eligible for the skills training workshop.

2. *Skill training workshop:* Participants get hands-on training in resuscitation skills on workstations using manikin and other equipment and supplies. The skills of participants are assessed using a performance checklist and evaluation forms. On successful demonstration of required skills on the manikin by the participant the next step is a case-based simulation and debriefing exercise. Simulation and debriefing exercises focus on developing leadership roles, communication, and teamwork skills.

PLANNING AND PREPARATION FOR NRP COURSES

Careful planning and preparation are critical for a successful NRP course. The information provided in this section will help you plan and execute a successful NRP course.

The course must be registered at least 1 month before the date of the course. All the participants should be provided with prestudy material/online module link well in advance to prepare for the knowledge assessment part of the course. Availability of the manikin kit and other documents required for training should be confirmed before the course. Training is conducted on workstations; each workstation consists of a maximum of eight participants with one instructor. There should be an adequate distance (10 feet) between two workstations to prevent voice-over from one workstation to another.

Training must be conducted using adult learning principles. One must understand the unique learning requirements of adult learners to ensure that the training interventions are effective. For adults to learn effectively, training needs to be designed in a way that meets the following core principles of adult learning:

Self-directed Learning

Clearly define the benefits, values, and purposes of the NRP course at the beginning of the course. The participants need to know why they are learning and what they are learning. If they cannot appreciate the purpose or value, they will be reluctant to engage in the learning process.

Learn by Doing

Adults learn through direct experience; therefore, their training and learning processes must include active and practical participation and offer implementable techniques and methodologies that will immediately improve their everyday work life.

Relevant

The content of the program should be meaningful and relevant to adult learners. They must very clearly see why and how this is important to them personally and how it applies to their workplace. If they cannot see how they can apply the learning in their setup, the motivation toward the training will be significantly reduced.

Experience

Adult learners need to be able to draw upon their past experiences to aid their learning. Training needs to be contextualized using language that they are familiar with. One needs to select case scenarios and examples that the participants can relate to their workplace experiences. This makes it more meaningful to the participants.

Practice

Adult learners are often engaged in learning because a problem needs to be solved. Practicing skills in a controlled environment allows them to build confidence and prepares them for the new tasks that they would have to perform independently outside of the learning environment. The participants must be allowed ample time to practice on a manikin at the workstations.

Documentation

After completion of the training, all evaluation forms, feedback forms must be scrutinized and preserved. They will be necessary for the required documentation that needs to be completed and submitted to the appropriate authority.

STRATEGIES TO IMPROVE SKILL RETENTION AFTER NRP TRAINING

At present the certification after initial NRP training, remains valid for 2 years and thereafter retraining is required. However, retention of skills and knowledge after initial neonatal resuscitation has remained a challenge. Studies have shown that after the initial NRP course there is a steady decline that is faster for skills than knowledge.[2-4] Even some studies have shown that skill deteriorates to an unsatisfactory level after 3 months.[5] The decline in skill is variable and it depends on various provider characteristics. These include:

- The type of facility where the provider works. Facilities with high birth load, provide increased opportunities for using resuscitation skills lead to better retention of skills than facilities with low birth load.

- Other factors that affect skill decline are the quality of initial training and prior resuscitation training.

Different strategies have been proposed to improve retention of skills and knowledge. Of these, spaced learning, or low-dose high-frequency (LDHF) training after the initial training is gaining importance.[6] For LDHF training, resuscitation skill stations with manikin kits are provided at the facility. After initial instructor-led training, participants are encouraged to self-practice on workstation biweekly for 10–15 minutes. Participants are provided with different tasks covering all the skills required for neonatal resuscitation. Participants must perform the given task and record it which can then be sent to trainers for their comments and feedback. Studies have shown the positive impact of LDHF training on the retention of skills and knowledge but the optimal LDHF training frequency and the optimal interval between formal instructor-led education sessions remain unclear.[7,8]

Another important intervention is to include quality improvement (QI) cycles along with LDHF training to improve the outcome[9,10] and now the World Health Organization has also recommended the inclusion of QI cycles in NRP training.

Capacity Development

The United Nations development group defines *"capacity"* as the ability of people, organizations, and society to manage their affairs successfully and *"capacity development"* as the process whereby people, organizations, and society unleash, strengthen, create, adapt, and maintain capacity over time, to achieve results.[11]

Capacity development can be grouped into three levels: (1) Individual; (2) Organizational; and (3) Enabling environment, which altogether are interdependent and mutually reinforcing. This section summarizes capacity development as it applies to NRP at these three levels.

1. *Individual:* Improving individual skills, knowledge, and performance of neonatal resuscitation through training, taking measures to retain the skill and knowledge as discussed earlier, and motivating the healthcare workers.

2. *Organizational:* Many organizations along with the Government of India are involved in improving neonatal outcomes and are helping in imparting neonatal resuscitation training. For better results, all the stakeholders must partner and make strategies for the future. Also, all the stakeholders must be on the same page while deciding on the curriculum and implementation plan for the program. IAP has done this by associating with NNF and the Government of India in conducting courses. Also for basic NRP, IAP and NNF have helped the Government of India in developing the training material and the same is now being used for basic NRP training in both the private and public sector across the country. However, there is still scope for better coordination, partnership, and deciding roles and responsibilities of involved organizations.

3. *Enabling environment:* It relates to political commitment and vision, and the inclusion of the community in decision making. Educating individuals regarding the benefits of the NRP program helps them to transform from passive recipients of services to active participants in a process of change. All the health organizations should do advocacy at the national, state, and community levels to explain the benefits and role of NRP training in decreasing neonatal mortality and morbidity. This will eventually help in making of a better policy, rules, and a higher provision of funds for the program.

■ CONCLUSION

Starting from 1990 when NRP training was first introduced in our country, we have come a long way. We know we are on the right path, but our journey is not finished until we achieve our target of having a healthcare provider trained in neonatal resuscitation for every birth.

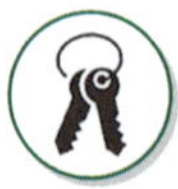 **KEY POINTS**

1. There are two levels of courses for neonatal resuscitation—basic and advanced.
2. Each course has a knowledge and a skill component.
3. Adult learning principles must be used for all training courses.
4. Meticulous planning is required to make a course useful to participants.
5. For skill retention, low-dose high-frequency (LDHF) method can be adopted.

■ REFERENCES

1. Deorari AK, Paul VK, Singh M, Vidyasagar D. The National Movement of Neonatal Resuscitation in India. J Trop Pediatr. 2000;46(5):315-7.

2. Kamath-Rayne BD, Berkelhamer SK, Kc A, Ersdal HL, Niermeyer S. Neonatal resuscitation in global health settings: an examination of the past to prepare for the future. Pediatr Res. 2017;82(2):194-200.

3. Reisman J, Arlington L, Jensen L, Louis H, Suarez-Rebling D, Nelson BD. Newborn resuscitation training in resource-limited settings: a systematic literature review. Pediatrics. 2016;138.pii:e20154490.

4. Bang A, Patel A, Bellad R, Gisore P, Goudar SS, Esamai F, et al. Helping Babies Breathe (HBB) training: what happens to knowledge and skills over time? BMC Pregnancy Childbirth. 2016;16(1):364.

5. Musafili A, Essen B, Baribwira C, Rukundo A, Persson LA. Evaluating Helping Babies Breathe: training for healthcare workers at hospitals in Rwanda. Acta Paediatr. 2013;102:e34-8.

6. Mduma E, Ersdal H, Svensen E, Kidanto H, Auestad B, Perlman J. Frequent brief on-site simulation training and reduction in 24-h neonatal mortality: an educational intervention study. Resuscitation. 2015;93:1-7.

7. Cavicchiolo ME, Cavallin F, Bertuola F, Pizzol D, Segafredo G, Wingi OM, et al. Effect of a low-dose/high-frequency training on real-life neonatal resuscitation in a low-resource setting. Neonatology. 2018;114(4):294-302.

8. Haynes J, Rettedal S, Perlman J, Ersdal H. A randomised controlled study of low-dose high-frequency in-situ simulation training to improve newborn resuscitation. Children (Basel). 2021;8(12):1115.

9. Bang A, Bellad R, Gisore P, Hibberd P, Patel A, Goudar S, et al. Implementation and evaluation of the Helping Babies Breathe curriculum in three resource-limited settings: does Helping Babies Breathe save lives? A study protocol. BMC Pregnancy Childbirth 2014;14:116.

10. Kc A, Wrammert J, Nelin V, et al. Evaluation of Helping Babies Breathe Quality Improvement Cycle (HBB-QIC) on retention of neonatal resuscitation skills six months after training in a low-income setting like Nepal. BMC Pediatr. 2017;17:103.

11. United Nations Development Group. (2017). Capacity Development: UNDAF Companion Guidance. [online] Available from: https://unsdg.un.org/sites/default/files/UNDG-UNDAF-Companion-Pieces-8-Capacity-Development.pdf. [Last Accessed January, 2023].

Annexures

ANNEXURE I
PERFORMANCE CHECKLISTS

The purpose of a performance checklist is to provide the learner with a step-by-step outline of the procedure for use during the practice phase of the lesson. It also provides the instructor with a checklist for evaluating the learner's performance of the skill. This section has 7 performance checklists starting from 'Preparation for Birth' up to 'Vascular Access'.

Important Note for Learners

The learner should have read the checklist thoroughly and use it to practice the procedure until it can be performed smoothly, correctly, and without hesitation. Learners should talk through the procedure as they perform on the manikin. The learner may ask any relevant question(s) seeking information about the baby's condition as they progress through the performance checklist. In real-life situations, one would have to assess the condition of the newborn by oneself.

Performance Checklist 1
PREPARATION FOR BIRTH

You have been called in the labor room for delivery of a baby. How would you prepare for birth of the baby?

- Assesses perinatal risk factors
  - Checks for expected gestational age
  - Checks if there is single or multiple fetuses
  - Checks for additional risk factors
- Discusses umbilical cord management with the obstetrician. If the baby is breathing or crying, the umbilical cord clamping would be delayed for at least one minute but if the baby does not breath after drying, then the umbilical cord would be clamped and cut immediately and the baby would be handed over to the person who would be resuscitating the baby.
- Assembles team according to risk factors
- *Pre-resuscitation team briefing:* Discusses possible outcomes according to perinatal history obtained. Chooses a team leader and delegates tasks to each member, i.e., who would receive the baby and do initial assessment, who would perform Positive Pressure Ventilation (PPV), Intubation, Chest Compression or Medication as required. Team members should arrange all the required equipment and supplies and discuss whom to call in emergency and where to shift the baby if need arises.
- Washes hands with soap and water for 40–60 seconds along with the team
- Checks all equipment and supplies
- Checks the functioning of bag and using the following three steps:
  1. Fits mask onto the bag and delivers test breaths against the palm of the hand. Learner should feel the pressure over the palm as the bag is squeezed.
  2. Forms an air-tight seal between the mask and the palm of the hand. Squeezes the bag hard enough for the pop-off (pressure release) valve to open which can be recognized by the hissing noise as the air escapes through the valve.
  3. Checks that the bag re-inflates quickly when it is released after squeezing the bag.

Performance Checklist 2
BIRTH AND ROUTINE CARE

You have come to attend a delivery. You have already prepared for birth. The baby may be born anytime. Demonstrate how you would evaluate and take care of this baby. You may ask any question you would like to know about the newborn condition as you progress. *(Instructor announces that the baby has been born)*

- Places baby on the mother's abdomen and starts drying
- Evaluates the baby for breathing as the baby is dried *(Instructor says, "yes, the baby is breathing")*
- Dries the baby, removes wet linen
- Places the baby prone with head turned to one side
- Clears secretions, if needed
- Delays the umbilical cord clamping by at least 60 seconds (1–3 minutes)
- Covers the baby and mother with warm linen
- Continues ongoing evaluation of breathing, heart rate, color, activity, and temperature
- Advices mother to initiate breastfeeding

Performance Checklist 3
BIRTH AND INITIAL STEPS

You have come to attend a delivery. You have already prepared for birth. The baby may be born anytime. Demonstrate how you would evaluate and take care of this baby. You may ask any question you would like to know about the newborn baby's condition as you progress. ***(Instructor announces that the baby has been born)***

- Places baby on mother's abdomen and starts drying
- Evaluates the baby for breathing as the baby is dried ***(Instructor says "The baby is not breathing")***
- Cuts the cord and receives baby at radiant warmer: Dries the baby and removes wet linen
- Positions Airway
- Stimulates the baby by rubbing its back
- Suctions mouth and nose, if baby has still no breathing
- Assesses breathing ***(Instructor says "Yes the baby is breathing")***
- Assesses heart rate ***(Instructor: "Heart rate 120 bpm")***
- Monitors breathing, and color ***(Instructor: "Baby appears cyanotic at 5 min")***
- Checks breathing ***(Instructor: "Baby is breathing")***
- Auscultates heart rate ***(Instructor: "Heart rate is 140 bpm")***
- Attaches pulse Oximeter correctly ***(Instructor: "SpO_2 is 72%")***
- Administers free flow oxygen using correct technique and concentration
- Monitors oxygen saturation and takes appropriate action
- If baby is maintaining oxygen saturation on room air, breathing well with heart rate >100 bpm, plans for observational care with mother

Performance Checklist 4
POSITIVE PRESSURE VENTILATION (PPV)

The baby has just been born and has been provided with initial steps of resuscitation. Demonstrate what you would do for this baby.

- Evaluates the baby for breathing and assistant if available can assess for heart rate *(Instructor: "Baby not breathing, heart rate not assessed/70 bpm")*
- Indicates need for PPV and initiates PPV within 60 seconds
- Calls for help if not available
- Selects appropriate size mask
- Applies mask correctly covering the mouth and the nose without jamming onto the eyes
- Starts PPV with appropriate FiO_2 (room air in term baby and 21–30% for preterm <35 weeks) within 60 seconds of birth
- Requests assistant to place pulse-oximeter probe on the baby's right hand
- As PPV is being provided, after 15 seconds of starting PPV, assistant checks heart rate
- Takes appropriate action based on heart rate and chest rise
  - *If Instructor says, "Heart rate is increasing"* → participant declares effective PPV and PPV is continued for 30 seconds from initiation of PPV (15 more seconds)
  - *If instructor says, "Heart rate not increasing"* → participant looks for chest rise with PPV
  - If learner observes chest rise on the manikin with PPV → learner declares effective PPV and PPV is continued for 30 seconds from initiation of PPV (15 more seconds)
- If there is no chest rise (in manikin), takes ventilation corrective steps
  - Mask adjusted to provide airtight seal
  - Repositions the head and neck
  - Gives 5 breaths and assesses Chest moment
- If there is no chest rise, takes the next ventilation corrective steps
  - Suctions the mouth and nose
  - Opens the mouth
  - Gives 5 breaths and assesses Chest moment
- If there is no chest rise (in manikin), takes the next ventilation corrective steps
  - Increases pressure by squeezing the bag harder
  - Provides 5 breaths and assess for chest movement

- If there is no chest rise (in manikin), takes the next ventilation corrective steps
    - Alternate airway—endotracheal intubation
- Provides effective PPV for 30 seconds
- Assesses heart rate, breathing and SpO_2 after 30 seconds of effective PPV *(Instructor: "Heart rate is 120 bpm, SpO_2 is 68%, respiration—few breaths or no breaths")*
- Continues ventilation, adjusts oxygen concentration as per target oxygen saturation table; evaluates every 30 seconds for heart rate, SpO_2 and respiratory effort *(Instructor: "The baby has spontaneous respiratory effort, heart rate is 145/min, SpO_2 is 75% at 3 minutes)*
- Gradually discontinuous PPV with ongoing evaluation *(Instructor: "Heart rate is 140 bpm, SpO_2 is 72% and baby has continuous respiratory effort")*
- Assesses need for free flow oxygen to maintain oxygen saturation within target range, initiates free flow oxygen correctly
- Assesses heart rate and oxygen saturation and respiratory effort *(Instructor: "Heart rate is 140 bpm, SpO_2 is 90% , the baby has good respiratory effort")*
- Weans and discontinuous free flow oxygen
- Plans post-resuscitation care
- The team leader debriefs the resuscitation team

Performance Checklist 5
INTUBATION

Demonstrate how you would prepare for and intubate a newborn baby.

Role of operator	Role of assistant
• Prepares for intubation, requests correct size tube and laryngoscope blade	• Checks laryngoscope light and prepares tape for securing tube
• Instructs assistant to inform when it is 30 seconds or if there is deterioration in the baby's condition	• Notes the timer and monitors the baby for any further deterioration
• Holds laryngoscope correctly in left hand	
• Opens baby's mouth with right index finger and inserts blade to base of tongue	
• Lifts blade correctly (no rocking motion)	
• Identify landmarks, takes corrective action to visualize glottis	• Assistant provides cricoid pressure if asked by the person who intubates
• Inserts appropriate size endotracheal tube (ETT) from the right corner of the mouth without obstructing the vision	• Provides ET tube with or without the stylet as instructed
• Aligns vocal cord guide of the ETT with vocal cords	
• Removes laryngoscope while firmly holding tube against baby's palate	• Assistant connects the PPV source to ET
• Hold tube against baby's palate	
• Administers PPV	• During PPV, Observes for symmetrical chest movements. Assistant auscultates for bilateral air entry if it is equal and absent air entry over epigastrium
• Fixes the ET at NTL+1 cm against the lip	• Assistant checks nasal-tragus length
• If the chest is not moving and heart rate is not increasing, then removes the endotracheal tube and resumes PPV by bag and mask	• Assistant secures the ET tube by tape if ET tube is in correct position
• Repeats intubation attempt as above	
• Observes chest movement. (*Instructor: "Chest movement present, air entry present bilaterally"*)	• Assistant checks air entry, heart rate
• Continues PPV in room air for 30 seconds	
• Reassesses for breathing, heart rate and saturation and takes appropriate action	

Performance Checklist 6
CHEST COMPRESSION AND MEDICATION

The baby has just been born and the baby has been provided with initial steps of resuscitation and effective PPV with bag and mask ventilation for 30 seconds. Demonstrate what you would do for this baby.

- Evaluates for breathing, heart rate and SpO_2 (***Instructor: "Heart rate is <60 bpm, baby not breathing, no signal in pulse oximeter"***)
- Indicates the need for intubation and provides effective PPV for 30 seconds in room air
- Evaluates for breathing, heart rate and SpO_2 (***Instructor: "Heart rate is <60 bpm, baby not breathing, no signal in pulse oximeter"***)
- Indicates the need for chest compression
- Calls for additional help
- Requests assistant to increase oxygen to 100%
- Administers chest compressions coordinated with ventilation (provides 3 chest compressions to one ventilation every 2 seconds)
- Continues coordinated chest compression and ventilation for 60 seconds
- Assesses heart rate after 60 second (***Instructor: "Heart rate is 30 bpm, pulse oximeter has no signal"***)
- Requests another assistant to prepare umbilical venous catheterization *(See PCL7)*
- Requests estimated baby weight (***Instructor: "Estimated baby weight is 3 kg"***)
- If venous access is delayed, requests assistant to provide 3 mL (1 mL/kg) epinephrine (1:10,000 dilution) via endotracheal tube
- Team uses closed loop communication with confirmation of medication
- Assistant provides the desired amount of epinephrine and announces that ET dose of 3 mL of epinephrine given (closed loop communication)
- Continues coordinated chest compression and ventilation for 60 seconds
- Assesses heart rate and SpO_2 after 60 second (***Instructor: "Heart rate is 30 bpm, pulse oximeter has no signal"***)
- Assistant places umbilical venous catheter in place
- Requests for injection epinephrine 0.6 mL (0.2 mL/kg)) and 3 mL of normal saline
- Team uses closed loop communication
- Assistant delivers 0.6 mL epinephrine by umbilical vein and flushes cannula with 3 mL NS and announces the same *"0.6 mL of epinephrine given followed by 3 mL flush of normal saline"*

- Assesses heart rate after 60 second *(Instructor: "Heart rate is 50 bpm, pulse oximeter has no signal, the baby is pale")*
- Checks for chest rise with PPV, airway secured with ETT, rate and depth of chest compression, inspired oxygen concentration delivered is 100%
- Continues coordinated chest compression and ventilation
- Checks for history of blood loss/pneumothorax using transillumination of the chest *(Instructor: "Retroplacental retroplacental clot present/antepartum hemorrhage")*
- Requests 30 mL of NS to be given in 5–10 min by UVC
- Assistant initiates NS bolus via umbilical lines
- Assesses HR every 60 seconds *(Instructor: "Heart rate is 80 bpm, pulse oximeter 67%")*
- Discontinues chest compressions and continues PPV
- Assesses heart rate, breathing and saturation after 30 seconds *(Instructor: "Heart rate is 100 bpm, pulse oximeter 80%, no spontaneous respiration")*
- Continues PPV and adjusts oxygen concentration as per saturation target
- Assesses heart rate, breathing and saturation after 30 seconds *(Instructor: "Heart rate is 130 bpm, pulse oximeter 92%, some spontaneous respiration present")*
- Supports baby with PPV and supplemental oxygen as per target oxygen saturation table
- Prepares to move baby to post-resuscitation care setting
- Counsels parents and inform them of next steps
- Team has a debriefing session on the resuscitation performed

Performance Checklist 7
VASCULAR ACCESS

Demonstrate how you would prepare for and insert umbilical venous cannula in a newborn baby.

- Procedure is carried out with all aseptic precautions
- Wears new sterile gloves
- Attaches 3-way stopcock to umbilical venous catheter
- Flushes catheter and stopcock with normal saline and closes stopcock to catheter
- Cleans lower segment of umbilical cord with skin antiseptic solution
- Ties umbilical tape loosely at base of cord
- Cuts cord about 1–2 cm above base
- Identifies the umbilical vein and inserts catheter into vein (approximately 2-4 cm) just until a free backflow of blood is seen, when the attached syringe with a 3-way stopcock is aspirated. Flushes catheter and closes stopcock towards catheter
- Ensures catheter is being held in place; may secure with clear adhesive dressing
- Announces vascular access is ready

ANNEXURE II
PERFORMANCE EVALUATION TEST

The learner is given a case scenario and evaluated for the skill. The performer is asked to perform all the steps of NRP. There should not be any interruptions until the case scenario concludes. At the end of the case scenario, the instructor should decide if the performer can be passed or needs remediation followed by evaluation.

Item	0	1	2
Assesses perinatal risk, organizes team if necessary, checks equipment and supplies			
Delivers baby on mother's abdomen and dries the baby			
Evaluates the baby for its breathing *(Instructor: "Baby is not breathing")*			
Provides initial steps on radiant warmer (position, stimulates and suction if required)			
Assesses breathing and heart rate *(Instructor: "Baby is not breathing and heart rate is 80 bpm" if assessed for heart rate by another participant)*			
Indicates need of PPV, requests for pulse oximeter			
Applies mask correctly and starts PPV within 60 seconds of birth			
After 15 seconds of beginning PPV, as the PPV is continued, checks for effective PPV: • Requests to check heart rate to assess if heart rate is increasing *(Instructor: "Heart rate is not increasing")* • Observes the manikin for chest rise with PPV			
Takes ventilation corrective steps when chest rise is not observed with PPV			
Ventilation corrective steps: Mask adjustment, reposition gives 5 breaths and assess for chest rise with PPV			
If no chest rise with PPV, then suctions, ventilates with open mouth, gives 5 breaths and assess chest rise			
If no chest rise with PPV, increases pressure by squeezing bag harder, gives 5 breaths, assesses chest rise			
If no chest rise with PPV, correctly intubates the baby, gives 5 breaths and assesses chest rise			
Provides 30 seconds of effective PPV at a rate 40–60 breaths/min			
Assesses for breathing and HR and SpO_2 *(Instructor: "Baby not breathing, heart rate is 50 bpm, pulse oximeter has no signal")*			
Indicates the need for chest compressions coordinated with ventilation and calls for additional help			
Intubates if not done already, administers 100% oxygen, prepares for UVC insertion			
Provides chest compressions for 60 seconds, coordinated with ventilation at the ratio of 3 CC:1 PPV over 2 seconds			
After 60 seconds of coordinated chest compression and ventilation assesses heart rate *(Instructor: "Heart rate is 50 bpm")*			
If no vascular access, requests epinephrine 1 mL/kg of 1:10,000 to be given by ET			

Contd...

Contd...

Item	0	1	2
If vascular access available, requests to administer epinephrine 0.2 mL/kg of 1:10,000 followed by 3 mL saline flush			
Continues chest compression with ventilation and assesses after 60 seconds *(Instructor: "Baby not breathing, heart rate is 50 bpm, pulse oximeter has no signal, baby is pale")*			
Continues coordinated chest compression and ventilation and requests 10 mL/kg of NS to be given in 5–10 min through umbilical venous line			
Assesses heart rate after 60 second *(Instructor: "Heart rate is 80 bpm, pulse oximeter 67%")*			
Discontinues chest compressions, continues PPV			
Assesses heart rate, breathing and saturation after 30 seconds *(Instructor: "Heart rate is 100 bpm, pulse oximeter 80%, no spontaneous respiration")*			
Continues PPV and adjusts oxygen concentration as per pulse oximetry			
Assesses heart rate, breathing and saturation after 30 seconds *(Instructor: "Heart rate is 130 bpm, pulse oximeter 92%, some spontaneous respiration present")*			
Supports baby with PPV and supplemental oxygen as per target oxygen saturation table			
Prepares to move baby to post-resuscitation care setting, updates family. Debriefs the team on resuscitation			

In your view has the participant demonstrated all the steps required in neonatal resuscitation correctly:
Yes…………….. No…………....

Pass……………………………….		**Re-evaluate**…………………………….

Name of Instructor							**Signature**

Chapter 1

1. d   **2.** d   **3.** c.   **4.** a. False
b. True   c. False   d. True   e. True   f. False   g. True.

Chapter 2

1. b   **2.** c   **3.** d   **4.** d   **5.** d   **6.** d
7. a. False   b. False   c. True   d. False.
8. Gestation of pregnancy, single/multiple births, any other risk factor.
9.
   i. Check with obstetrician about gestation, number of fetuses, and other risk factors.
   ii. Identify team for resuscitation.
   iii. Conduct preresuscitation briefing (as team leader allots roles and responsibilities to team members, review risk factors, discuss anticipated problems, and proposes plan of action).
   iv. Conduct equipment checklist (see **Table 4**).

Chapter 3

1. False   **2.** True   **3.** False   **4.** True   **5.** False   **6.** False
7. True   **8.** Position, stimulation, clear secretions (if needed).
9. 10, 30
10. Baby must be monitored for breathing, heart rate, color, and temperature for at least 1 hour.

Chapter 4

1. b   **2.** c   **3.** d   **4.** c   **5.** c   **6.** a
7. d   **8.** d   **9.** b   **10.** b   **11.** b

Chapter 5

1. a, b, d   **2.** c   **3.** d, c, b, a
4. a. False; b. False; c. True; d. False.

Chapter 6

1. True   **2.** False   **3.** 2.5 mm ID
4. Nasotragal length +1 and gestational age-based charts
5. As an alternative airway, for prolonged positive pressure ventilation, before chest compression, for tracheal suction
6. (d) Use of stylet is optional.

7. (d) Initiate chest compression and give adrenaline through umbilical route.

8. Vocal cords   **9.** (c) Shock   **10.** 30

Chapter 7

1. 60
2. initiate PPV alone
3. take ventilation corrective steps
4. 100%
5. two thumbs with hands encircling the chest
6. lower one-third of sternum
7. 3:1 ratio, 60, 120.
8. (b) Chest compressions are stopped and only PPV is continued.
9. True.
10. True.

Chapter 8

1. 60
2. 0.02 mg/kg (0.01–0.03 mg/kg)
3. 3.0 mL, normal saline
4. 0.1 mg/kg (0.05–0.1 mg/kg)
5. (a), (b), (d)
6. 5–10 minutes
7. 20 minutes

Chapter 9

1. a. Compliant rib cage with weak muscles of the chest wall; b. Deficiency of surfactant; c. Frequent hypothermia developing during resuscitation.
2. a. Polythene bag/wrap; b. Preterm mask; c. Laryngoscope blade 0 and 00; d. T-piece resuscitator; e. Oxygen blender.
3. b. At 30 sec to 1 minute
4. b. Same as term neonates
5. a. 21–30% oxygen
6. b. CPAP

Chapter 10

1. Pneumothorax or pleural effusion
2. Decreased
3. Transillumination
4. Lighting up of hemithorax
5. 4th

Chapter 11

1. Choanal atresia   **2.** c   **3.** d   **4.** d   **5.** d
6. a

Chapter 12

1. b   **2.** c   **3.** b

Chapter 13

1. False **2.** False **3.** True **4.** False **5.** False   **6.** False
7. False **8.** True **9.** False **10.** False

Chapter 14

1. Such a neonate must be nursed with the mother. This is known as observational care. Initiate breastfeeding and monitor this neonate for temperature, heart rate, breathing, and activity every 30 minutes for 2 hours.

2. Such neonates require admission to special newborn care unit (SNCU)/neonatal intensive care unit (NICU) for receiving post-resuscitation care.

3. Neonates requiring postresuscitation care must be assessed for temperature, airway, breathing, perfusion, blood sugar, and neurological status. Provide supportive care and organ-specific management as required. If the neonate fulfills the criteria for therapeutic hypothermia and if facilities exist, the same must be provided.

4. This neonate requires therapeutic hypothermia, besides the management for postresuscitation care.

5. Such parents must be counseled for regular follow-up and the need for early intervention besides routine discharge counseling.

Chapter 15

1. b   **2.** c   **3.** d   **4.** c

5. The use of preheated radiant warmers, plastic wraps, thermal mattress, prewarmed transport incubator, increased ambient delivery room temperature to >23°C, hats, warm humidified blended oxygen have been found to decrease the incidence of hypothermia in the premature neonates.

Chapter 16

1. a   **2.** b

3. Advanced steps of resuscitation (e.g., method of chest compression, use of intraosseous route, and dose and route of epinephrine) are based on observational data, animal experiments or Manikin studies. Due to relative rarity of the need of these interventions, unanticipated need and little time to obtain consent, it is difficult to conduct randomized controlled trials.

Chapter 18

1. (a) False   (b) False   (c) True

2. a. *Autonomy:* Patient (parents in case of babies) has the right to refuse or choose their (beloved baby) treatment.

b. *Beneficence:* The decision on clinical interventions should be in the best interest of baby.

c. *Non-maleficence:* Primum non-nocere (first, do no harm) is imbibed in our Hippocratic oath and remains the guiding principle.

d. *Justice:* Car should be equal and fair to all human beings irrespective of their background.

e. *Dignity:* Patient/neonate and all caregivers must be dealt with mutual respect.

f. *Truthfulness and honesty:* Decisions and events should be based communicated to all involved in a transparent manner.

3. CEASE = Clinical Features, Effectiveness, Ask, Stop, Explain

4. (d)

5. 1. Success rate of available therapies

2. The risks involved with the therapy

3. Increment in quality of life with the therapy

4. Duration of life gained with the therapy

5. The pain, discomfort and cost associated

6. a. Review antenatal history and re-confirm gestational age with available data.

b. Discusses the situation with the team and takes the opinion.

c. Communicate the parents about baby's condition in a transparent and honest manner in simple language after obtaining good rapport on following aspects.

d. Senior most person in the team should lead communications.

e. Inform about the condition of the neonate and anticipated immediate problems.

f. Explain about the chances of survival and long-term neuro-developmental outcomes based on local data with aggressive management.

g. Explain about the facilities and level of care available at their center and alternatives available.

h. Help the parents to take the decision about continuation/withdrawal of care and facilitates the same.

i. If parents opted for withdrawal, consent will be taken with them and plan bereavement counseling.

j. Team meeting will be called for to discuss about the situation and debriefing will be done by the senior member of the team.

k. Baby will be given comfort care if parent wishes the same.

Chapter 19

1. This baby has extensive brain hemorrhage which will affect the long-term intact survival and probably will be left with extensive residual damage. So in this case the parents/family members must be explained in clear simple terms about the condition and possible poor outcome and counseled for shifting from life-sustaining treatment to palliative or end-of-life care.
2. Parents are the surrogate decision makers for babies and therefore have a shared role in deciding about end-of-life care.

Chapter 21

1. One-fourth   2. One-fifth or 20%   3. Single digit
4. c   5. d   6. c   7. d   8. d   9. a
10. d

Chapter 22

1. d   2. a   3. d

Chapter 23

1. SMART—Specific, Measurable, Achievable, Relevant, and Timely
2. c
3. False. This is a process indicator
4. Time series chart or Run chart
5. PDSA cycle—Plan, Do, Study, Act
6. d

Index

Page numbers followed by *b* refer to box, *f* refer to figure, and *t* refer to table.